T0275892

An introduction to
pharmaceutical sciences

Woodhead Publishing Series in Biomedicine

Published by Woodhead Publishing Limited

Published by Woodhead Publishing Limited

Published by Woodhead Publishing Limited

Published by Woodhead Publishing Limited

Published by Woodhead Publishing Limited

Woodhead Publishing Series in Biomedicine: Number 6

An introduction to pharmaceutical sciences

Production, chemistry, techniques and technology

Jiben Roy

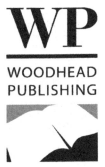

WP

WOODHEAD
PUBLISHING

Oxford   Cambridge   Philadelphia   New Delhi

Published by Woodhead Publishing Limited

Woodhead Publishing Limited, 80 High Street, Sawston, Cambridge, CB22 3HJ, UK
www.woodheadpublishing.com
www.woodheadpublishingonline.com

Woodhead Publishing, 1518 Walnut Street, Suite 1100, Philadelphia, PA 19102-3406, USA

Woodhead Publishing India Private Limited, G-2, Vardaan House, 7/28 Ansari Road,
Daryaganj, New Delhi – 110002, India
www.woodheadpublishingindia.com

First published in 2011 by Biohealthcare Publishing (Oxford) Limited; republished in 2012 by Woodhead
Publishing Limited
ISBN: 978-1-907568-52-7 (print) and ISBN: 978-1-908818-04-1 (online)
Woodhead Publishing Series in Biomedicine ISSN 2050-0289 (print); ISSN 2050-2097 (online)

Published by Woodhead Publishing Limited

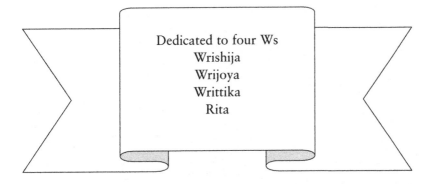

Dedicated to four Ws
Wrishija
Wrijoya
Writtika
Rita

Published by Woodhead Publishing Limited

Contents

Published by Woodhead Publishing Limited

Published by Woodhead Publishing Limited

Published by Woodhead Publishing Limited

Published by Woodhead Publishing Limited

Preface

During my career I have switched between teaching and undertaking other work in the pharmaceutical industry a couple of times. This book is a reflection of my ten years of work experience in the industry and 15 years of teaching experience. I have worked with many pharmaceutical consultants and visited many pharmaceutical industries around the world. Although I am not an expert in pharmaceutical sciences, my teaching experience is a testament to my ability to communicate what I know successfully.

This book is organized according to my understanding of pharmaceutical sciences, and it should give readers a good comprehension of this very important field. It is not comprehensive like *Remington's Pharmaceutical Sciences*, but covers essential information for twenty-first-century beginners.

Students and instructors will find a large amount of chemistry in the book as I wanted to employ my knowledge and experience of teaching organic chemistry, a science that is intimately connected with the origin and development of medicines. When I started my career in the pharmaceutical industry in 1985, there was no process analytical technology (PAT) or quality by design (QbD) but students today will see plenty of new concepts like these in the book.

Why this book?

There are hundreds of books on pharmaceutical science, so why write another book covering production, chemistry, techniques, and technology in pharmaceutical science? The reason is that one can hardly find a textbook on pharmaceutical sciences for a one or two semester course that covers all the essential aspects of the twenty-first-century's pharmaceutical industry, but is one-quarter the length of *Remington's Pharmaceutical Sciences*. In order to keep it affordable for students, the graphics are in black and white.

Published by Woodhead Publishing Limited

What materials are covered?

This book covers many activities and concepts in the pharmaceutical sciences (Figure P.1). It is a story about medicines – a biography of medicines – and uses figures to illustrate all the key concepts.

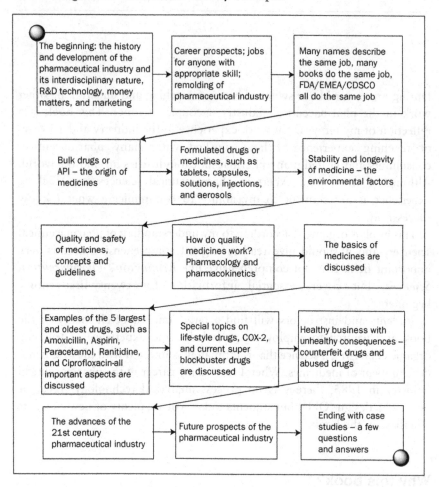

Figure P.1 Outline of subjects covered in this book

Future editions

Future editions of this text will have many more case studies. Please send your questions and comments to the author at jroy@as.muw.edu or royjiben@yahoo.com

Published by Woodhead Publishing Limited

Acknowledgements

The job of the publisher is to publish, but Glyn Jones of Biohealthcare Publishing (Oxford) Limited did much more. He not only encouraged me during the writing of this book, but made many suggestions and kept in touch with me until the end. I am very grateful to Glyn. I am also indebted to the copy editor of my book, Susannah Wight, who made a splendid job of organizing the book.

Ed Dechert of Mississippi State University also made the book happen. He worked hard with me by editing the book chapter by chapter. My sincere thanks to him.

When I worked in Square Pharmaceuticals Ltd of Bangladesh, the company was not approved by any top regulatory agency, but it is now approved by the Medicines and Healthcare Products Regulatory Agency (MHRA), UK. The company now produces insulin dosage forms and will soon apply for approval by the Food and Drug Administration (FDA), USA. I feel proud to have worked with them. Many of the pictures and documents included in this text were provided by Square Pharmaceuticals. Permission to reproduce material owned by Square Pharmaceuticals Limited, Dhaka, Bangladesh, is gratefully acknowledged. I thank them and wish them well.

In writing, constant inspiration is required otherwise it is hard to make good progress. I was always encouraged by talking and getting a helping hand from many colleagues, friends, former students, family members, and family friends in particular: my colleagues – Druba Adikari, Michael Elioff, Dionne Fortenberry, Ganashyam Heda, Dorothy Kerzel; my friends – Sabornie Chatterjee, Anup Das, Nathenial Das, Ayan Dey, Avijit Kar, Amitava Moitra, Reza Mustafa; my former students – Sharif Ahmed, Pijus Saha, Kakon Nag; Square Group's Tapan Chowdhury, Muhammadul Hoque, Anjan Paul, Ahmed Kamrul Alam, Jahidur Rashid; Bob Linton of IMS; family members Wrishija, Wrijoya, Writtika and Rita (Mithu); and family friends – Scott and Becky Rogers.

Finally, I would appreciate hearing from any students, instructors, or readers with suggestions or comments for the improvement of this text.

Jiben Roy

Published by Woodhead Publishing Limited

List of figures and tables

Figures

Published by Woodhead Publishing Limited

Published by Woodhead Publishing Limited

Published by Woodhead Publishing Limited

Published by Woodhead Publishing Limited

Published by Woodhead Publishing Limited

Published by Woodhead Publishing Limited

Published by Woodhead Publishing Limited

Published by Woodhead Publishing Limited

Published by Woodhead Publishing Limited

Published by Woodhead Publishing Limited

Published by Woodhead Publishing Limited

Tables

Published by Woodhead Publishing Limited

Published by Woodhead Publishing Limited

Published by Woodhead Publishing Limited

Abbreviations

6-APA	6-aminopenicillanic acid
7-ADCA	7-aminodeacetoxycephalosporanic acid
△9-THC	delta-9-tetrahydrocannabinol
ADME	absorption, distribution, metabolism, excretion
ADR	adverse drug reaction
AIDS	Acquired Immune Deficiency Syndrome
ANDA	abbreviated new drug application
API	active pharmaceutical ingredient
ASA	acetylsalicylic acid
AUC	area under curve
BBB	blood brain barrier
BCS	Biopharmaceutical Classification Systems
BHA	butylated hydroxyanisole
BHT	butylated hydroxytoluene
bid	twice a day
BP	British Pharmacopoeia
BP/USP	BP or USP specification
BPC	bulk pharmaceutical chemical
CAP	cellulose acetate phthalate
CDSCO	Central Drugs Standard Control Organization, India
CEO	chief executive officer
CFC	chlorofluorocarbon
cGMP	current good manufacturing practice
CNS	central nervous system
COX	cyclooxygenase
COX-2 drug	cyclooxygenase-2 inhibitor

DEG	diethylene glycol
DPI	dry powder inhaler
DRIFTS	Diffuse Reflectance Infrared Fourier Transform Spectroscopy
ED	effective dose
EG	ethylene glycol
EMEA	European Medicine Evaluation Agency
EU	European Union
FCC	Food Chemical Codex
FDA	Food and Drug Administration, USA
FTIR	Fourier transform infrared
GC	gas chromatography
GC-MS	gas chromatography – mass spectrometry
GHB	gamma-hydroxybutyric acid
GIT	gastrointestinal tract
GMP	good manufacturing practice
GTI	genotoxic impurity
HAART	highly active antiretroviral treatment
HIV	Human Immunodeficiency Virus
HMG-CoA	3-hydroxyl-3-methylglutaryl-CoA
HMGCoAR	hydroxymethylglutaryl coenzyme A reductase
HMGCR	HMG-CoA reductase
HPLC	high performance liquid chromatography
HPMCP	hydroxypropyl methylcellulose phthalate
HR	human resources
ICH	International Conference on Harmonization of Technical Requirements for Registration of Pharmaceuticals for Human Use
ID	intradermal
IM	intramuscular
IMS	Intercontinental Marketing Services
IND	investigational new drug
IQ	installation qualification
IR	infrared
ISO	International Organization for Standardization
IUPAC	International Union of Pure and Applied Chemistry

IV	intravenous
IVIVC	*in-vitro in-vivo* correlation
JP	Japanese Pharmacopoeia
LAL	limulus amebocyte lysate
LD	lethal dose
LIBS	laser-induced breakdown spectroscopy
LIF	light-induced fluorescence
LSD	lysergic acid diethylamide
MDI	metered dose inhaler
MDMA	3,4-methylenedioxymethamphetamine
Meth	methamphetamine
MHRA	Medicines and Healthcare Products Regulatory Agency, UK
mRNA	messenger ribonucleic acid
NAPQI	N-acetyl-p-benzoquinoneimine
NDA	new drug application
NF	National Formulary
NHS	National Health Service, UK
NIR	near infrared
NMR	nuclear magnetic resonance
NSAID	non-steroidal anti-inflammatory drug
OQ	operation qualification
OTC	over the counter
PAP	p-aminophenol
PAT	process analytical technology
PDF5	phosphodiesterase-5 enzyme
Pen G	penicillin G or benzylpenicillin
Pen V	penicillin V or penoxymethylpenicillin
Ph. Eur.	European Pharmacopoeia
Ph. Int.	International Pharmacopoeia
PhRMA	Pharmaceutical Research and Manufacturers of America
PIC	Pharmaceutical Inspection Convention
PIC/S	Pharmaceutical Inspection Co-operation Scheme

Published by Woodhead Publishing Limited

PMDA	Pharmaceutical and Medical Devices Agency, Japan
pMDI	pressurized metered dose inhaler
PNCB	p-nitrochlorobenzene
PNP	p-nitrophenol
POM	prescription-only medicine
PQ	performance qualification
QA	quality assurance
QbD	quality by design
QC	quality control
qid	four times a day
QMS	quality management system
R&D	research and development
RFID	radio-frequency identification
RNAi	ribonucleic acid interference
SC	subcutaneous
siRNA	short interfering ribonucleic acid
SK&F	Smith, Kline & French laboratories
SNP	single nucleotide polymorphism
TAMC	total aerobic microbial counts
tbl	tablespoon
TCYMC	total combined yeast and mold counts
THC	tetrahydrocannabinol
tid	three times a day
TLC	thin layer chromatography
TPS	terahertz-pulsed spectroscopy
tsp	teaspoon
US FDA	US Food and Drug Administration
USAN Council	US Adopted Name Council
USP	US Pharmacopoeia
USP-NF	US Pharmacopeia-National Formulary
UV-VIS	ultra-violet visible spectrophotometer
WFI	water for injection
WHO	World Health Organization
XR	extended release
XRF	X-ray fluorescence

About the author

Following his college education at Notre Dame College, Dhaka, Jiben Roy attended Dhaka University to complete his BSc Honors in Chemistry and MSc in Organic Chemistry. As an MSc student, he started teaching at Holy Cross College, which was the beginning of his teaching career. After finishing his Master's Degree, he joined Dhaka University as a lecturer in 1976 and by 1979 he wrote his first textbook on organic chemistry for college students, which has undergone a number of editions in Bangladesh.

Jiben received his PhD in 1983 from the University of Saskatchewan, Canada, and did his post-doctoral fellowship at the University of Hawaii at Manoa. He then went back to Bangladesh and joined Gonoshasthaya Pharmaceuticals in the Department of Quality Control. That was a new career, and Jiben successfully pioneered the development of Bangladesh's first antibiotic drug manufacturing plant in 1988 as the project director and principal researcher. He enthusiastically embraced the new discipline and went back to academia to teach pharmaceutical sciences at the newly formed Department of Pharmacy at Jahangirnagar University in 1990, where he chaired the department. Later on Jiben joined Square Pharmaceutical Ltd, the largest pharmaceutical manufacturer in Bangladesh, as head of R&D and Technical Services. He worked with many international consultants and visited many pharmaceutical companies in India, China, the Netherlands, Germany, and Switzerland. In 2001, Jiben came to the USA with a faculty position at Salem International University, West Virginia.

Jiben has published research articles on pharmaceutical sciences in several internationally reputed journals such as *AAPS PharmSciTech*; *World Health Forum*; *Bulletin of the World Health Organization*; *BMJ*; *Drug Development and Industrial Pharmacy*; *Australian Journal of Rural Health*; *Journal of Pharmaceutical Science*; *Indian Drugs*; *Current Medicinal Chemistry*; and *African Journal of Traditional, Complementary and Alternative Medicines*. He has co-edited a special issue of *Current Medicinal Chemistry* on natural medicine.

Published by Woodhead Publishing Limited

Jiben Roy is currently an associate professor in the Department of Sciences and Mathematics at Mississippi University for Women where he teaches chemistry courses and pharmaceutical sciences as a special topics course. Jiben and his wife Rita (Mithu) are the parents of three daughters, Writtika, Wrijoya, and Wrishija.

The author may be contacted at:

Department of Sciences and Mathematics
1100 College Street, W-100
Mississippi University for Women
Columbus, MS 39701, USA
Email: jroy@as.muw.edu

Published by Woodhead Publishing Limited

1

Introduction

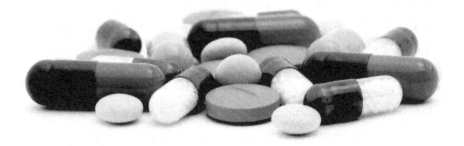

Learning objective

This introductory chapter provides students with a description of pharmaceutical science and its major components: pharmaceuticals and the pharmaceutical industry. There is a discussion of the gradual development of the industry, its multidisciplinary nature, its economics and technology, its impact on global health, and its ethical nature. Some pharmaceutical industries and their contributions to human life expectancy around the globe are briefly presented.

The mission of pharmaceutical science is to improve global health by discovering, developing, and producing quality medicines that are safe, appropriate, effective, affordable, and cost-effective, and widely distributing them around the world (Figure 1.1).

Published by Woodhead Publishing Limited

Key concept terms

Absorption: movement of a drug from the site of entry into the blood circulation system

ACE inhibitor: angiotensin-converting enzyme

Administration: how a drug is taken

AIDS: Acquired Immune Deficiency Syndrome

API: active pharmaceutical ingredient

Apothecary: a pharmacist

Biopharmaceutical: biotechnology-based drugs, biologics

Blockbuster drug: a drug that has made more than US$1 billion/year

Bulk drug: API in bulk

Chronotherapy: administering a drug to work in coordination with a body's biological clock

Distribution: the circulation of a drug in the body once absorbed

Dosage form: the physical form of a drug, such as tablet, capsule, ointment, and liquid injection

Elimination: removal of a drug from the body

Ethics: concepts of correct conduct

Excipient: non-active pharmaceutical ingredient

Formulated drug: dosage form of drugs made from APIs mixed with excipients

GMP: good manufacturing practice

HIV: Human Immunodeficiency Virus

IMS Health: Intercontinental Marketing Services, an information company

Injectable: intravenous or intramascular shot

Longevity: how long a person lives

Orange Guide: a book on GMP guidelines published by the Medicines and Healthcare Products Regulatory Agency

Parenteral: injectable

Pharmaceutical: synthetic chemical used as drugs

US FDA: US Food and Drug Administration

Published by Woodhead Publishing Limited

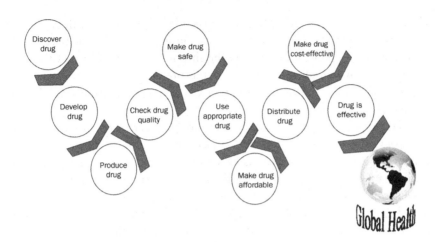

Figure 1.1 The mission of pharmaceutical science

Pharmaceutical science is a multidisciplinary science combining many areas of the basic and applied sciences, such as chemistry, biochemistry, biology, mathematics, statistics, physics, medical sciences, and engineering.

1.1 The theme of the book

This book has been developed as a unified approach to topics ranging from bulk drugs to formulated medicines based on a course offered by the author as a special topic within the physical sciences at the Mississippi University for Women. The theme of the book is similar to the course theme: to explain what students should know about pharmaceuticals.

Staying in good health is important to most people, but many people become ill or have injuries at some time in their lives. Therefore, pharmaceuticals have a role in curing people or helping them return to good health. The importance of pharmaceuticals to the US population's longevity cannot be understated.

Several books have been written on pharmaceutical topics, including pharmaceutical production, medicinal chemistry, drug design, dosage forms, pharmaceutical technology, quality assurance and control of pharmaceuticals, pharmaceutical research, and pharmaceutical marketing.

Published by Woodhead Publishing Limited

These books are all specialized and very useful. This book is a little different as it is a biography of medicine. Beginning with the discovery of pharmaceutical applications, continuing through the manufacture of active pharmaceutical ingredients (APIs) and the preparation of various dosage forms, and finally marketing to patients, it explains pharmaceutical and medicinal chemistry.

It encompasses many topics relevant to pharmacy students, industrial pharmacy students, pharmacy research students, newly appointed pharmaceutical employees, and anyone who seeks general health information and prefers to read one comprehensive book rather than several narrowly focused texts.

General chemistry is taught widely at college and university as an introduction to various sub-disciplines of chemistry. Similarly, since we teach courses in various aspects of pharmaceutical sciences, there is a need for a book about applied general pharmaceutical sciences covering production, chemistry, techniques, technology, and so on. This book brings a unified approach to topics ranging from bulk drugs to formulated medicines.

Let us take an example of a fictional medicine called 'cure all'. This book tells the story of how 'cure all' was discovered and then converted from lab scale to manufacturing scale. What is the role of the regulatory agency in regulating the drug? What reaction chemistry is involved in producing it? What motivated the discovery of 'cure all'? How were experimental difficulties in its production overcome? Once the bulk 'cure all' is made, it goes to a formulation factory and is formed into various dosages, such as tablets, capsules, and liquid dosage or parenteral forms. Why are there so many dosage forms? Do dosage forms make any difference to the way a drug

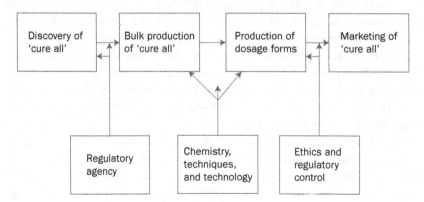

Figure 1.2 Steps involved in discovering 'cure all' and making it available for use by the public

Published by Woodhead Publishing Limited

acts in our bodies? How is the quality of 'cure all' maintained? How does the manufacturer tell what the expiration date of 'cure all' would be? Figure 1.2 shows the steps involved in discovering 'cure all', which also apply to discovering other medicines.

The book will also help students understand the exciting career opportunities in the pharmaceutical industry. This book is intended for 2nd to 4th year undergraduate students or postgraduate students who have already taken organic chemistry. Topics include:

- possibilities of having a career in this industry
- the manufacturing of APIs
- different dosage forms
- what bulk drugs and formulated drugs are
- critical factors in the development of pharmaceutical formulations in relation to the principles of chemistry
- good manufacturing practice
- quality assurance
- interdisciplinary science networks – the usefulness of teamwork in science
- the regulation of pharmaceuticals by government agencies.

A large number of students in chemistry, biochemistry, biology, microbiology, and pharmacy are interested in the pharmacy profession, health science careers, or pharmaceutical industrial jobs. This book is intended for them.

1.2 Development of the pharmaceutical industry and its impact

This industry is gigantic. Many people recognize the big name pharmaceutical companies or their logos, such as Abbott, Amgen, Astra-Zeneca, Bayer, Bristol-Myers Squibb, Eisai, Eli Lilly, GlaxoSmithKline (GSK), Johnson & Johnson, Merck, Novartis, Pfizer, Roche, Sanofi-aventis, Schering-Plough, or Wyeth (Figure 1.3). Some of these companies were either small pharmacy shops on a street corner or nonexistent 100 years ago.

In the early 1600s in Europe, street corner pharmacies or apothecaries used to make galenicals (medicines based on herbs or vegetable matter), decoctions, or balms using botanicals or herbs, in addition to powder, or pills, some of which contained very toxic compounds such as antimony and mercury salts. Some of them became profitable pharmaceutical industries.

The first pharmacopoeia (a book describing drugs and medicinal preparations) containing a list of useable drugs appeared in 1546 in

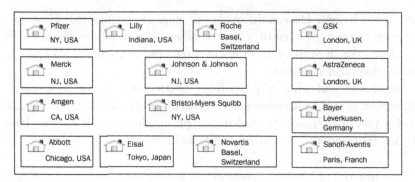

Pfizer NY, USA	Lilly Indiana, USA	Roche Basel, Switzerland	GSK London, UK
Merck NJ, USA	Johnson & Johnson NJ, USA		AstraZeneca London, UK
Amgen CA, USA	Bristol-Myers Squibb NY, USA		Bayer Leverkusen, Germany
Abbott Chicago, USA	Eisai Tokyo, Japan	Novartis Basel, Switzerland	Sanofi-Aventis Paris, Franch

Figure 1.3 Some global pharmaceutical companies

Nürnberg, Germany. In England, the first nationally recognized pharma-copoeia was the London pharmacopoeia (*pharmacopeia Londinensis*), which became mandatory for the preparation of medicines in 1618 (Figure 1.4). The US pharmacopeia, with a national formulary containing 217 drugs, was published in 1820. Pharmacopoeias in different countries helped to develop pharmaceutical industries in Europe and the USA.

During the early 1800s, Germany was the center of the development of the dye industry, and the chemistry of the dye industry helped Germany to be an early leader in the development of the pharmaceutical industry, later continued by well-known companies such as Boehringer Ingelheim, Hoechst, Bayer, Kalle, and Agfa. Swiss companies also emerged, some of which are still thriving. In the early 1800s, French chemists Pelletier and Caventou developed a method to isolate pure quinine from imported

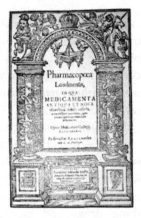

The *pharmacopoeia Londinensis*, written in Latin and first published by the Royal College of Physicians in May 1618, is recognized as Europe's first national pharmacopoeia. It included 712 compound remedies and 680 crude drugs, the origin of which were plants, animals, salts, and metals. However, it was immediately withdrawn from circulation; a new edition with more items was published in December 1618.

Figure 1.4 The cover page of the first edition of *pharmacopoeia Londinensis*, issued by the Royal College of Physicians in 1618

Published by Woodhead Publishing Limited

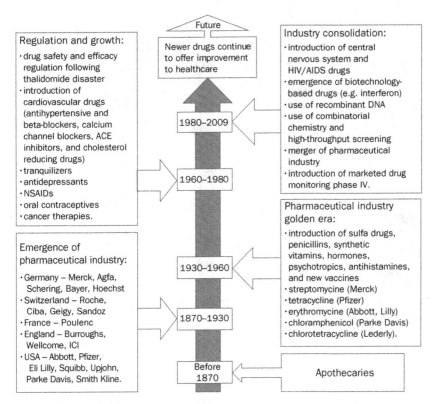

Figure 1.5 The development of the pharmaceutical industry since 1870

Source: Arthur A. Daemmrich and Mary Ellen Bowden[1]

cinchona bark and set up a factory in Paris for quinine extraction in 1826. In the UK there were family-owned pharmacy shops and small firms. Many corporate entities surfaced in the USA around the mid-1800s. Figure 1.5 illustrates the development of the pharmaceutical industry since 1870.

Most pharmaceutical companies originated in the 1870s, especially in the UK, the USA, Germany, Switzerland, and France (Figure 1.6).

Many of the giant pharmaceutical companies of today started as small pharmacy shops, which grew into small companies and then expanded further. Figures 1.7–1.11 illustrate the development of some well-known pharmaceutical companies: Pfizer, Merck, GlaxoSmithKline, Roche, and Bayer.

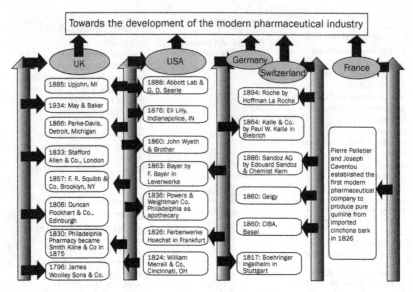

Figure 1.6 The development of the pharmaceutical industry in the UK, the USA, Germany, Switzerland, and France

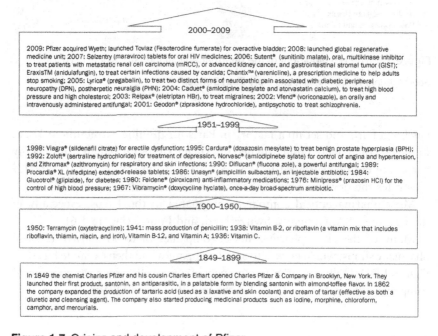

Figure 1.7 Origins and development of Pfizer

Source: Pfizer website[2]

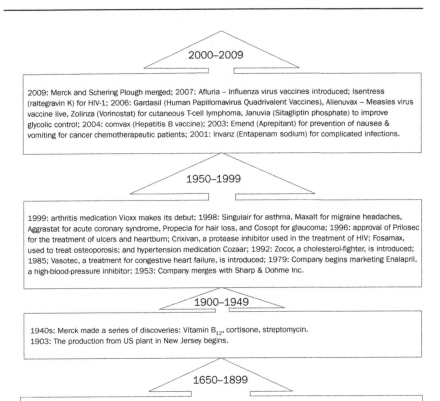

Figure 1.8 Origins and development of Merck

Source: Merck website[3]

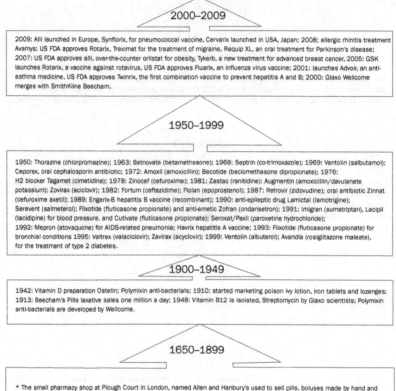

2000–2009

2009: Alli launched in Europe, Synflorix, for pneumococcal vaccine, Cervarix launched in USA, Japan; 2008: allergic rhinitis treatment Avamys; US FDA approves Rotarix, Treximet for the treatment of migraine, Requip XL, an oral treatment for Parkinson's disease; 2007: GSK approves alli, over-the-counter orlistat for obesity, Tykerb, a new treatment for advanced breast cancer, 2005: GSK launches Rotarix, a vaccine against rotavirus, US FDA approves Fluarix, an influenza virus vaccine; 2001: launches Advoir, an anti-asthma medicine, US FDA approves Twinrix, the first combination vaccine to prevent hepatitis A and B; 2000: Glaxo Wellcome merges with SmithKline Beecham.

1950–1999

1950: Thorazine (chlorpromazine); 1963: Betnovate (betamethasone); 1968: Septrin (co-trimoxazole); 1969: Ventolin (salbutamol); Ceporex, oral cephalosporin antibiotic; 1972: Amoxil (amoxicillin); Becotide (beclomethasone dipropionate); 1976: H2 blocker Tagamet (cimetidine); 1978: Zinocef (cefuroxime); 1981: Zastac (ranitidine); Augmentin (amoxicillin/davulanate potassium); Zovirax (aciclovir); 1982: Fortum (ceftazidime); Flolan (epoprostenol); 1987: Retrovir (zidovudine); oral antibiotic Zinnat (cefuroxime axetil); 1989: Engerix-B hepatitis B vaccine (recombinant); 1990: anti-epileptic drug Lamictal (lamotrigine); Serevent (salmeterol); Flixotide (fluticasone propionate) and anti-emetic Zofran (ondansetron); 1991: Imigran (sumatriptan), Lacipil (lacidipine) for blood pressure, and Cutivate (fluticasone propionate); Seroxat/Paxil (paroxetine hydrochloride); 1992: Mepron (atovaquone) for AIDS-related pneumonia; Havrix hepatitis A vaccine; 1993: Flixotide (fluticasone propionate) for bronchial conditions 1995: Valtrex (valaciclovir); Zavirax (acyclovir); 1999: Ventolin (albuterol); Avandia (rosiglitazone maleate), for the treatment of type 2 diabetes.

1900–1949

1942: Vitamin D preparation Ostelin; Polymixin anti-bacterials; 1910: started marketing poison ivy lotion, iron tablets and lozenges; 1913: Beecham's Pills laxative sales one million a day; 1948: Vitamin B12 is isolated, Streptomycin by Glaxo scientists; Polymixin anti-bacterials are developed by Wellcome.

1650–1899

* The small pharmacy shop at Plough Court in London, named Allen and Hanbury's used to sell pills, boluses made by hand and tinctures by maceration. That was the beginning of today's Glaxo Wellcome in 1715.
*In 1830 John K Smith opened his first drugstore in Philadelphia, USA. Thomas Beecham introduced laxative pills in England. Businesswise it was a great success.
*Joseph Nathan in 1873 opened a general trading company in Wellington, New Zealand, which laid the foundation of Glaxo Company later on. In 1880 Henry Wellcome and Silas Burroughs established their company in London.

Figure 1.9 Origins and development of GlaxoSmithKline

Source: GlaxoSmithKline website[4]

Published by Woodhead Publishing Limited

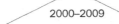

2000–2009

2009: EU & US FDA approves actemra-humanized anti II-6 receptor monoclonal antibody for rheumatoid arthritis; US FDA approves Influenza A/H1N1 diagnostic kit; 2007: Mircera, anemia product; 2005: Boniva/Bonviva, osteoporosis treatment; 2004: Tarceva, lung cancer treatment; Avastin, colon cancer treatment; 2003; Fuzeon, HIV treatment; Bondronat, osteoporosis & cancer treatment; 2001: Xeloda, colorectal cancer drug; Valcyte, treatment for AIDS-related CMV retinitis; Pegasys, hepatitis C treatment; 2000: Kytril, antiemetic drug used in chemotherapy.

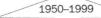

1950–1999

1999: Herceptin, breast cancer treatment; Tamiflu, influenza drug; 1996: Invirase, Roche's first protease inhibitor HIV antiviral drug (launched 1995 in USA); 1995-98: CellCept, transplant rejection drug; Vesanoid, leukaemia; Mabthera/Rituxan, cancer; Posicor, angina; Tasmar, Parkinson's disease; Zenapax, transplantation; Fortovase, HIV infection; Viracept, HIV infection; Xeloda, breast cancer; Xenical, obesity; 1993: Pulmozyme, genetically engineered drug for cystic fibrosis; 1992: Hivid, Roche's first HIV antiviral drug; Quinodis and Globocef, both for bacterial infections; 1991: Loceryl, fungal infections; Neupogen, adjuvant cancer chemotherapy agent; 1990: Aurorix, antidepressant; Inhibace, antihypertensive drug; 1987; Anexate, anaesthesia; Tilcotil, anti-inflammatory agent; 1986: Roferon-A (interferon alfa-2a),, Roche's first genetically engineered drug; 1985: Lariam and Fansimef, two antimalarial drugs; 1982: Rocephin, antibiotic drug of the cephalosporin class; 1981: Pretuval, cold and flu remedy; Benical, cough syrup; 1978: Rocaltrol, osteodystrophy drug; 1975: Rohypnol, tranquilliser; 1973: Madopar, drug against Parkinson's disease; 1971: Fansidar (pyrimethamine sulfadoxine), antimalarial drug; 1969: Bactrim, antiinfective agent; Berocca, nerve tonic Vitamin B complex/Vitamin C; 1965: Mogadon, insomnia agent; 1964: Cai-C-Vita, Vitamin C and calcium preparation; 1963: Valium Roche, tranquillizer; 1962: Fluoro-uracil Roche, the company's first anticancer drug; 1960: Librium, the first benzodiazepine drug for emotional, psychosomatic and muscular disorders; other benzodiazepine drugs: Librax (1961), Mogadon (1965), Limbitrol (1967), Nobrium (1968), Dalmadorm (1972), Lexotanil (1974); 1953: Konakion, hemorrhagic disorders (a synthetic Vitamin KI); 1952: Rimifon (Isoniazid), antituberculosis drug.

1900–1949

1944: Bepanthen (dexpanthenol), skin care product; 1938: Industrial synthesis of Vitamin A, Vitamin B group, Vitamin E, Vitamin K; 1933: Industrial synthesis of Vitamin C and introduction of Saridon, analgesic drug containing phenacetin; 1920: Allonal (first synthetic product), as analgesic sedative and hypnotic; 1909: Pantopon (opium alkaloids) remedy for pain, colic, spasms, cough, anxiety and excitation states; 1904: Digalen, purified digitals preparation containing all the cardiac glycosides of the purple fox-glove leaf.

1650–1899

In 1896 Fritz Hoffmann La-Roche established 'Roche' pharmaceutical company in Basel, Switzerland. In the same year Roche introduced first product Aiodin as thyroid preparation. The other products included Airol, an antiseptic wound-healing powder, and Sirolin, a cough syrup.

Figure 1.10 Origins and development of Roche

Source: Roche website[5]

Published by Woodhead Publishing Limited

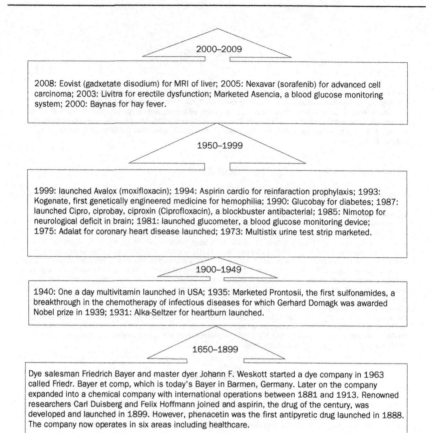

2000–2009

2008: Eovist (gadxetate disodium) for MRI of liver; 2005: Nexavar (sorafenib) for advanced cell carcinoma; 2003: Livitra for erectile dysfunction; Marketed Asencia, a blood glucose monitoring system; 2000: Baynas for hay fever.

1950–1999

1999: launched Avalox (moxifloxacin); 1994: Aspirin cardio for reinfarction prophylaxis; 1993: Kogenate, first genetically engineered medicine for hemophilia; 1990: Glucobay for diabetes; 1987: launched Cipro, ciprobay, ciproxin (Ciprofloxacin), a blockbuster antibacterial; 1985: Nimotop for neurological deficit in brain; 1981: launched glucometer, a blood glucose monitoring device; 1975: Adalat for coronary heart disease launched; 1973: Multistix urine test strip marketed.

1900–1949

1940: One a day multivitamin launched in USA; 1935: Marketed Prontosii, the first sulfonamides, a breakthrough in the chemotherapy of infectious diseases for which Gerhard Domagk was awarded Nobel prize in 1939; 1931: Alka-Seltzer for heartburn launched.

1650–1899

Dye salesman Friedrich Bayer and master dyer Johann F. Weskott started a dye company in 1963 called Friedr. Bayer et comp, which is today's Bayer in Barmen, Germany. Later on the company expanded into a chemical company with international operations between 1881 and 1913. Renowned researchers Carl Duisberg and Felix Hoffmann joined and aspirin, the drug of the century, was developed and launched in 1899. However, phenacetin was the first antipyretic drug launched in 1888. The company now operates in six areas including healthcare.

Figure 1.11 Origins and development of Bayer

Source: Bayer website[6]

1.2.1   The impact of pharmaceutical industries on human lives

Life expectancy throughout the world increased from an average of 30–40 years in the early twentieth century to an estimated 66.12 years in 2009.[7] In the USA, life spans increased from an average of 47 years in 1950 to 78.06 years today, and US life expectancy continues to grow (Figure 1.12).

Research data suggest there is a correlation between life expectancy and the development of the pharmaceutical industry. Using aggregate time series data, Dr Frank R. Lichtenberg, a researcher at Columbia University, studied the impact of new drug approval by the US Food and Drug Administration (FDA) on US lifespan longevity. The results show that a 40% increase in life expectancy can be attributed to new medicines (Figure 1.13). According

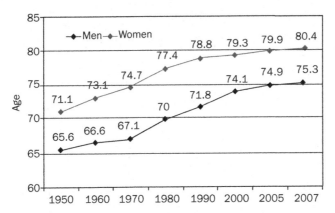

Figure 1.12 US life expectancy in the USA, 1950–2007

Source: Department of Health and Human Services, CDC, US, and Innovation.org[8]

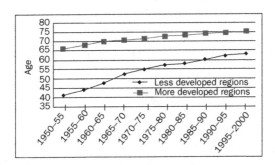

Figure 1.13 Life expectancy in more and less developed regions of the USA, 1950/55–1995/2000

Source: Frank R. Lichtenberg[9]

to another study, by innovation.org and the Pharmaceutical Research and Manufacturers of America (PhRMA), the new drugs reduce the risk of death (Figure 1.14).

Alan Sheppard of IMS Health made an effective correlation between life expectancy and drug use in an aging Europe after collecting data from the United Nations and an IMS market prognosis (Figure 1.15).

The effect that drugs have in countering disease is exemplified by data on HIV/AIDS cases. In the 1980s there were only one or two drugs available to treat AIDS patients, but the number and availability of newer medicines

Published by Woodhead Publishing Limited

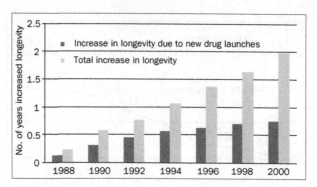

Figure 1.14 Total increase in longevity compared with increase in longevity resulting from new medicines, USA, 1988–2000

Source: Frank R. Lichtenberg[10]

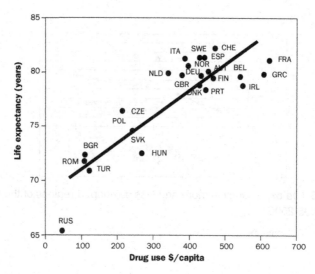

Figure 1.15 Correlation between life expectancy and drug expenditure per capita in Europe, 2005–2010

Source: IMS Heath[11]

increased dramatically since 1996, when highly active antiretroviral treatment (HAART) was introduced, which had an immediate effect (Figure 1.16).

During the last decade, the US FDA approved more than 300 new medicines in various disease categories, for example cancer and cardiovascular disease, which have increased patients' survival rates and longevity, and decreased disability.

Published by Woodhead Publishing Limited

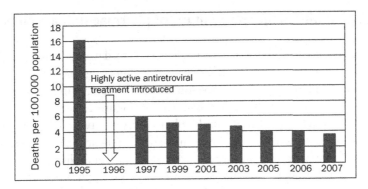

Figure 1.16 Mortality rate 1995–2007, showing effect of introducing highly active antiretroviral treatment in 1997 for AIDS patients in the USA

Source: PhRMA[12]

1.3   Important milestones in the introduction of pharmaceuticals

In the twentieth century alone, major breakthroughs in the treatment of diseases occurred when new pharmaceuticals were introduced. A timeline of major events is shown in Figure 1.17.

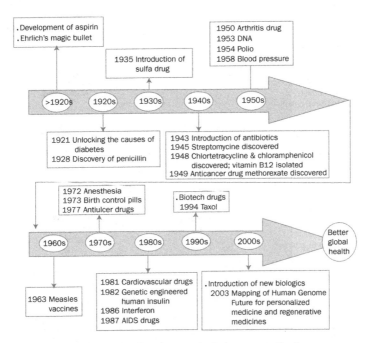

Figure 1.17 Milestones in the development of pharmaceuticals

Published by Woodhead Publishing Limited

1.4 The multidisciplinary nature of pharmaceutical sciences

The primary goal of pharmaceutical sciences is to develop drugs and drug delivery systems, using chemistry, chemical engineering, biology, statistics, economics, and marketing to develop drugs to treat, cure, and prevent diseases. It is truly a multidisciplinary science (Figure 1.18).

Pharmaceutical scientists and pharmacists have different jobs. Pharmaceutical scientists are involved in the development of drugs, concerned with their administration, absorption, distribution, metabolism, elimination, safety and toxicology; pharmacists work with the application of existing drugs and patients. Some pharmacists are also pharmaceutical scientists, but pharmaceutical scientists can only become pharmacists if they are professionally certified.

Although the pharmaceutical industry is based on scienctific research, it requires employees from non-science disciplines too. Success in the industry involves more than discovering a drug, although this is the most important step; success comes from properly managing, positioning, pricing, advertizing, and marketing a discovered product. This calls for multidisciplinary team work. The functionality of core pharmaceutical sciences starts with the drug discovery unit and continues to marketing and sales (Figure 1.19).

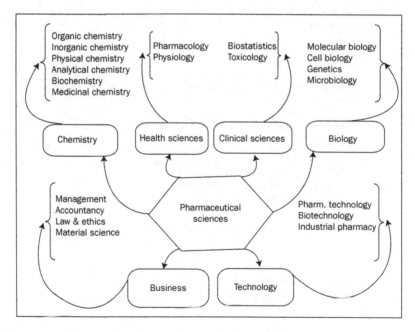

Figure 1.18 The multidisciplinary nature of pharmaceutical sciences

Published by Woodhead Publishing Limited

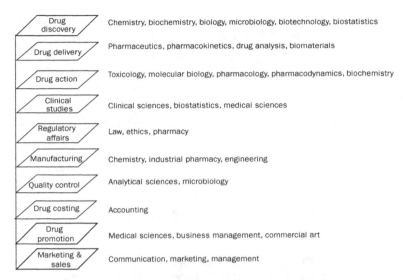

Figure 1.19 The core functionality of pharmaceutical sciences

1.5 Medicinal trees

A medicinal tree is a tree or plant that produces a certain medicine. In ancient societies people depended on medicinal plants to cure their ailments. There are also many modern medicines in nature, though some are not currently in use. Recently, very important medicines such as taxol, vincristine, and vinblastine have been isolated from medicinal plants. In most cases isolated medicinal compounds from plants are synthesized in laboratories and the products – medicines – used to cure and take care of humans. Figure 1.20 illustrates some medicinal trees.

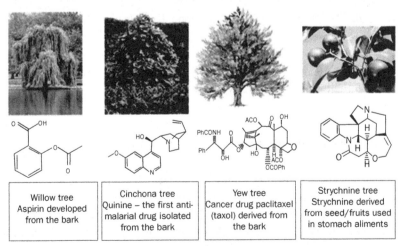

| Willow tree Aspirin developed from the bark | Cinchona tree Quinine – the first anti-malarial drug isolated from the bark | Yew tree Cancer drug paclitaxel (taxol) derived from the bark | Strychnine tree Strychnine derived from seed/fruits used in stomach aliments |

Figure 1.20a Medicinal trees: willow, cinchona, yew, and strychnine

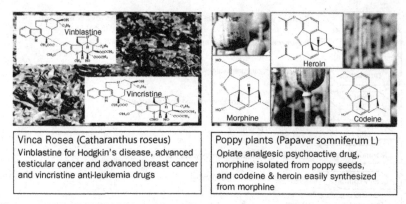

Vinca Rosea (Catharanthus roseus)
Vinblastine for Hodgkin's disease, advanced
testicular cancer and advanced breast cancer
and vincristine anti-leukemia drugs

Poppy plants (Papaver somniferum L)
Opiate analgesic psychoactive drug,
morphine isolated from poppy seeds,
and codeine & heroin easily synthesized
from morphine

Figure 1.20b Medicinal trees: Vinca Rosea and poppy plants

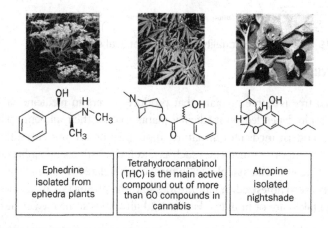

Ephedrine
isolated from
ephedra plants

Tetrahydrocannabinol
(THC) is the main active
compound out of more
than 60 compounds in
cannabis

Atropine
isolated
nightshade

Figure 1.20c Medicinal trees: ephedrine, cannabis, and nightshade

The World Health Organization (WHO) attributes the success of the pharmaceutical industry to many entities (Figure 1.21).

1.6   Pharmaceutical research and development

The pharmaceutical industry is research-based. If there were no research, there would be no new molecular entity. The top ten pharmaceutical companies in the world spent close to US$50 billion in 2009 on research and development (R&D).[13] The USA's pharmaceutical and biotechnology research companies invested an estimated US$65.3 billion in R&D in 2009.[14] The

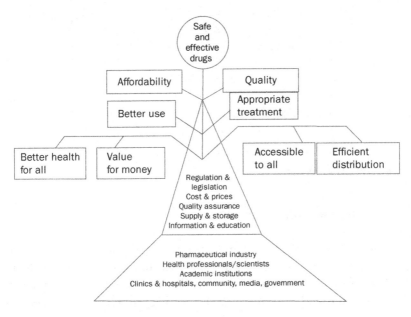

Figure 1.21 Entities the pharmaceutical industry depends on to make drugs safe and effective

Source: World Health Organization[15]

leading pharmaceutical company Pfizer continues to invest more than US$20 million every business day in discovering and developing new medicines.[16]

In 1980, PhRMA member companies invested US$2 billion on R&D to develop new medicines, and since then have steadily increased the amount they invest in R&D.[17] Figure 1.22 shows the expenditure of US biopharmaceutical companies on R&D from 2004 to 2009. As a result, the US FDA approved 34 new drugs and biologics in 2009 and more than 2,000 medicines are in the development pipeline. It is estimated that 90,712 personnel are employed in pharmaceutical R&D in the USA and that the total global expenditure on pharmaceutical R&D is about 16% of the sales.[18]

According to the Association of British Pharmaceutical Industry, UK pharmaceutical companies invested £4.3 billion on R&D in 2008,[19] which is almost 30% of total pharmaceutical sales. This was more than £10 million per day, and on average the investment in pharmaceutical R&D has been greater than investments on R&D of other British manufacturing sectors. Investment on pharmaceutical R&D in other countries, especially the fast growing Asian countries such as China, India, Singapore, and Korea, is also encouraging.

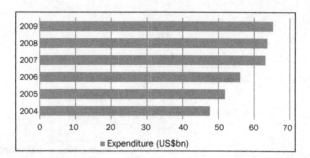

Figure 1.22 US expenditure on pharmaceutical R&D, 2004–2009[20]

1.7   Pharmaceutical technology

Injectable dosage forms have some advantages, but needle injections are uncomfortable and can be scary for children and some adults, so many people benefit from needleless injections (Figure 1.23). Such injections are only possible through technology, an engineering process by which scientific needs are met.

Pharmaceutical production is highly automated and depends on technology, which helps to address the unmet medical needs of patients. As a result of technology the patch form developed, which is the most comfortable dosage form for patients.

Tablets usually take time to dissolve so therapeutic action is delayed; this form of medication is slower than liquid dosage forms. The pharmaceutical industry uses different technologies, such as freeze drying, spray drying, and

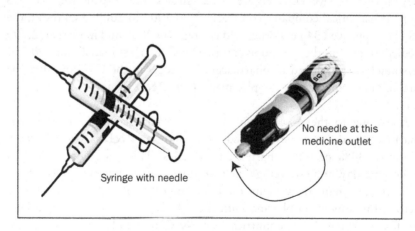

Figure 1.23 Needle and needleless injectors[21]

Published by Woodhead Publishing Limited

sublimation, to formulate fast dissolving or mouth dissolving tablets. There are also tablets on the market with a combination of immediate and controlled release. There is a new dosage form under development called chronotherapeutic technology, which would control drug release according to circadian rhythms and the timing of the symptoms of certain diseases, such as ulcers, asthma, and cardiovascular disease. This drug delivery technology will deliver the appropriate drug when symptoms occur.

1.8 Pharmaceutical economics

The pharmaceutical industry is based on research, technology, investors, and ethics, and is the most profitable industry in the world. Even in the poor economic environment of 2008–2009, the overall profit margin of the world's 13 leading pharmaceutical companies was 24.9% in the first quarter of 2009. which was slightly higher (0.7%) than in the first quarter of 2008. In the same period, the top six biotech companies recorded a 32.4% profit.[22] An article in *Fortune Magazine* described the pharmaceutical industry as a 'star industry' whose average profit margin has been two times greater than the median for all industries in the Fortune 500 in the 1970s and 1980s.[23] The industry has been criticized for its marketing and pricing practices, especially in developing countries. When Viagra was introduced in the USA in 1998 it had an average wholesale price of US$8.75 per pill.[24] In most countries, including the USA, government-run health insurances do not cover Viagra purchases.

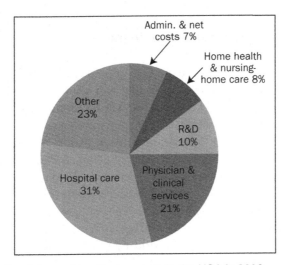

Figure 1.24 Breakdown of healthcare costs in the USA in 2006

Source: Centers for Medicare and Medicaid, 'National Health Expenditures'[25]

Published by Woodhead Publishing Limited

The pharmaceutical R&D accounts for 10% of the total cost of overall healthcare costs in the USA; other costs include the services of physicians, hospital care, and administration (Figure 1.24). Similarly, medicines account for only around 10% of the total National Health Service (NHS) costs in the UK.[26]

Though the cost of prescription drugs is only one-tenth of overall health costs, for many people who do not need hospitalization drug costs can become a major healthcare expense. However, as innovation comes at a cost, there must be incentives for it. Whatever policy a country adopts, pharmaceutical economics will be in good condition as long as human innovation stays on course and patent protection exists. These are some future pharmaceutical market trends according to consulting firm, Urch Publishing, Ltd:

- The global pharmaceutical market is expected to grow to US$929 billion in 2012.
- About one-third of the pharmaceutical market by value is accounted for by blockbuster drugs. A blockbuster drug is one that generates more than US$1 billion in revenue each year.[27]

In 2007 Pfizer earned US$12.2 billion from the sale of its super drug Lipitor (generic name Atorvastatin). In the same year there were 111 blockbuster drugs on the market, which generated more than US$250 billion in revenue.[28] Some blockbuster drugs and their sales figures for three consecutive years are shown in Figure 1.25.

1.9   The world pharmaceutical market

The worldwide pharmaceutical market grew steadily until 2008, but in 2008 and 2009 it slowed down, probably as a result of the recession. IMS Health shows that this market was valued at more than US$800 billion in 2009 (Figure 1.26).[29] The market was expected to grow by 4–5% in 2010.

In contrast, pharmaceutical markets in Asia, Africa, Australia, and Latin America, including the emerging markets of China, India, Singapore, South Korea, Russia, Brazil, Turkey, and Mexico, grew by double digits in 2009 (Figure 1.27). Double digits growths are expected in future too.

The world pharmaceutical market and its growth also reflect the individual markets of the world's leading companies. The top ten leading pharmaceutical industries in the world by sales in billions of dollars are shown in Figure 1.28.

Published by Woodhead Publishing Limited

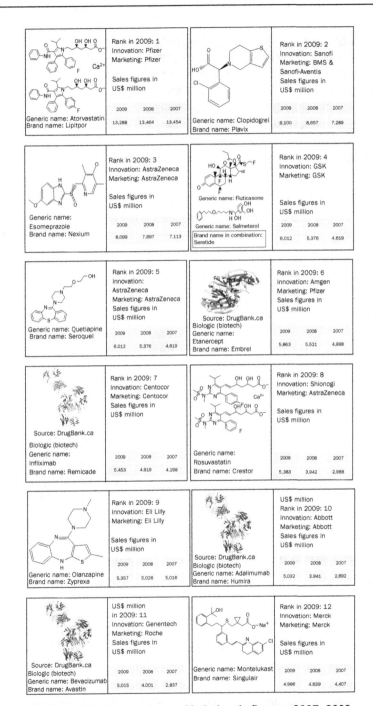

Figure 1.25 Some blockbuster drugs with their sale figures, 2007–2009

Source: IMS Health website[30]

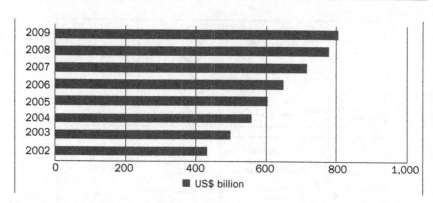

Figure 1.26 The size of the global pharmaceutical market, 2002–2009 (US$ billion)

Source: IMS Health[31]

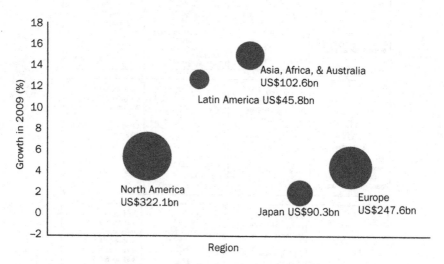

Figure 1.27 Percentage growth of the world pharmaceutical market in 2009

Source: IMS Health[32]

The world market for medicine comprises two sectors, pharmaceutical and biopharmaceutical, but so far no distinction is made between the two at the company level. Most leading companies have pharmaceutical and biopharmaceutical facilities, but there are also categorically biopharmaceutical companies such as Amgen and Genzyme.

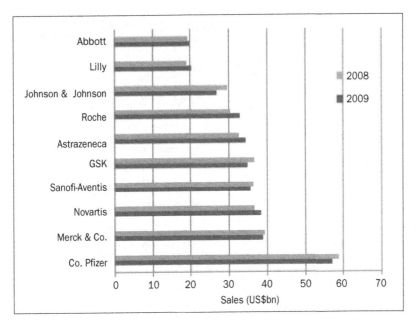

Figure 1.28 The world's top leading pharmaceutical companies by sales, 2008–2009

Source: IMS[33]

1.10 Embedded ethics in the pharmaceutical industry

The most important and unique characteristic of pharmaceutical operations is the industry's adherence to ethical guidelines. Embedded in the production and marketing of pharmaceutical products are norms, rules, and regulations. The industry's entire operation is regulated; even factory packaging workers have a dress code and need to follow good manufacturing practice (GMP) in their duties (Figure 1.29).

GMP guidelines are well accepted and practiced in the pharmaceutical industry all over the world. Most countries follow the WHO's GMP guidelines, though every country has its own guidelines also. In the UK the official rules and guidance for pharmaceutical manufacturers and distributors is popularly referred to as the Orange Guide.[34] Figure 1.30 illustrates the close connection between the production and marketing of pharmaceuticals, GMP, and ethics.

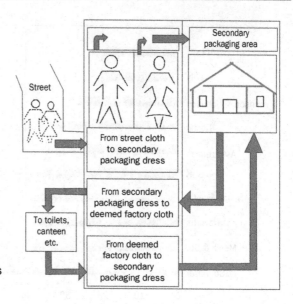

Figure 1.29 How good manufacturing practice applies to dress changes of packaging workers

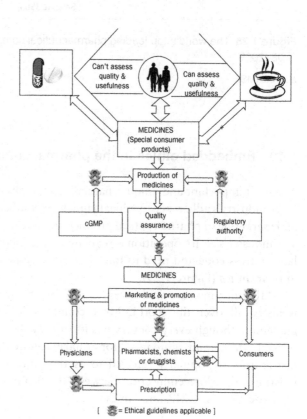

Figure 1.30 The connection between the production and marketing of pharmaceuticals, GMP and ethics

Practice questions

1. Why do GMP guidelines not allow personnel to enter a factory in street clothes?
2. Why do we use medicines?

Answers to practice questions

1. To avoid contamination.
2. To treat, cure, or prevent diseases.

Notes

1. Arthur A. Daemmrich and Mary Ellen Bowden, 'Pharma since 1870: a rising drug industry', *Chemical and Engineering News*, Vol. 83, Issue 25, June 20, 2005, pp. 28–42.
2. See www.pfizer.com/home/.
3. See www.merck.com/.
4. See www.gsk.com/.
5. See www.roche.com/index.htm.
6. See www.bayer.com/.
7. Central Intelligence Agency, *The World Factbook*, 2008, https://www.cia.gov/library/publications/the-world-factbook/geos/xx.html (accessed December 20, 2010); and Oded Galor and Omer Moav, 'Natural selection and the evolution of life expectancy', http://sticerd.lse.ac.uk/seminarpapers/dg09102006.pdf (accessed December 20, 2010).
8. US National Center for Health Statistics, *Health, United States, 2008, with Chartbook*, Hyattsville, MD: US Department of Health and Human Services, 2009; M. Heron et al., 'Deaths: final data for 2006', *National Vital Statistics Reports*, Vol. 57, No. 14, April 17, 2009, www.cdc.gov/nchs/data/nvsr/nvsr57/nvsr57_14.pdf (accessed February 16, 2011); and Innovation.org, 'Charts', www.innovation.org/index.cfm/ToolsandResources/Charts (accessed February 16, 2011).
9. Frank R. Lichtenberg, 'The impact of new drug launches on longevity: evidence from longitudinal, disease-level data from 52 countries, 1982–2001', National Bureau of Economic Research Working Paper No. 9754, Cambridge, MA: NBER, June 2003, cited in PhRMA, *Value of Medicines: Facts and Figures 2006*, www.innovation.org/documents/Value%20of%20Medicine%20FINAL%200712061.pdf (accessed July 7, 2010).
10. Ibid.
11. Alan Sheppard, 'Medicines: essential contributors to the long-term health of society', IMS Health, www.imshealth.com/imshealth/Global/Content/Document/Market_Measurement_TL/Generic_Medicines_GA.pdf (accessed October 15, 2010).
12. PhRMA, *Pharmaceutical Industry Profile*, 2010, p. 3, www.phrma.org/sites/default/files/159/profile_2010_final.pdf (accessed December 28, 2010).

Published by Woodhead Publishing Limited

13. Drugs.com, 'Top 20 pharma's R&D spending topped $86 billion in 2009, December 22, 2010, www.drugs.com/news/top-20-pharma-s-r-amp-d-spending-topped-86-billion-2009-28542.html.
14. PhRMA, *Pharmaceutical Industry Profile*, 2010, www.phrma.org/sites/default/files/159/profile_2010_final.pdf (accessed February 16, 2011).
15. World Health Organization, 'How to develop and implement a national drug policy: guidelines for developing national drug policy', 1988; and issues of WHO's *Essential Drug Monitor*.
16. See www.pfizer.com.
17. PhRMA, *Pharmaceutical Industry Profile*, 2010, www.phrma.org/sites/default/files/159/profile_2010_final.pdf (accessed February 16, 2011).
18. Ibid.
19. Association of the British Pharmaceutical Industry, *Annual Report*, 2009/10, www.abpi.org.uk/publications/pdfs/AnnualReport0910.pdf (accessed February 16, 2011).
20. Burrill & Co., analysis for PhRMA, 2005–2010; and *PhRMA Annual Member Survey*, Washington, DC: PhRMA, 1981–2010; cited in PhRMA, *Profile: Pharmaceutical Industry*, 2010, www.phrma.org/sites/default/files/159/profile_2010_final.pdf (accessed February 16, 2011).
21. Medisize, www.medisize.com/development.asp?cat_id=16&subcat_id=94&case_id=59 (accessed April 18, 2011).
22. Maureen Rouhi, 'Pharma is for the long term', *Chemistry & Engineering News*, Vol. 87, No. 23, June 8, 2009, p. 3, http://pubs.acs.org/cen/editor/87/8723editor.html (accessed February 23, 2011).
23. Quoted in John Mullins, 'A recent history of the pharmaceutical industry – based on all five forces', *The New Business Road Test*, August 2007, www.venturenavigator.co.uk/content/154 (accessed February 15, 2011).
24. Alison Keith, 'The economics of Viagra', *Health Affairs*, Vol. 19, No. 2, 2000, pp. 147–57.
25. Centers for Medicare and Medicaid, 'National health expenditure data', January 7, 2008, www.cms.hhs.gov/NationalHealthExpendData (accessed February 23, 2011).
26. 'Facts and statistics from the pharmaceutical industry', www.abpi.org.uk/statistics/section.asp?sect=4 (accessed February 10, 2011).
27. Urch Publishing, *Pharmaceutical Market Trends, 2008–2012*, www.urchpublishing.com/publications/market_trends/pharmaceutical_market_trends_2008_-_2012.html (accessed February 16, 2011).
28. MarketResearch.com, 'Emerging blockbusters: 2009's most promising drugs and the future of the blockbuster model', December 16, 2008, www.marketresearch.com/product/display.asp?productid=2066398 (accessed November 27, 2010).
29. 'IMS forecasts global pharmaceutical market growth of 4–6% in 2010; predicts 4–7% expansion through 2013', www.imshealth.com/portal/site/imshealth/menuitem.a46c6d4df3db4b3d88f611019418c22a/?vgnextoid=500e8fabedf24210VgnVCM100000ed152ca2RCRD&vgnextfmt=default (accessed June 10, 2010).
30. IMS Health, www.imshealth.com/portal/site/imshealth; redrawn with permission.
31. IMS Health, Market Prognosis, March 2010; redrawn with permission.
32. Ibid.
33. IMS Health, Midas, December 2009; redrawn with permission.
34. Medicines and Healthcare Products Regulatory Agency, *Rules and Guidance for Pharmaceutical Manufacturers and Distributors*, the Orange Guide, London: Pharmaceutical Press, 2007.

2

Career prospects in the pharmaceutical industry

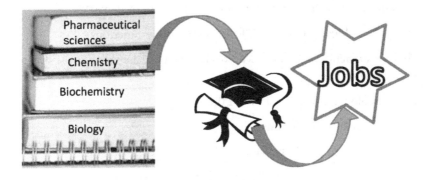

Learning objective

This chapter discusses job prospects in the pharmaceutical industry. Regardless of your chosen major, if you have a strong desire to work in the health industry, including the pharmaceutical industry, you can successfully find a specific career provided you are adequately prepared. After reading this chapter you will know what to do to prepare yourself, where to look, and how to get yourself ready, and have an idea of the global opportunities available to you.

Published by Woodhead Publishing Limited

Key concept terms

API: active pharmaceutical ingredient

Biopharmaceutical: drug made from a living system; biotech drugs or biologics

Biostatistics: application of statistics to medical and pharmaceutical data

Bulk drug: API in bulk

Epidemiology: disease related information in the population

Fermentation: act of a microorganism or enzyme producing desirable products

Generic: drug with a nonproprietary name or no trademark

Pathophysiology: physiology of disordered body functions

Pharmacokineticist: a person who deals with what happens to the drugs inside bodies

Pharmacology: a drug's action on the body

PharmD: doctor of pharmacy

Therapeutic: medically treated

Translational medicine: evidence-based medicine

2.1 Job opportunities in the pharmaceutical industry

Figure 2.1 shows three real job advertisements, which show the multidisciplinary nature of pharmaceutical jobs. For a high-level job with a six figure salary, you need to have well-rounded qualifications, but even mathematicians can have jobs in medicine development.

Imagine you have discovered a drug that will ensure each human being a hundred years of active life. You are not only making your own life better, but you are making the lives of 6 billion people better. It is definitely a good feeling. If Fleming had not discovered penicillin in 1928, there would have been thousands more deaths during World War II due to infectious diseases. At the same time, the introduction of life-style drugs (e.g. Viagra) has given millions of senior citizens higher-quality lives. A career in drug discovery,

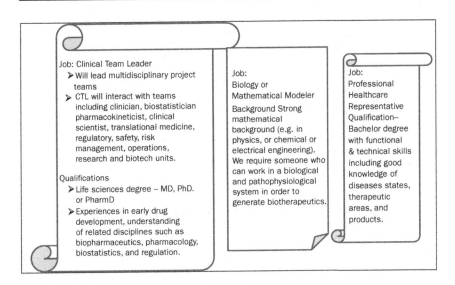

Figure 2.1 Excerpts from pharmaceutical job advertisements

drug production, or drug formulation is always exciting as you are working to improve the health of millions of people.

The pharmaceutical industry makes health better for all; it is completely different from other industries as the quality of its product cannot be judged by sight, touch, or taste. As discussed in Chapter 1, there are dozens of associated industries, institutions, and organizations throughout the world to support and regulate this industry, for example the Food and Drug Administration (FDA) in the USA and the Medicines and Healthcare Products Regulatory Agency (MHRA) in the UK. All these supporting industries employ a large number of professionals (e.g. scientists, researchers, chemists, biochemists, biologists, physicians, statisticians, physicists, mathematicians, engineers, and technicians) and administrators (e.g. office clerks, workers, drivers, and cleaners). See Figure 2.2.

2.1.1 Types of pharmaceutical industries

There are main four types of pharmaceutical companies:

- research-based pharmaceutical companies with facilities for bulk drugs and formulation, including generic subsidiaries
- generic pharmaceutical industries

Published by Woodhead Publishing Limited

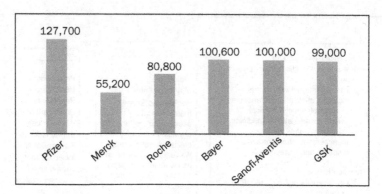

Figure 2.2 The number of employees in six leading pharmaceutical industries in 2009

Source: Companies' websites

- small start-up research companies
- bulk drug manufacturers.

Research-based pharmaceutical companies like Pfizer, Merck, GSK, Roche, Bayer and Sanofi-Aventis are corporate-based and often become larger through mergers and acquisitions. These companies are also known as drug discovery companies. They complete research to discover a noble drug (one that is effective), and then market it. Under patent law, no other company can make and market a patented drug until its patent expires after 20 years.

As soon as a drug's patent expires, generic versions of the drug appear on the market produced by other companies, with one condition: the generic drug has to be bioequivalent to the originator. There are many generic pharmaceutical companies in several countries, such as Teva, Mylan, and Barr Pharmaceuticals in the USA; Arrow Generics and Actavis UK in the UK; and Dr Reddys and Ranbaxy in India.

Small start-up research companies are special disease-based companies that initiate research to find a lead compound and start clinical trials. In most cases, if the clinical trial is successful, the companies collaborate or sell it to a larger company. There are hundreds of these types of companies. Bulk drug companies are chemical companies that only produce bulk drugs and sell them to the formulation companies.

The healthcare industry, especially pharmaceutical companies, has been a good source of jobs around the world, including in developing countries. Data shows that the industry directly provided almost 700,000 jobs in the

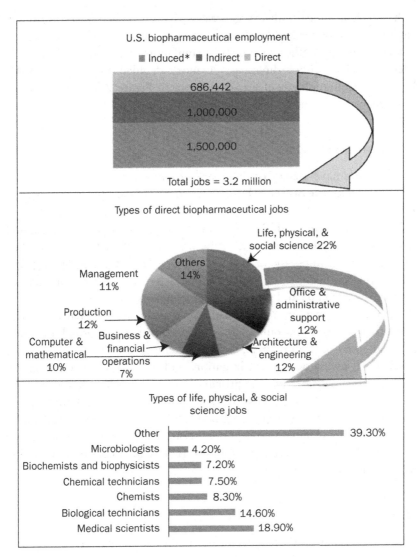

Figure 2.3 Jobs in the biopharmaceutical sector in USA, 2006

*When a job opportunity is provided at a local daycare facility.

Source: L. R. Burns[1]

USA in 2009, and created another 2.5 million jobs in other sectors as well.[2] In the UK, the industry employed around 72,000 people and generated another 250,000 jobs in related industries in 2009.[3] Most pharmaceutical companies in the USA are in California, Illinois, Texas, Indiana, New Jersey, New York, North Carolina, Pennsylvania, and Florida.

The pharmaceutical industry generally pays good salaries and provides benefits, with jobs for highly educated scientists and researchers as well as for technicians and other workers in manufacturing areas who have only college or high school diplomas. A more detailed breakdown of US pharmaceutical employment areas is shown in Figure 2.3. Some areas of employment are discussed briefly below.

2.1.1.1   Administration

All companies have a chair of the board of management, board members, and a chief executive officer (CEO). Divisional heads usually report directly to the CEO.

The human resources (HR) department is responsible for recruiting and managing people in a company, attracting highly skilled staff, and then training and retaining them. It is also responsible for negotiating and determining compensation and benefits. The department of finance manages the accounts and finances of the company.

The most important and critical department for a pharmaceutical company is its legal and public affairs department. Professional attorneys handle all sorts of legal matters, such as patents and trademarks, business transactions, regulatory affairs, litigation, and compliance. The regulatory affairs professionals become the primary liaison between the company and the regulatory authority. Those who are interested in regulatory affairs must have skills in analysis, communication, organization, leadership, writing, time-management, and presentation, and adequate knowledge of law and ethics. Information technology (IT) is an integral part of any pharmaceutical company.

2.1.1.2   Clinical areas

Researchers design and study clinical trials to determine the safety and efficacy of a product, develop study protocol, and execute and manage it. These researchers also analyze data and write reports that document the clinical trials.

2.1.1.3   Marketing and sales

Marketing personnel plan and develop marketing strategies, including advertisements, promotion, and branding for a particular pharmaceutical product. They train and support the sales representatives. The sales professionals are partly responsible for turnover of the pharmaceutical company. Pharmaceutical sales professionals should have clinical knowledge and analytical and communication skills. As frontline spokespersons for a company, sales representatives work hard to disseminate the company's products to physicians and other prescribers. These sales representatives often earn lucrative salaries; the median annual earnings for a sales representative were US$59,000–70,000 in the USA in 2010 (Figure 2.4).

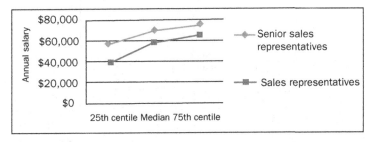

Figure 2.4 Median annual salaries of pharmaceutical sales representatives in the USA, 2010

Source: salary.com[4]

2.2 Education and training

To have a successful career your interest is as important as your skill. If you are interested to know more about medicine, or are excited to hear news of a drug being discovered that may cure cancer or Alzheimer's, you will be more likely to learn as much as possible about it. As your knowledge increases, your skill will develop as well. The pharmaceutical field is a good choice for people who like science, want to work in laboratories, and want to ensure the good health of people. There is a wide variety of jobs; your education and training will depend on the career you decide to pursue, and include a certain amount of on-the-job training.

Figure 2.5 illustrates the wealth of career opportunities in different areas within the pharmaceutical industry and Figure 2.6 shows the probable work areas within the pharmaceutical industry by type of degree and subject specialty.

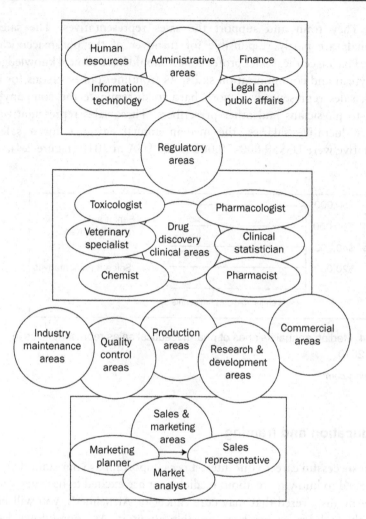

Figure 2.5 Employment opportunities in the pharmaceutical industry

Published by Woodhead Publishing Limited

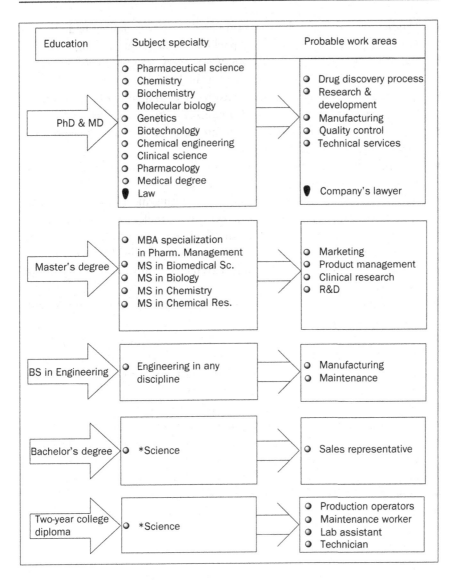

Figure 2.6 How level of education, subject specialty, and type of degree lead to certain work areas within the pharmaceutical industry

2.3 Various departments of a pharmaceutical company

An ideal pharmaceutical industrial unit requires the following departments to run the pharmaceutical business efficiently:

Published by Woodhead Publishing Limited

- *production* – deals with production according to a daily schedule
- *packaging* – deals with primary packing to shipment packing
- *quality control* – tests and analyzes every sample including raw materials, in-process samples, and finished products
- *quality assurance and auditing* – ensures overall quality of the products, environment, and facilities, and organizes in-house inspection systems
- *engineering and maintenance* – operates and maintains factory utilities, machinery, and instruments
- *product management* – deals with product selection, product brochures, promotion, literature, packing, and design
- *technical services* – selects and supplies an arrangement of machinery and spares, coordinates product development, and handles product complaints
- *medical services* – deals with medical-related support services, such as organizing clinical meetings and disseminating medical information
- *clinical services* – conducts clinical trials, bioequivalence studies, and other clinically related research
- *regulatory services* – handles and coordinates regulatory affairs with the drug authority.
- *R&D* – deals with drug discovery and development, process development, and formulated product development activities
- *personnel and administration* – manages and implements industry policy and takes care of overall administration
- *human resources* – recruits, trains, and places staff
- *marketing and sales* – plans and implements marketing strategies
- *marketing research* – deals with market surveys and monitors competitors' activities
- *distribution* – ensures the supply of medicines to hospitals and retailers
- *commercial* – handles imports and exports
- *accounts and finance* – manages company's finances
- *information technology* – deals with the usage and management of computer technology.

If your education and training are in sciences or pharmaceutical sciences, you can apply for a job at a pharmaceutical company, but it is better to have an advanced degree in a related field, such as chemistry, pharmacy, pharmaceutical sciences, pharmaceutical technologies, biotechnology, biology, microbiology, medicine, or engineering. It is also possible to work in laboratories as an analyst or scientist; pharmaceutical scientists usually earn high salaries and work to develop new drugs or research and develop other areas. There are also plenty of careers in the manufacturing or quality control units. If you aren't interested in a laboratory oriented or manufacturing job, you can still find a lucrative job in marketing and sales, regulatory affairs, or product management. Even someone with a non-science major, such as graduates of commerce, economics, marketing, business, marketing, or international relations, would be able to find an exciting job in a pharmaceutical company.

2.4   Mergers and acquisitions in the pharmaceutical industry

Mergers and acquisitions are unique and common occurrences in the pharmaceutical sector. They result in the takeover of one company by another – the difference is in the detail of how they are financed. A merger is the combination of two companies of equal size to become a single company. An acquisition is the taking over by a big company of a smaller one, and the financing involves cash, stocks, or other forms of company equity.

The current pharmaceutical giants – Pfizer, Merck, GlaxoSmithKline, Sanofi-Aventis, and Roche – all owe their size to mergers and acquisitions (Figures 2.7–2.11). In 2009 there were two important deals: the takeover of Wyeth by Pfizer, and the takeover of Schering Plough by Merck.

There are several reasons for these mergers and acquisitions:

- to make larger companies, which leads to a more reputable image and a bigger presence in the market
- to reduce costs, especially in R&D and work forces
- to develop and strengthen a new product line
- to promote global business
- to boost shareholders' confidence.

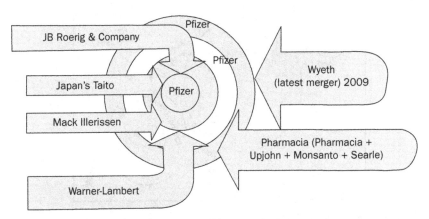

Figure 2.7 Mergers and acquisitions of Pfizer until 2009

Published by Woodhead Publishing Limited

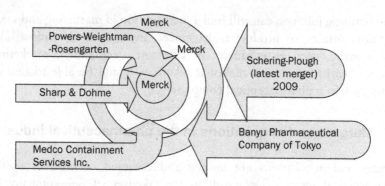

Figure 2.8 Mergers and acquisitions of Merck until 2009

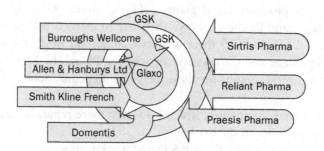

Figure 2.9 Mergers and acquisitions of Glaxo until 2009

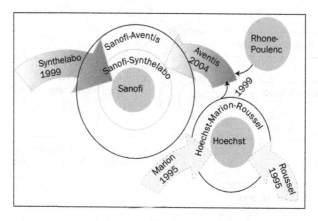

Figure 2.10 Mergers and acquisitions of Sanofi-Aventis, 1995–2004

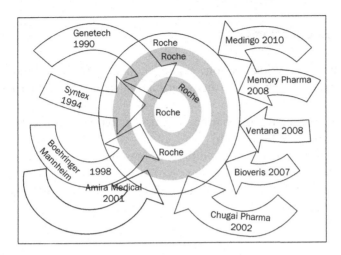

Figure 2.11 Mergers and acquisitions of Roche, 1990–2010

Mergers and acquisitions always have some impact on jobs. Often there are job cuts in some common areas of the two companies, but experienced and skilled personnel can usually find a job with another company if they are made redundant.

2.5   Careers for pharmaceutical physicians

The pharmaceutical industry provides challenging careers for doctors. According to the Association of British Pharmaceutical Industry, there are over 1,000 physicians working for different pharmaceutical companies. In the UK, doctors interested in working in the industry can obtain a Diploma in Pharmaceutical Medicines, which has been offered since 1976 by the Faculty of Pharmaceutical Medicine at the Royal College of Physicians. Physicians are increasingly interested in non-practicing jobs in the industry, in any of the following areas:

- drug discovery and clinical R&D
- marketing and post-marketing surveillance
- regulatory and legal affairs
- drug safety
- clinical pharmacology
- medical education
- pharmaco-economics
- epidemiology.

Published by Woodhead Publishing Limited

Practice questions

1. What kind of jobs can one expect in the pharmaceutical industry?
2. Is there any difference between pharmacists and pharmaceutical scientists?
3. Describe the job of pharmaceutical sales representatives. How do they prepare for the job?
4. Is it true that there is no difference between selling medicines and selling ball point pens? If not, explain.
5. Explain how the pharmaceutical industry is a work place of multidisciplinary careers.

Answers to some practice questions

2. Pharmacists can become pharmaceutical scientists by doing research but pharmaceutical scientists cannot become pharmacists without a professional certificate.

Notes

1. Adapted from L. R. Burns, *The Biopharmaceutical Sector's Impact on the U.S. Economy: Analysis at the National, State, and Local Levels*, Washington, DC: Archstone Consulting, 2009.
2. PhRMA, *Pharmaceutical Industry Profile*, 2009, www.interfarma.org.br/site2/images/SiteInterfarma/Informacoesdosetor/Publicacoes/PhRMA2009Profile FINAL.pdf (accessed February 24, 2011).
3. ABPI, *Prescription for Innovation*, London: Association of British Pharmaceutical Industry, 2009/10.
4. Salary.com, 'Salary Wizard', www.salary.com/salary/index.asp (accessed Apr 3, 2011).

3

Drugs, medicines, and regulatory authorities

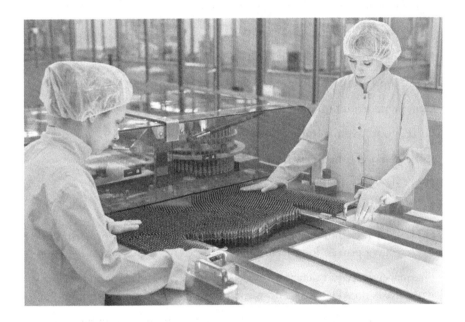

Learning objective

This chapter looks at the common terms used for drugs – medicines, brand names, generic names, chemical names, prescription drugs and over-the-counter drugs – and at how drugs are developed. It describes how regulatory agencies regulate the quality of generic drugs and the role of pharmacopoeias (Figure 3.1).

Key concept terms

Bioequivalency: *in-vivo* equivalency between brand name and generic name drugs regarding pharmacokinetic profiles

Blockbuster drug: a drug whose annual sale is US$1 billion or more

Brand name: trade or proprietary name

CDSCO: Central Drug Standard Control Organization

Chemical name: based on IUPAC nomenclature

Clinical trial: testing of a drug on humans

Drug: active pharmaceutical ingredient

EMEA: European Medicine Evaluation Agency

FDA: Food and Drug Administration

Generic name: international non-proprietary name

GMP: good manufacturing practice

IND: investigational new drug

IVIVC: *in-vivo in-vitro* correlation

Medicine: formulated drug

OTC: over the counter; OTC drugs can be bought without prescription as they have proven long term safety

Pharmaceutical equivalency: equivalency between brand name and generic name drugs on APIs, dosage forms, dose, and route of administration

Pharmacopoeia: a book for the use of pharmaceutical industry on specifications and methodologies of testing of APIs or dosage forms

POM: prescription-only medicine; these medicines cannot be purchased without a doctor's prescription

Preclinical trial: *in-vivo* animal model study to determine drug activity, safety, and toxicity

Regulatory agency: agency that regulates manufacturing of medicines, enforces good manufacturing practice, and approves importation, promotion, marketing and labeling of medicines.

Published by Woodhead Publishing Limited

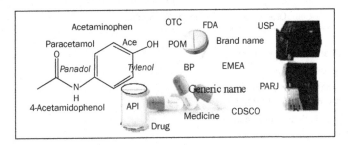

Figure 3.1 The talking points of Chapter 3

3.1 Drugs and medicines: brand names and generic names

The terms 'drug' and 'medicine' essentially mean the same thing. 'Drug' is used more often than 'medicine' in the USA as the US Food and Drug Administration (FDA) uses this term. In Europe 'medicine' is more common as it is the term agencies such as the Medicine and Healthcare Products Regulatory Agency (MHRA) in the UK and the European Medicine Evaluation Agency (EMEA) use. Most often, especially in the USA, the term 'drug' refers to psychoactive products that produce pleasurable sensations. The non-medical use of illicit psychoactive products is a big social problem around the world.

The Federal Food, Drug, and Cosmetic Act 1938 defines drugs as 'articles intended for use in the diagnosis, cure, mitigation, treatment, or prevention of disease' and 'articles (other than food) intended to affect the structure or any function of the body of man or other animals'.[1] Here 'articles' is used to refer to any substances, whether chemical substances or biologics. In this book, 'drug' and 'medicine' are used interchangeably to refer to the same item, although strictly speaking 'drug' refers to active pharmaceutical ingredients (APIs), which are always embedded with certain information, such as pharmacological effects, safety, and usefulness.

Figure 3.2 shows the embedded information of a drug. Information about medicines is vital, which is why every medicine has an insert with full details about it in its packaging (Figure 3.3).

A 'medicine' is simply a formulated drug made using APIs and excipients (non-APIs). The excipients are also chemical substances but have no pharmacological function and help to produce a particular dosage form, such as a tablet or capsule (Figure 3.4).

In the market place there are two categories of drugs: prescription-only drugs and non-prescription drugs. A prescription drug or prescription-only

Drug = API + embedded information

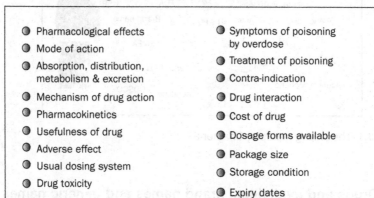

- ● Pharmacological effects
- ● Mode of action
- ● Absorption, distribution, metabolism & excretion
- ● Mechanism of drug action
- ● Pharmacokinetics
- ● Usefulness of drug
- ● Adverse effect
- ● Usual dosing system
- ● Drug toxicity
- ● Symptoms of poisoning by overdose
- ● Treatment of poisoning
- ● Contra-indication
- ● Drug interaction
- ● Cost of drug
- ● Dosage forms available
- ● Package size
- ● Storage condition
- ● Expiry dates

Figure 3.2 The embedded information of a drug

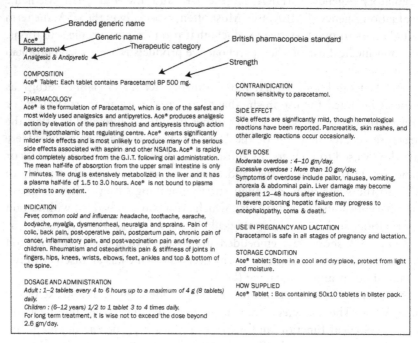

Branded generic name
Ace®
Generic name
Paracetamol
Therapeutic category
Analgesic & Antipyretic
Strength
British pharmacopoeia standard

COMPOSITION
Ace® Tablet: Each tablet contains Paracetamol BP 500 mg.

PHARMACOLOGY
Ace® is the formulation of Paracetamol, which is one of the safest and most widely used analgesics and antipyretics. Ace® produces analgesic action by elevation of the pain threshold and antipyresis through action on the hypothalamic heat regulating centre. Ace® exerts significantly milder side effects and is most unlikely to produce many of the serious side effects associated with aspirin and other NSAIDs. Ace® is rapidly and completely absorbed from the G.I.T. following oral administration. The mean half-life of absorption from the upper small intestine is only 7 minutes. The drug is extensively metabolized in the liver and it has a plasma half-life of 1.5 to 3.0 hours. Ace® is not bound to plasma proteins to any extent.

INDICATION
Fever, common cold and influenza: headache, toothache, earache, bodyache, myalgia, dysmenorrheal, neuralgia and sprains. Pain of colic, back pain, post-operative pain, postpartum pain, chronic pain of cancer, inflammatory pain, and post-vaccination pain and fever of children. Rheumatism and osteoarthritis pain & stiffness of joints in fingers, hips, knees, wrists, elbows, feet, ankles and top & bottom of the spine.

DOSAGE AND ADMINISTRATION
Adult : 1–2 tablets every 4 to 6 hours up to a maximum of 4 g (8 tablets) daily.
Children : (6–12 years) 1/2 to 1 tablet 3 to 4 times daily.
For long term treatment, it is wise not to exceed the dose beyond 2.6 gm/day.

CONTRAINDICATION
Known sensitivity to paracetamol.

SIDE EFFECT
Side effects are significantly mild, though hematological reactions have been reported. Pancreatitis, skin rashes, and other allergic reactions occur occasionally.

OVER DOSE
Moderate overdose : 4–10 gm/day.
Excessive overdose : More than 10 gm/day.
Symptoms of overdose include pallor, nausea, vomiting, anorexia & abdominal pain. Liver damage may become apparent 12–48 hours after ingestion.
In severe poisoning hepatic failure may progress to encephalopathy, coma & death.

USE IN PREGNANCY AND LACTATION
Paracetamol is safe in all stages of pregnancy and lactation.

STORAGE CONDITION
Ace® tablet: Store in a cool and dry place, protect from light and moisture.

HOW SUPPLIED
Ace® Tablet : Box containing 50x10 tablets in blister pack.

Figure 3.3 Details about paracetamol provided in the packaging

Source: Square Pharmaceuticals Ltd

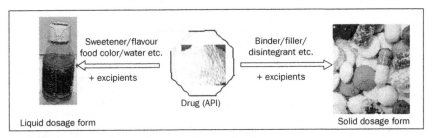

Figure 3.4 Liquid and solid dosage forms of a drug

Source: Square Pharmaceuticals Ltd

medicine (POM) is only available with a doctor's prescription. These drugs are safe and appropriate if a doctor prescribes them. For example, antibiotics, steroids, and cardiovascular drugs are all POMs. Non-prescription drugs, commonly known as over-the-counter drugs (OTCs), are available without prescriptions. The long-term safety of OTC drugs has been established, so they can be sold over the counter. Paracetamol and aspirin have long been OTC drugs, and ranitidine (Zantac) is a recent addition to the OTC list.

3.2 Drug names

Drugs names are sometimes confusing and hard to understand. For example, Tylenol, a fever reducer or antipyretic medicine, is very common but there is no difference between Tylenol and paracetamol, acetaminophen, or Panadol. This product is an OTC medicine, so pharmacies commonly sell paracetamol (acetaminophen, Tylenol, or Panadol). In England and Australia these products are available as Panadol.

These different names are based on one root and only one chemical compound. The Merck Index or International Union of Pure and Applied Chemistry (IUPAC) provides different chemical names, such as 4-Acetamidophenol, p-Acetamidophenol, N-(4-hydroxyphenyl)ethanamide, N-(4-hydroxyphenyl)-acetamide, and N-acetyl-para-aminophenol. Chemical compounds named or categorized as drugs eventually have a chemical name, a generic name, and a brand name. The chemical name relates to the nomenclature system formulated by the IUPAC, and is usually long and difficult, derived from the structure of the drug. See Figure 3.5.

Published by Woodhead Publishing Limited

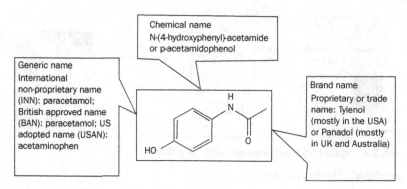

Chemical name
N-(4-hydroxyphenyl)-acetamide
or p-acetamidophenol

Generic name
International
non-proprietary name
(INN): paracetamol;
British approved name
(BAN): paracetamol; US
adopted name (USAN):
acetaminophen

Brand name
Proprietary or trade
name: Tylenol
(mostly in the USA)
or Panadol (mostly
in UK and Australia)

Figure 3.5 Example of the generic, chemical, and brand names of a drug

3.2.1 Generic drugs

The generic name of a drug is the chemical equivalent of a brand name drug whose patent has expired. The original manufacturer of a drug can produce and sell the drug for a 20-year patent, but once the patent expires, other manufacturers can produce and sell the drug. These manufacturers use a generic or branded generic name, which is usually a shorter version of the chemical name. The brand name is known as the trade name or proprietary name. The original manufacturer can name the discovered drug anything that might boost the sale of the drug. When the antipyretic acetaminophen (paracetamol) was developed in the 1950s it was marketed in the USA only under the name Tylenol, and there were no acetaminophen drugs with alternate names available. Today there are dozens of generic versions of Tylenol available on the market.

As generic drugs are marketed by many generic pharmaceutical companies, branded generic names are used to differentiate them from each other. Figure 3.3 shows that paracetamol is marketed as 'Ace' by Square Pharmaceuticals Ltd in Bangladesh. In general, the pharmaceutical company that discovers a drug assigns it an internal code number once the lead compound's structure is confirmed and can assign the chemical name at the same time. If the compound will ultimately pass the the US FDA approval process, the company can create any brand name it wishes. Simultaneously, the US Adopted Name (USAN) Council selects a generic name through the US Pharmacopeial Convention based on the compound's structure and activities.

Let's take the example of Viagra. In 1985, Pfizer in the UK started research using a code name of the discovered compound UK-92480, whose chemical name is 5-[2-ethoxy-5-(4-methylpiperazin-1-ylsulfonyl) phenyl.]-1-methyl-3-propyl-1,6-dihydro-7H-pyrazolo[4,3-d.]pyrimidin-7-one. Eventually the compound was given the trade or brand name Viagra, whose generic name is sildenafil citrate.

Published by Woodhead Publishing Limited

3.3 Drug discovery and the drug development process

Chapter 1 described how drug discovery is a very lengthy and extremely risky process, and even after spending billions of dollars and ten to 12 years in research, a drug still may not ultimately succeed. The withdrawal of Vioxx from the market at the phase IV level is an example of this. A close look at pharmaceutical companies on the stock market shows that a single-day price of a company's stock might jump by three or four times because of the success of phase III clinical trials or the US FDA's approval of a drug, but there are far more failures than successes in different stages of drug development. The stock price of a pharmaceutical company can plummet by half or a quarter because of an unsuccessful clinical trial data or disapproval by the US FDA.

Figure 3.6 shows how much Roche estimates the company spends to develop one drug.

Figure 3.7 shows how much Tufts University's Tufts Center for the Study of Drug Development estimated spent on developing one drug in 1995, using some different drug development measures. It shows its average cost of developing one medicine was not much different from the Roche estimate.

Investment, time, and risk are all parts of the drug development process. Lipitor (generic name atorvastatin), a cholesterol-reducing drug, began to be marketed in 1997 and since then has become an instant blockbuster drug, earning over US$13 billion for Pfizer in 2009,[2] but there is no guarantee that after spending almost US$1 billion a drug will be successful like Lipitor. Most lead drugs do not see the market, but one that makes it

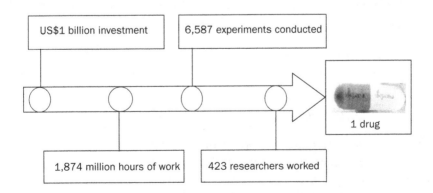

Figure 3.6 Figures from Roche on the investment required to develop a drug

Source: Roche website[3]

Published by Woodhead Publishing Limited

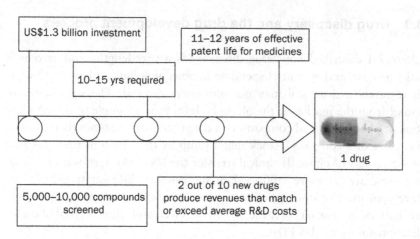

Figure 3.7 Figures from Tufts University on the investment required to develop a drug

to the market and becomes a blockbuster drug, such as Lipitor, Zantac, or Viagra, can bring a company large profits.

3.3.1 Phases in the drug development process

Drug development research is a never-ending process, which starts with drug discovery. The process can be divided into the following phases:

- drug discovery
- preclinical
- application to be an investigational new drug
- clinical trials phases 1–3
- filing to be a new drug application
- post-marketing survey.

3.3.1.1 The drug discovery phase

Understanding how a disease works is the first step towards drug discovery. A team of researchers tries to find out the cause of the disease, which could be enzyme activity, a lack of enzyme, or the presence of a new pathogen. Researchers can include pharmacologists, chemists, biochemists, biostatisticians, and computer programmers who screen thousands of compounds to find promising lead compounds.

Published by Woodhead Publishing Limited

3.3.1.2 The preclinical phase

The objective of this phase is to make *in-vitro* experiments in cell cultures and *in-vivo* animal model testing to determine a drug's activity, safety, and toxicity. At this stage the studies include a pharmacological profile of the drug and its short-term toxicity in animals. When it has positive results, the pharmaceutical company files two applications: a patent application to secure 20 years' protection and an investigational new drug (IND) application to the US FDA.

3.3.1.3 Applying to be an investigational new drug

The company makes an IND application to the US FDA for it to continue to develop the drug by pursuing human trials. The IND package should contain:

- the chemistry of the drug
- animal test results – pharmacology and safety data
- manufacturing information and stability
- the rationale for carrying out clinical studies in human and clinical protocols.

The US FDA's Center for Drug Evaluation & Research reviews the IND application and makes a decision.

3.3.1.4 Clinical trials to test the drug on humans

There are three phases of clinical trials to test the drug on humans:

- *Phase 1* The drug is tested in a small group of normal, healthy volunteers (20–100 people) to find out drug safety, pharmacology (absorption, distribution, metabolism, and excretion), and dose range.
- *Phase 2* For the first time the investigational drug is tested at the patient level. The phase 2 placebo-controlled clinical trials provide information on the efficacy of the drug. The trial is conducted on approximately 100–500 volunteer patients.
- *Phase 3* This is an extension of the phase 2 trial with a larger-scale patient population (1,000–5,000 people). The placebo-controlled and double-blinded (randomized) phase 3 clinical trials provide statistically significant data on the efficacy, safety, and side effects of the drug.

3.3.1.5 Filing a new drug application

After analyzing all the experimental data, if the drug is found to be effective and safe with few adverse effects, a new drug application (NDA) is filed with the US FDA for approval. Typically the NDA contains details of:

- the chemistry of the drug
- its manufacturing processes
- its pharmacology and pharmacokinetics
- clinical trials data
- its toxicity
- labeling information.

Once the US FDA approves the drug, the company starts marketing it, but the FDA's requirements still need to be fulfilled, which is known as phase 4 post-marketing surveillance.

3.3.1.6 Phase 4 studies

Phase 4 post-marketing surveys evaluate the long-term effects of the drug.

3.3.2 Summary of the drug development process

The complete drug development process is shown in Figures 3.8 and 3.9.

The long journey to new medicine development does not usually go smoothly. There are many obstructions and setbacks throughout the journey that need to be carefully analyzed. The developer has to move forward while making the right decisions.

3.4 Marketing of generic drugs in the USA or Europe

We have seen that drug development and bringing a drug to the market can be a long process. The innovator company can have the patent for 20 years, but the innovator company gets only ten to 15 years of market monopoly with its brand name drug because the company applies for a patent immediately after initial development. After the expiration of the patent, any pharmaceutical company can bring the same drug to the market, but the company must go through the registration process. Figure 3.10 illustrates the process of developing and marketing brand name drugs.

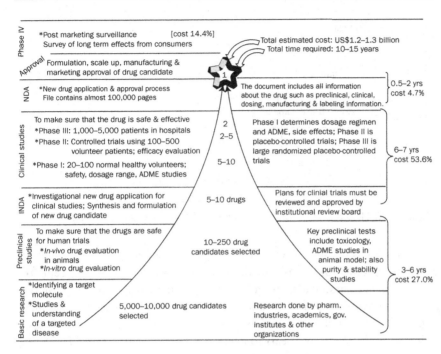

Figure 3.8 Summary of the drug development process 1[4]

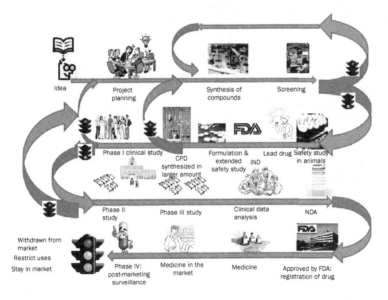

Figure 3.9 Summary of the drug development process 2

Source: Redrawn with permission from a presentation by Jorkasky[5]

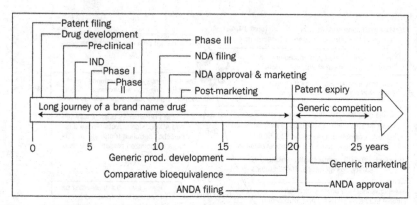

Figure 3.10 How a generic drug is developed from a brand name drug

The FDA has requirements for the development of generic drugs. Generic drug companies should have all the information about a drug except for bioequivalence data. The team members of a generic drug company use the available information of the brand name drug to make their own product. Figure 3.11 shows the drug review processes for brand and generic drugs.

It takes only one to two years to develop a generic drug compared with ten years or more to develop a brand name drug. The art of drug formulation is crucial when developing generic drugs. A good formulation can bring necessary bioequivalence, and the only experimental clinical step is undertaken.

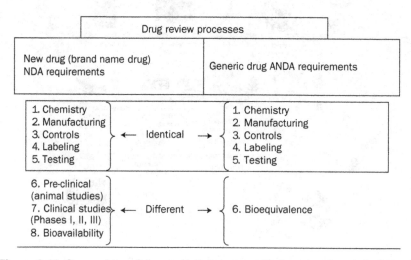

Figure 3.11 Comparison of drug review processes for brand and generic drugs

Published by Woodhead Publishing Limited

3.4.1 Bioequivalence

The Center for Drug Evaluation and Research, which is part of the US FDA, defines bioequivalence as 'pharmaceutical equivalents whose rate and extent of absorption are not statistically different when administered to patients or subjects at the same molar dose under similar experimental conditions'.[6] More simply, bioequivalence is *in-vivo* equivalence. There is another equivalence called pharmaceutical equivalence or *in-vitro* equivalence. The equivalence relationships between brand name and generic drugs are shown in Figure 3.12.

If there is pharmaceutical equivalence, it is likely there will be bioequivalence between two products. Bioequivalent products can be substituted for one another, and as a whole they show therapeutic equivalence to each other. To establish bioequivalence, the rate and extent of drug absorption in the innovator's drug and the generic drug must be comparable, so both products must have similar Cmax (maximum concentration) and corresponding Tmax (time for maximum concentration) (as an index of rate of absorption) and area under curve (AUC) (as an index of the extent of absorption

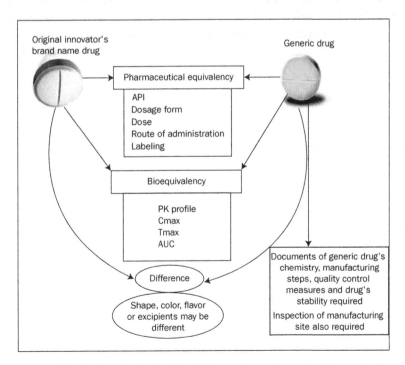

Figure 3.12 Equivalence relationships between brand name and generic drugs

Published by Woodhead Publishing Limited

determined by the trapezoidal method). Figure 3.13 shows how drug plasma concentration changes over time.

The data should be statistically significant: using two one-sided procedures, 90% confidence intervals of Cmax and AUC must fit between 80% and 125%. The bioequivalence studies are carried out on normal healthy volunteers, preferably male and female, but patients can be included as study subjects too. The US FDA prefers single dose, fasting and fed bioequivalence studies for most of the oral solid dosage forms unless there are labeling restrictions in the innovator's drug. There are also biowaivers (waivers of *in-vivo* testing) for certain dosage forms or formulations such as intravenous solutions, other parenteral solutions, oral solutions, inhalation anesthetics, and topical (skin) solutions.

An Abbreviated New Drug Application (ANDA) is an application for approval to market a generic drug in the USA. The company making the application reviews its completeness, and then seeks plant inspection by the US FDA. The bioequivalence data is evaluated along with other related information. The FDA's flow sheet for the approval process for generic drugs is shown in Figure 3.14.

There are no requirements for bioequivalence studies for generic drugs marketed in most developing countries. Regulatory agencies or companies in developing countries have to ensure the bioavailability of the drugs they

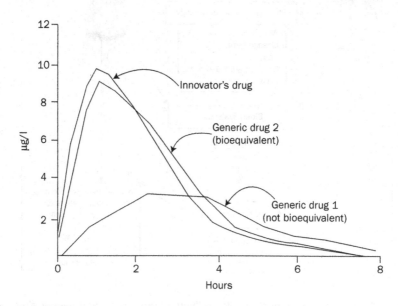

Figure 3.13 Drug plasma concentration over time

Published by Woodhead Publishing Limited

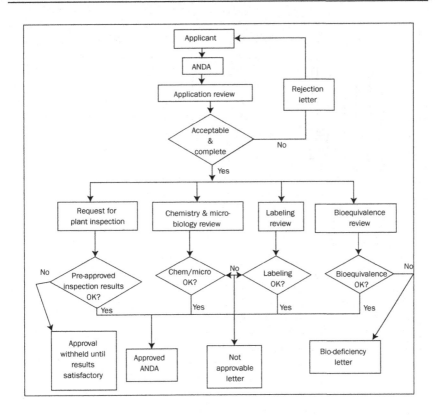

Figure 3.14 The US FDA's approval process for generic drugs

Source: US FDA website[7]

market. Local manufacturers usually compare the results of the *in-vitro* dissolution of the solid dosage forms with those of the innovator's drug before marketing. *In-vitro* dissolution helps develop an optimum formulation of oral solid dosage forms and maintain batch-to-batch quality control of the products. *In-vitro in-vivo* correlation (IVIVC) is becoming more important because researchers believe it may serve as a substitute for *in-vivo* studies. The US FDA defines IVIVC as 'a predictive mathematical model describing the relationship between an *in-vitro* property of a dosage form and an *in-vivo* response'.[8] Dissolution rate and dissolution efficiency can be correlated with the Cmax, Tmax and AUC of *in-vivo* studies. The IVIVC relationship is depicted in Figure 3.15.

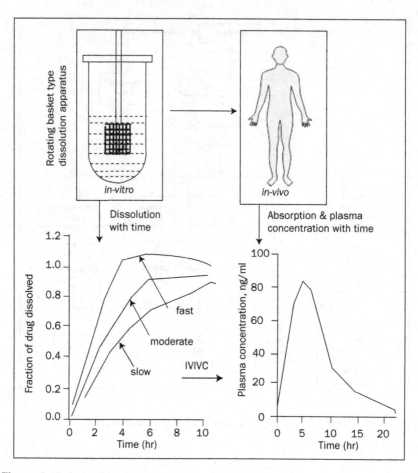

Figure 3.15 *In-vitro in-vivo* correlations of solid dosage forms

3.4.2 Pricing of generic drugs

During the patent period, the original discovery company has a monopoly on business and the price of the drug is expensive, but after the patent expires a generic drug is available at a much lower price. The US FDA describes a generic drug as 'identical to their brand-name drug in dosage, safety, and strength, how it is taken, quality, performance, and intended use'.[9]

Table 3.1 Cost of 20 brand name drugs provided by Blue Cross Blue Shield of Michigan compared with their generic counterparts, February 2009

Brand name and strength*	Generic name	Quantity drugs required for a 30-day supply	Cost for a 30-day supply of brand name drug**	Cost for a 30-day supply of generic drug***	Savings when use generic drug for 30 days
Adderall 20 mg	Amphetamine Mixture	60	$185.40	$24.00	$161.40
Altace® 10 mg	Ramipril	30	$64.64	$18.10	$46.54
Ambien® 10 mg	Zolpidem Tartrate	30	$160.09	$3.00	$157.09
Coreg® 25 mg	Carvedilol	60	$148.16	$9.00	$139.16
Coumadin® 5 mg	Warfarin Sodium	30	$33.06	$5.10	$27.96
Glucophage® XR 500 mg	Metformin Hcl	90	$106.96	$11.70	$95.26
Imitrex® 100 mg^	Sumatriptan Succinate	12	$335.28	$228.60	$106.68
Lotrel® 10/20 mg	Amlodipine Besylate/ Benazepril	30	$133.71	$65.40	$68.31
Norvasc® 5 mg	Amlodipine Besylate	30	$82.22	$6.00	$76.22
Paxil CR® 25 mg	Paroxetine Hcl	30	$119.00	$80.21	$38.79
Prilosec® 40 mg	Omeprazole	30	$261.34	$166.41	$94.93
Requip® 1 mg^	Ropinirole Hcl	60	$182.78	$31.64	$151.13
Risperdal® 1 mg	Risperidone	60	$333.45	$204.75	$128.70
Ritalin® 20 mg	Methylphenidate Hcl	90	$126.82	$25.71	$101.11
Tenormin® 50 mg	Atenolol	30	$558.97	$3.00	$555.97
Valium® 5 mg	Diazepam	60	$177.77	$1.82	$175.94
Wellbutrin XL® 150 mg	Bupropion Hcl	30	$189.53	$90.80	$94.73
Xanax® 0.5 mg	Alprazolam	90	$158.58	$4.50	$154.08
Zocor® 40 mg	Simvastatin	30	$150.79	$7.50	$143.29
Zoloft® 100 mg	Sertraline Hcl	30	$120.80	$7.50	$113.30

* Most common strength dispensed for BCBSM members.
** Brand name cost based on average wholesale price obtained from various data sources (Feb 25, 2009)
*** Generic cost based on BCBSM maximum allowable cost schedule or discounted average wholesale price (Feb 27, 2009)
^ Newly available generic medication

Source: BCBSM[10]

Published by Woodhead Publishing Limited

Generic drugs are always less expensive than brand name drugs, and the consumer can save money by choosing a generic version of any drug available on the market. Table 3.1 shows the cost of the top 20 brand-name drugs provided by Blue Cross Blue Shield of Michigan with any generic counterparts. A new drug has no generic version until the patent expires. According to IMS Health, global sales of generic drugs increased from US$29 billion in 2003 to US$78 billion in 2008.[11] In developing countries the drug market is predominantly generic.

The FDA lists the following facts about generic drugs:

- The FDA requires generic drugs to have the same quality and performance as the brand name drugs.
- Research shows that generics work just as well as brand name drugs.
- There is a big difference in price between generic and brand name drugs. On average, the cost of a generic drug is 80–85% lower than the brand name product.
- The FDA recently evaluated 2,070 human studies conducted between 1996 and 2007. The average difference in absorption into the body between the generic and the brand name drug was only 2.3%. Some generics were absorbed slightly more, some slightly less.
- There is no evidence that people who switch to using a generic drug after having used a brand name drug are risking treatment failure.
- Generic manufacturers are able to sell their products for lower prices not because the products are of lesser quality, but because generic manufacturers generally do not engage in costly advertising, marketing and promotion, or significant research and development.
- The FDA's aggressive action in this case demonstrates the high standards to which all prescription drugs – generic and brand name – are held.
- The FDA receives very few reports of adverse events about specific generic drugs. Most reports of adverse events are related to side effects of the drug ingredient itself.
- The FDA is actively engaged in making all regulated products – including generic drugs – safer.[12]

A recent survey by IMS Health indicates that about 69% of all prescriptions in the USA today are filled using generic drugs.[13]

3.5 The role of pharmacopoeias

A pharmacopoeia is a book containing information on specifications and the methodology of qualitative and quantitative standards of APIs and the dosage forms of medicines. It is published by the authority of a government, pharmaceutical board or commission. The nations with the most medicine consumers have their own pharmacopoeias, such as the US Pharmacopoeia (USP), British Pharmacopoeia (BP), Japanese Pharmacopoeia (JP) or the collective European Pharmacopoeia (Ph. Eur.). The global International Pharmacopoeia (Ph. Int.) is published by the World Health Organization (WHO). The medicines produced by some developing countries are labeled as BP/USP. Paracetamol BP/USP means that the paracetamol produced conforms to BP or USP specifications. The pharmacopoeia provides guidelines for producing safe, effective, and quality medicines. In any country there are many pharmaceutical industries, which vary in size. They usually follow the national pharmacopoeia, if there is one; otherwise they use BP or USP, which is universally accepted around the world. A brief history of the development of pharmacopoeias is shown in Figure 3.16.

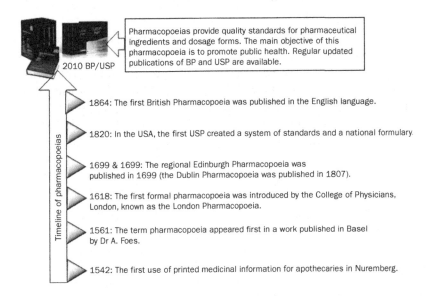

Figure 3.16 The development of pharmacopoeias, 1542–2010

Published by Woodhead Publishing Limited

3.6 Regulatory agencies

There is a drug, medicine, or pharmaceutical regulatory agency or administration in most countries responsible for:

- regulating the manufacture of medicines in the country, enforce good manufacturing practice (GMP), and ensuring that safe, effective, and quality medicines are produced
- approving importation, promotion, marketing, labeling, and use of drugs.

Each pharmaceutical company has its own regulatory affairs department, which interacts with regulatory agencies. These are some of the main regulatory agencies:

- the Food and Drug Administration (FDA), USA
- the European Medicines Evaluation Agency (EMEA), Europe
- the Medicines and Healthcare Products Regulatory Agency (MHRA), UK
- the Pharmaceutical and Medical Devices Agency (PMDA), Japan
- the Central Drugs Standard Control Organization (CDSCO), India.

3.6.1 The Food and Drug Administration

The FDA is a regulatory agency run by the US Department of Health and Human Services. It regulates foods, food additives, dietary supplements, infant formulas, human drugs, vaccines, blood products, medical devices, veterinary products, cosmetics, and tobacco products. It consists of six product centers, one research center, and two offices (Figure 3.17). The FDA has a comprehensive website (www.fda.gov), which provides detailed information about the agency.

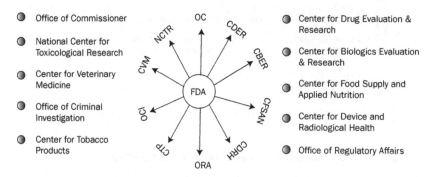

Figure 3.17 The administrative structure of the US FDA

Published by Woodhead Publishing Limited

The US FDA's Center for Drug Evaluation and Research regulates everything related to prescription drugs, OTC drugs, and generic drugs. In 2010 it had 2,889 staff members out of a total 11,516 FDA employees.[14] The agency has many technical and scientific advisory committees from which it seeks advice on challenging drug-related issues.

3.6.2 The European Medicine Evaluation Agency

The EMEA requires one application from the pharmaceutical company for scientific evaluation of medicines and makes recommendations to the European Commission for use in the European Union. The agency has six different committees (Figure 3.18), each of which assesses the quality, safety, and efficacy of medicine and submits opinions to the European Commission, which makes decisions based on these recommendations.

The EMEA represents the European Union (EU), which in 2011 consisted of 27 member states and three European Economic Areas. The EMEA evaluates applications from pharmaceutical companies and gives its opinion to the European Commission, which ultimately delivers a decision (Figure 3.19).

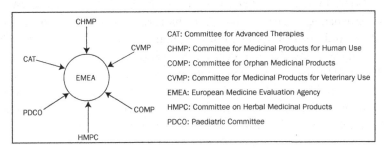

Figure 3.18 The administrative structure of the EMEA

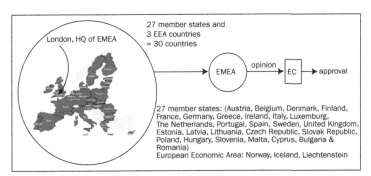

Figure 3.19 The role of the EMEA in making decisions about drugs in Europe

Companies applying for authorization to market human drugs (new or generic) in more than one country in the EU must use either a centralized procedure administered by the EMEA or a mutual recognition procedure, where assessments are made in one member state and, if approved, recognized by other member states. Another decentralized procedure starts with filling out a pre-submission meeting request form to the EMEA.

There is not much difference in the required scientific information for registering a drug with the US FDA or the EMEA; in fact there are common technical documents that are acceptable in the USA, the EU, and Japan.

3.6.3 Pharmaceutical administration and regulation in Japan

Japan has the second largest individual drug market in the world. The longevity of Japanese people is currently above 80 years and, according to the US Census Bureau, one in five Japanese is at least 65 years old.[15] As older people tend to consume more medicines than younger ones availability of drugs in Japan is important.

Medicines are highly regulated and it takes a long time for new products to be approved in comparison with other developed countries. Structurally, the PMDA in Japan is a counterpart to the US FDA. The PMDA – an independent body – is primarily responsible for approving new pharmaceutical products and medical devices, but the Japanese Ministry of Health, Labour and Welfare makes the final decision to approve new products.

The PMDA does not accept applications for registering a drug that has been imported or manufactured and sold in Japan unless clinical trials are carried out in Japan. Figure 3.20 shows the different bodies responsible for pharmaceutical administration and regulation in Japan.

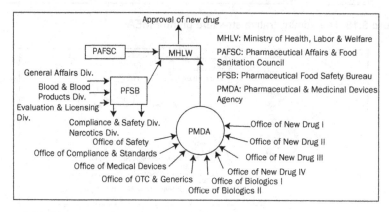

Figure 3.20 Pharmaceutical administration and regulation in Japan

3.6.4 The Central Drugs Standard Control Organization

The CDSCO is the Indian drug regulatory agency within the Health Ministry of India, with headquarters in New Delhi. There are two

Table 3.2 Generic and brand names of new drugs developed by Indian research institutes or companies approved by the CDSCO

Generic name	Brand name	Uses	Developed by	Marketed by
Arteether	E-Mal	A blood schizontocidal antimalarial	Central Drug Research Institute (CDRI)	Themis Chemicals
Bacosides enriched standardized extract of Bacopa	Memory Sure	A standardized herbal memory enhancer	CDRI	Lumen Marketing Co
Bulaquin	Aablaquin	An antirelapse antimalarial	CDRI	Nicholas Piramal
Centbucridine	Centoblok	A local anaesthetic	CDRI	Themis Chemicals
Centchroman	Saheli Centron	A non-steroidal oral contraceptive, the first in the world	CDRI	Hindustan Latex Torrent Pharmaceuticals
Centpropazine		Antidepressant	CDRI	
Compound CDRI, 99/373		A new antiosteoporosis	CDRI	
Consap		Spermicidal cream	CDRI	
Gugulipid	Guglip	A hypolipidaemic	CDRI	Cipla
Isaptent	Dilex-C	A cervical dilator for medical termination of pregnancy	CDRI	Unichem Laboratories
Picroliv		Hepatoprotective	CDRI	

Published by Woodhead Publishing Limited

government agencies in India: the CDSCO at the central level and state drug controllers at the state level. The functions of the CDSCO are:

- to approve new drug and clinical trials
- to register and license products
- to amend drug and cosmetic acts and rules
- to test drugs
- to coordinate the activities of state drug controllers.

The state drug controllers regulate licensing and manufacturing, and monitor the quality of API and formulated drugs.

The CDSCO encourages global clinical trials in India, but phase I trials are not permitted if the new drug is developed outside India. This agency has so far approved a number of new drugs developed by the Central Drug Research Institute and marketed by Indian pharmaceutical companies. Table 3.2 lists the drugs approved by the CDSCO with their uses.

The CDSCO has recently adopted a common technical document format to cover the technical requirements for the registration of pharmaceutical products for human use.[16]

Practice questions

1. Can you buy antibiotics without a prescription?
2. Can you buy acetaminophen (paracetamol) tablets without a prescription?
3. If you work in the pharmaceutical industry can you take medicines without a physician's prescription? Explain.
4. Consider a hypothetical situation, where a doctor prescribed Tylenol for your headache. You have at home four bottles of medicines labeled acetaminophen, paracetamol, panadol, and Tylenol (expired). Will you buy Tylenol again? Explain.
5. 'Read the label when you take medicine.' Is this advice necessary? Explain.
6. Why does a 500 mg tablet of paracetamol weigh more than 500 mg?
7. The drug development process is lengthy. Explain the different stages involved.

8. After the expiration of a drug patent, any pharmaceutical company can manufacture the generic version of that drug. Is there any regulation of generic drugs? Do you think they are bioequivalent compared with brand name drugs?
9. What do 'pharmaceutical equivalency' and 'bioequivalency' mean? Are there any differences between bioavailability and bioequivalency?
10. Explain the differences between *in-vitro* and *in-vivo* testing of medicines.
11. Can you market a US FDA approved medicine to the European market directly without going through its regulatory body?

Answers to some practice questions

1. No. Antibiotics are prescription-only medicine.
2. Yes. Paracetamol is an over-the-counter medicine.
3. Yes and no. You can obtain over-the-counter medicines without a doctor's prescription but not prescription-only medicines. For the latter, you need a doctor's prescription whether you work in the pharmaceutical industry or not.

Notes

1. See Food, Drug, and Cosmetic Act, Chapter II – Definitions, www.fda.gov/RegulatoryInformation/Legislation/FederalFoodDrugandCosmeticActFDCAct/FDCActChaptersIandIIShortTitleandDefinitions/ucm086297.htm (accessed February 11, 2011).
2. IMS Health, Midas, December 2009, 'Top 15 global products, 2009, total audited markets', www.imshealth.com/deployedfiles/imshealth/Global/Content/StaticFile/Top_Line_Data/Top%2015%20Global%20Products_2009.pdf (accessed February 16, 2011).
3. See www.roche.com/index.htm (accessed September 10, 2010).
4. Association of the British Pharmaceutical Industry, *ABPI Annual Report*, 2009/10, www.abpi.org.uk/publications/pdfs/AnnualReport0910.pdf (accessed June 15, 2010).
5. Diane K. Jorkasky, 'Where do drugs come from?', presentation of Pfizer Global Research & Development, http://hcwbenefits.com/documents/Jorkasky.ppt (accessed February 15, 2011).
6. Dale P. Conner, 'General BA/BE issues', [n.d.], www.aapspharmaceutica.com/meetings/files/90/19Conner.pdf (accessed February 11, 2011).

Published by Woodhead Publishing Limited

7. See www.fda.gov (accessed December 23, 2010).

8. US Food and Drug Administration, Center for Drug Evaluation and Research, US Department of Health and Human Services, 'Guidance for industry: extended release oral dosage forms: development, evaluation and application of in vitro/in vivo correlations', September 1997, www.fda.gov/downloads/ Drugs/GuidanceComplianceRegulatoryInformation/Guidances/ucm070239. pdf (accessed February 23, 2011).

9. US Food and Drug Administration, 'Generic drug roundup: December 2010', www.fda.gov/downloads/ForConsumers/ConsumerUpdates/UCM237406.pdf (accessed February 15, 2011).

10. Blue Cross Blue Shield of Michigan, 'Brand-name vs. generic drug costs', 2011, www.bcbsm.com/pdf/ps_generic.pdf (accessed October 10, 2010). This price list for generic drugs is based on the BCBSM maximum allowable cost, which applies to Michigan Blue members only.

11. IMS Health, 'IMS health reports annual global generics prescription sales growth of 3.6 percent, to $78 billion', www.imshealth.com/portal/site/ imshealth/menuitem.a46c6d4df3db4b3d88f611019418c22a/?vgnextoid=2943 d52288d1e110VgnVCM100000ed152ca2RCRD&vgnextfmt=default (accessed February 15, 2011); and IMS Health, Midas, Market Segmentation, Mat, September, 2009, prescription-only drugs.

12. US Food and Drug Administration, 'Fact and myths about generic drugs', www.fda.gov/Drugs/ResourcesForYou/Consumers/BuyingUsingMedicineSafely/ UnderstandingGenericDrugs/ucm167991.htm (accessed February 12, 2011).

13. Linda Cahn, 'Don't pay too much for generic fills', *Managed Care Magazine*, November 2010, www.managedcaremag.com/archives/1011/1011.cahn_ genericfills.html (accessed February 12, 2011).

14. US Food and Drug Administration, 'How many people are employed by FDA and in what areas do they work?', www.fda.gov/AboutFDA/Transparency/ Basics/ucm213161.htm (accessed August 14, 2010).

15. US Census Bureau, International Statistics, www.census.gov/compendia/ statab/2011/tables/11s1333.pdf (accessed February 15, 2011).

16. See www.cdsco.nic.in.

Published by Woodhead Publishing Limited

4

Bulk drugs or active pharmaceutical ingredients

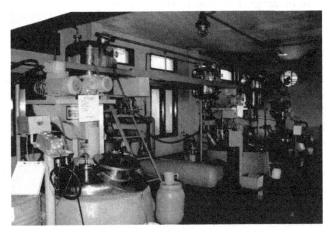

Source: Square Pharmaceuticals Ltd

Learning objective

Bulk drugs, or active pharmaceutical ingredients (APIs), are the key components of the medicines we consume. Without APIs, pills and tablets would simply be placebos, which are also used in clinical trials to determine the effectiveness of a drug. In this chapter there is a discussion of some important aspects of bulk drugs, ranging from their nomenclature to the drugs' analytical profiles. There is a description of the reactor where drug manufacturing takes place and some specific examples of production or analysis. Finally, the modern trend in bulk drug manufacturing of green chemistry and chiral drugs is described.

In this chapter, students will learn about:

● bulk drugs or APIs
● bulk drug plants
● scale ups

Published by Woodhead Publishing Limited

Key concept terms

Achiral: not chiral; molecule with a plane of symmetry

API: active pharmaceutical ingredient

Bulk drug: API in bulk

cGMP: current good manufacturing practice

Chiral: molecule with no plane of symmetry

Degradation of drug: breaking down of a drug

Enantiomer: non-superimposable mirror image stereoisomers

Green chemistry: environmentally friendly chemistry

Hydrogen bonding: dipole–dipole intermolecular attraction in which hydrogen with its partial positive charge is involved

Hydrophilicity: water loving

Hydrophobic: water hating

IR: infrared

Lab scale: gram level production

Lipophilicity: lipid loving

Lipophobic: lipid hating

Manufacturing scale: ton level (1,000 Kg)

Micronized: 1.0–10 mm

Nanosize: 0.5–1.0 mm (500–1,000 nm)

NMR: nuclear magenetic resonance

Pill: medicinal tablet

Pilot scale: production of API in small scale or at kilogram level

Racemic: a 50-50 mixture of d(+) isomer and l(–) isomer

Resolution: separation

Tablet: used as either a medicine or a non-medicinal solid form; mostly used in oral solid dosage form

Published by Woodhead Publishing Limited

- manufacturing tools – the reactor and production of cephalexin
- drug solubility
- chiral bulk drugs
- degradation and impurity profile
- critical factors in drug manufacturing
- the analytical profile of a drug
- green chemistry.

4.1   Bulk drugs and bulk drug plants

The term 'bulk drugs' refers to the API or active pharmaceutical raw material from which different dosage forms are made.

An API is defined by the International Conference on Harmonization of Technical Requirements for Registration of Pharmaceuticals for Human Use (ICH) guidance, Q7A, as:

> any substance or mixture of substances intended to be used in the manufacture of a drug product and that, when used in the production of a drug, becomes an active ingredient in the drug product. Such substances are intended to furnish pharmacological activity or other direct effect in the diagnosis, cure, mitigation, treatment or prevention of disease or to affect the structure and function of the body.[1]

Alternative names for API, such as drug substances, bulk drugs, pharmaceutical fine chemicals, and bulk pharmaceutical chemicals (BPCs), which refers to inactive ingredients. Large scale production or fermentation produces bulk drugs (Figure 4.1).

The most important criterion for API is its purity. The identities, purity, and stability of bulk drugs or APIs are essential. The quality of bulk drugs must conform to pharmacopoeial specifications. The API is used in the

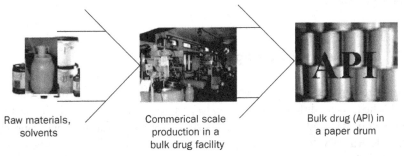

| Raw materials, solvents | Commerical scale production in a bulk drug facility | Bulk drug (API) in a paper drum |

Figure 4.1 The production of bulk drugs or APIs

Published by Woodhead Publishing Limited

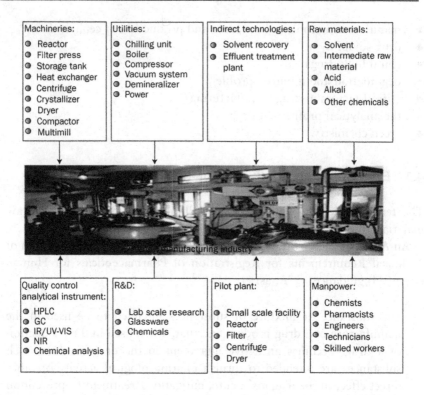

Figure 4.2 The bulk drug manufacturing industry

Source: Square Pharmaceuticals Ltd

production of formulated drugs, which the pharmacists, chemists, and druggists ultimately sell to customers. Thus the bulk drug industry is actually a chemical industry, built and operated according to pharmaceutical current good manufacturing practice (cGMP) (Figure 4.2).

'Bulk drugs' include synthetic and semi-synthetic chemical products, biological or biotechnological products, recombinant DNA products, and radioactive products.

4.2   Lab to manufacturing level scale-up

During research and development (R&D) of bulk drugs a synthetic route is established, using different glassware, to prepare the gram level of the desired compound. This lab scale is the important beginning for the long journey towards drug development. All the methods of trial and error are conducted in this lab scale. It is better to have failures in the lab scale than in the manufacturing

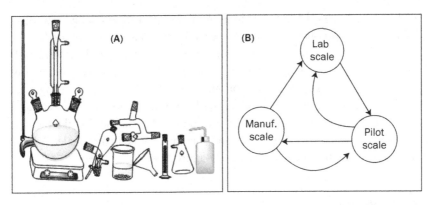

Figure 4.3 Lab glassware used in manufacturing scale, lab scale and pilot scale

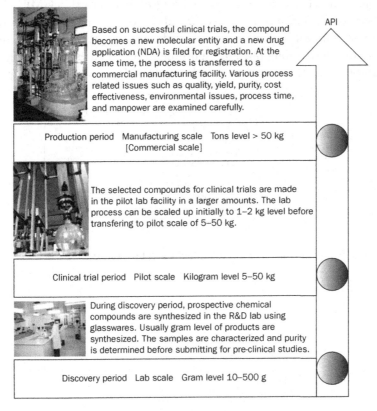

Based on successful clinical trials, the compound becomes a new molecular entity and a new drug application (NDA) is filed for registration. At the same time, the process is transferred to a commercial manufacturing facility. Various process related issues such as quality, yield, purity, cost effectiveness, environmental issues, process time, and manpower are examined carefully.

Production period   Manufacturing scale   Tons level > 50 kg
[Commercial scale]

The selected compounds for clinical trials are made in the pilot lab facility in a larger amounts. The lab process can be scaled up initially to 1–2 kg level before transfering to pilot scale of 5–50 kg.

Clinical trial period   Pilot scale   Kilogram level 5–50 kg

During discovery period, prospective chemical compounds are synthesized in the R&D lab using glasswares. Usually gram level of products are synthesized. The samples are characterized and purity is determined before submitting for pre-clinical studies.

Discovery period   Lab scale   Gram level 10–500 g

API

Figure 4.4 The development of bulk drugs on different scales

Source: Square Pharmaceuticals Ltd

Published by Woodhead Publishing Limited

scale later on. Any problem found in pilot or manufacturing scale goes back to the lab scale to find out a solution. Figure 4.3 shows lab glassware used.

In establishing a better synthetic route, many factors need to be considered. The route has to be cost-effective, non-hazardous, and environmentally friendly, and have good atom economy. The availability of starting raw materials and recyclable solvent along with a minimum number of steps and final product yield should be carefully evaluated. After a successful lab scale, the process is tested in a pilot scale and then a manufacturing scale. A brief description of each scale is provided in Figure 4.4.

4.3   Bulk drug manufacturing

Bulk drug manufacturing is the primary manufacturing mode for medicines, essentially a chemical industry with pharmaceutical cGMP. The manufacturing plant must be inspected, validated, and approved by a drug regulatory authority. Plants can be dedicated single-drug production facilities or, most commonly, multi-purpose drugs facilities. Depending on the nature of the API, bulk drugs can be made with chemical technology or

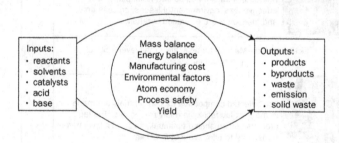

Figure 4.5 Factors involved in the manufacture of bulk drugs

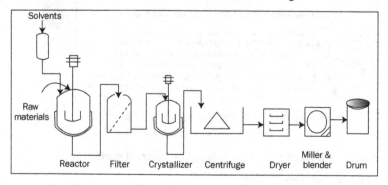

Figure 4.6 Typical steps and equipments involved in drug manufacturing

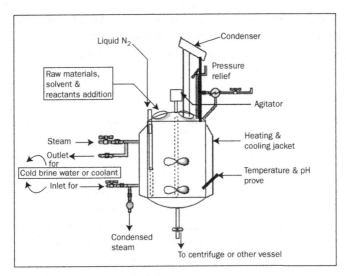

Figure 4.7 A schematic of a typical reactor

biotechnology. Most productions use batch operations, starting with certain inputs, such as reactants, solvents, and catalysts; ultimate outputs include products with some by-products and waste. Other issues, such as environmental impacts, atom economy, process safety, and product yield, are considered before finalization of the manufacturing route (Figure 4.5).

In chemical operations, the production lines usually include reactors, solvent or liquid reagents, feeding tanks, filters, crystallizers, centrifuge, dryers, millers and blenders, and storing containers (Figure 4.6).

The reactor size depends on the batch size. A reactor can be glass-lined or made of stainless steel, and typically has a capacity of 500–10,000 liters. The reactors are usually jacketed to allow coolant or steam circulation to control

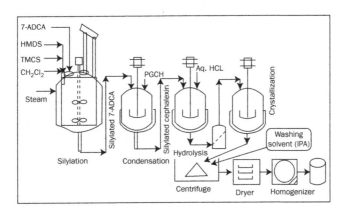

Figure 4.8 The manufacture of cephalexin

the temperature of the reaction inside. In some cases, liquid nitrogen is directly used to enable very low-temperature reactions. The reactors can also be operated under high-pressure, vacuum, or refluxing conditions. A schematic of a typical reactor is shown in Figure 4.7.

4.3.1 Manufacturing method used for cephalexin

As an example, a manufacturing method for cephalexin, a semi-synthetic cephalosporin, is described (Figure 4.8). The semi-synthetic cephalexin is manufactured from the intermediate, 7-aminodeacetoxycephalosporanic acid (7-ADCA) by introducing a side chain, phenylglycine.

To begin, solvent (methylene chloride) is added to the first reactor, and then the main raw material, 7-ADCA, is mixed. A suspension of 7-ADCA in

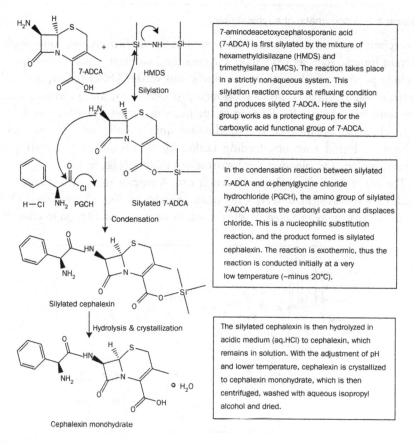

7-aminodeacetoxycephalosporanic acid (7-ADCA) is first silylated by the mixture of hexamethyldisilazane (HMDS) and trimethylsilane (TMCS). The reaction takes place in a strictly non-aqueous system. This silylation reaction occurs at refluxing condition and produces silyted 7-ADCA. Here the silyl group works as a protecting group for the carboxylic acid functional group of 7-ADCA.

In the condensation reaction between silylated 7-ADCA and α-phenylglycine chloride hydrochloride (PGCH), the amino group of silylated 7-ADCA attacks the carbonyl carbon and displaces chloride. This is a nucleophilic substitution reaction, and the product formed is silylated cephalexin. The reaction is exothermic, thus the reaction is conducted initially at a very low temperature (~minus 20°C).

The silylated cephalexin is then hydrolyzed in acidic medium (aq.HCl) to cephalexin, which remains in solution. With the adjustment of pH and lower temperature, cephalexin is crystallized to cephalexin monohydrate, which is then centrifuged, washed with aqueous isopropyl alcohol and dried.

Figure 4.9 Reaction chemistry of cephalexin production from 7-ADCA

Published by Woodhead Publishing Limited

methylene chloride is then silylated with the addition of trimethyl chlorosilane (TMCS) and hexamethyldisilazane (HMDS). The silylation reaction is exothermic, however reaction temperature is maintained around 350 °C. The silylated 7-ADCA is transferred to the next reactor to undergo a condensation reaction with phenylglycine chloride hydrochloride (PGCH). This reaction is highly exothermic, so the reaction must start at a very low temperature (–20 °C). This condensation reaction produces silylated cephalexin, which is then hydrolyzed to produce cephalexin. The solution of cephalexin is crystallized then centrifuged, washed, and dried. The reaction chemistry is described in Figure 4.9.

The production processes are carried out following cGMP. If an injectable product is desired, there are a few differences. First, the parenteral products (injectables) are sterile, so the production processes must ensure the sterility of the end product, and the product should be water soluble. A production process for injectable amoxicillin is shown in Figure 4.10. A solution of amoxicillin trihydrate is obtained in alcoholic triethylamine, which is then filtered through a 0.2 micron filter to get a sterile solution. At the same

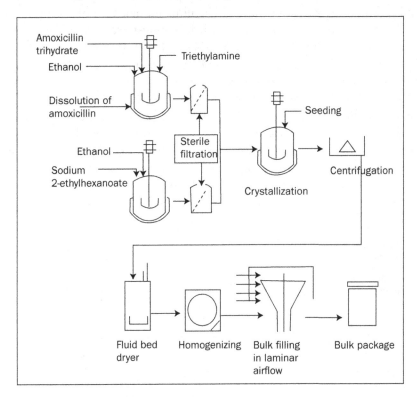

Figure 4.10 Production flow diagram of sterile amoxicillin

Published by Woodhead Publishing Limited

time, a solution of sodium salt of 2-ethylhexanoic acid is made in another reactor and filtered in a similar way, and finally both the sterile solutions are mixed together in a third reactor and crystallized by the addition of crystals of sodium amoxicillin. The crystalline product is then centrifuged, dried, and packed under laminar airflow. The whole operation is carried out in a closed system and aseptic environment.

4.4 Solubility of API

The 'solubility' of a drug is the amount of the drug that dissolves in a given volume of solvent, at a specific temperature. The item being dissolved is called the solute and the substance that does the dissolving work is called the solvent. When an API is dissolved in water the drug is the solute and water is the solvent.

The term 'miscibility' is used to describe the mixing of solute and solvent when both are liquids. The aqueous solubility characteristics of a drug are very important for the formulation in specific dosage forms and the biodisposition after administration. The ultimate objective of a drug is to be absorbed into the blood stream when administered enterally or even parenterally, and the solution form is preferable to the suspension form. Once the drug is ingested it must undergo dissolution into the aqueous buffer medium of the gastrointestinal tract.

The solubility of a drug can be either hydrophilic (aqueous soluble) or liphophilic (lipid or fat soluble). Though the body contains 60–70% water, the drug must still move through aqueous and lipid media. The biological membranes are composed of lipids, and the drug needs to cross through these biological membranes. There are also drugs of extreme solubility – either water-soluble only or fat-soluble only. However, most drugs, especially orally administered drugs, have some degree of solubility in aqueous and lipid media.

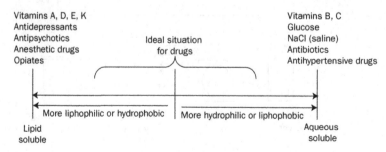

Figure 4.11 The hydrophilicity and lipophilicity of bulk drugs

Published by Woodhead Publishing Limited

There are drugs at both ends of the spectrum, such as anesthetic drugs, antidepressants, and antipsychotic drugs, that are all lipid-soluble drugs. These drugs need to cross the blood brain barrier, which is made up of lipids. These lipid-soluble drugs rapidly pass through the blood brain barrier and act rapidly. Drugs such as NaCl (saline), glucose, antibiotics, and cardiovascular drugs are mostly water-soluble.

Polar molecules are soluble in polar solvents, such as water, and non-polar molecules are soluble in non-polar solvents, such as vegetable oils (Figure 4.11). The solubility depends on the solute–solvent intermolecular interactions.

4.4.1 Dipole–dipole interaction (hydrogen bonding)

Dipole–dipole interaction is the most important intermolecular interaction and helps with solubilization of drugs in water. The dipole results from an unequal sharing of electron pairs in covalent bonding. The unequal sharing of electron pairs occurs because of the electronegativity difference between bonded atoms.

Hydrogen bonding is a special case of dipole–dipole intermolecular attraction, in which hydrogen, with its partial positive charge ($\delta+$), is involved (Figure 4.12). Thus, organic functional groups present in the drug molecule indicate the possibility of hydrogen bonding in aqueous solution.

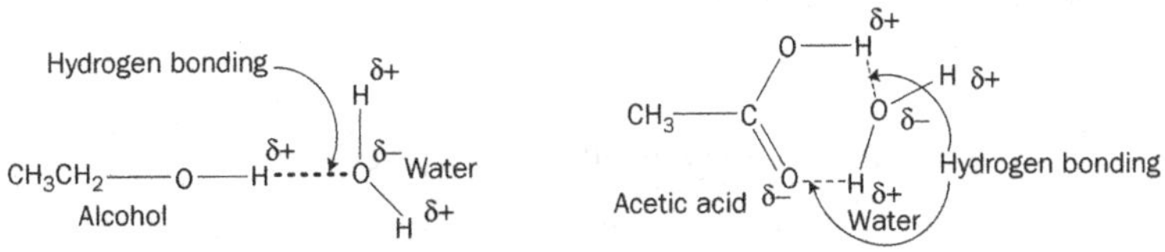

Figure 4.12 Intermolecular hydrogen bonding

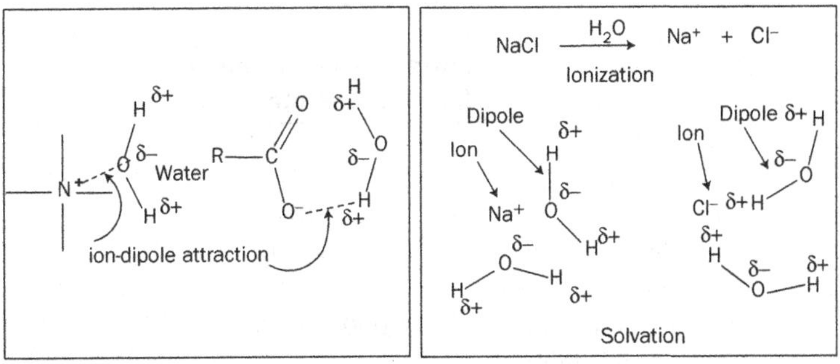

Figure 4.13 Ion–dipole interaction and solvation

Published by Woodhead Publishing Limited

4.4.2 Ion–dipole attraction (ionic bonding)

Ionic bonding is a common feature of inorganic compounds and the salts of organic molecules. When inorganic compounds or salts of organic molecules are mixed with water, there is always an ion–dipole attraction, which means the ions are solvated (hydrated) (Figure 4.13). Table salt (NaCl) undergoes this process when it is mixed with water.

In some cases, bulk drugs are produced as a non-toxic salt of the free acid or a free base to improve the water solubility. For example, atorvastatin (Lipitor) is a calcium salt and sildenafil (Viagra) is a citrate salt. Sometimes the counter ion can not only cause changes in the solubility but also improve the stability of the salt, relative to the original form.

4.4.3 Van der Waals attraction

This attraction, also called the induced dipole attraction, is very electrostatically weak in nature. It is common between non-polar molecules.

The US Pharmacopeia-National Formulary (USP-NF) defines drug solubility as the volume of solvent required to dissolve 1g of the drug at a specified temperature. *Remington's Pharmaceutical Sciences* uses a descriptive classification, which provides an approximate solubility. Table 4.1 shows the parts of solvent required for different solubilities.

4.4.4 The Biopharmaceutical Classification System

The Biopharmaceutical Classification System (BCS) is a scientific framework for classifying drugs according to their aqueous solubility and intestinal

Table 4.1 The parts of solvent required for different solubilities

Description	Parts of solvent required for 1 part solute
Very soluble	< 1
Freely soluble	1–10
Soluble	10–30
Sparingly soluble	30–100
Slightly soluble	100–1,000
Very slightly soluble	1,000–10,000
Practically insoluble or insoluble	> 10,000

Published by Woodhead Publishing Limited

permeability. The US Food and Drug Administration (FDA) and the European Medicine Evaluation Agency (EMEA) accept the BCS as an alternative to *in-vivo* bioequivalence studies. For immediate-release solid-oral dosage forms such as tablets and capsules the BCS accounts for dissolution rates, solubility, and permeability, which all regulate the rate and extent of drug absorption. According to the BCS, drugs can be classified in one of four classes:

- *class 1* – high solubility and high permeability
- *class 2* – low solubility and high permeability
- *class 3* – high solubility and low permeability
- *class 4* – low solubility and low permeability.

This suggests that the ideal drug falls in class 1, having high solubility and high permeability.

The BCS considers a drug substance to be:

- *highly soluble* – when the highest dose strength is soluble in < 250 ml water over a pH range of 1–7.5
- *highly permeable* – when the extent of absorption in humans is determined to be > 90% of an administered dose, based on mass-balance or in comparison to an intravenous reference dose
- *rapidly dissolving* – when > 85% of the labeled amount of drug substance dissolves within 30 minutes using USP apparatus I or II in a volume of < 900 ml buffer solutions.[2]

The drugs in classes 2 and 4 with low water-solubility usually have low oral-bioavailability in the body, but there are various techniques by which the solubility of drugs can be enhanced, some of which are shown in Figure 4.14.

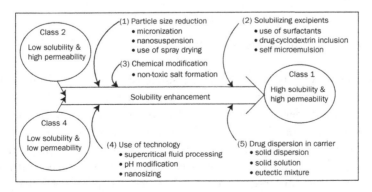

Figure 4.14 Solubility enhancement processes

Published by Woodhead Publishing Limited

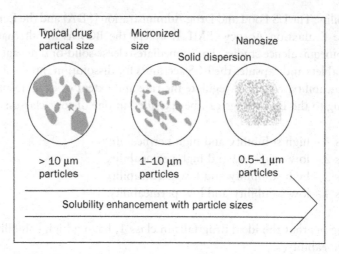

Figure 4.15 Solubility enhancement with particle sizes (relative sizes shown)

Nifedipine is practically insoluble in water. The solubilities at 37 °C in buffer solutions of different pH values are pH 4, 0.0058 g/L, pH 7, 0.0056 g/L, pH 9.0, 0.0078 g/L, and pH 13, 0.006 g/L. However, solubility enhancement and improved bioavailability of nifedipine was achieved by the application of push–pull osmotic pump technology (OROS technology), developed by ALZA. In 1989, the US Food and Drug Administration (FDA) approved Procardia (Nifedipine) XL tablets. The researchers were excited about the possibility of making insoluble drugs in action. Since then, many processes for solubility enhancement have been developed. The most important solubility enhancement technologies include particle size reduction (Figure 4.15), addition of surfactants, and inclusion in cyclodextrin-drug complexes, self-emulsifying systems, micronisation via nanoparticles, pH adjustment, and salting-in processes.

4.5 Stereoisomeric bulk drugs

'Stereochemistry' is the study of the three-dimensional aspects of a molecule; these are the spatial arrangements of its atoms. The action of a drug in the biological system depends on the spatial arrangements of atoms in the drug molecule. If one spatial arrangement works, either another will not or it will work in a different way. The concept of chirality, or asymmetry, is important in drug discovery and bulk drugs. When a carbon atom is bonded to four different atoms or groups, it produces two non-superimposable mirror images called enantiomers (Figure 4.16).

Published by Woodhead Publishing Limited

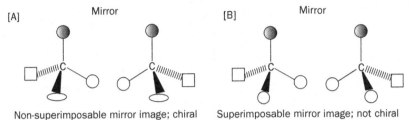

[A]   Mirror   [B]   Mirror

Non-superimposable mirror image; chiral   Superimposable mirror image; not chiral
(Enantiomers; has no plane of symmetry)   (No enantiomers; has plane of symmetry)

Figure 4.16 Enantiomers: chirality [A] and achirality [B]

The molecule with no plane of symmetry is chiral or has a non-superimposable mirror image, and these two structures are non-identical (Figure 4.16 [A]). Molecules with a plane of symmetry (Figures 4.16 [B] and 4.17) are not chiral, have a superimposable mirror image, and these two structures are identical (Figures 4.16 [B] and 4.17).

Whenever a drug is chiral with one chiral center, it has two stereoisomers: one rotates plane polarized light clockwise [d or (+) sign used], the other rotates counter clockwise [l or (−) sign used]. The two enantiomers are thus best characterized by their optical rotation and absolute configuration (R and S system). There is a rule to determine the R and S configuration of a chiral molecule. Again, R and S will be a non-superimposable mirror image. If one stereoisomer is R then its mirror image will be S. However, when a molecule contains two chiral carbon or centers, there are four possible stereoisomers or two pairs of enantiomers. The number of stereoisomers depends on the number of chiral centers:

Number of stereoisomers = 2^n where n = number of chiral centers

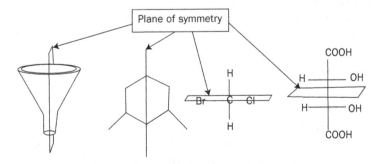

Figure 4.17 Achiral molecules with a plane of symmetry

Published by Woodhead Publishing Limited

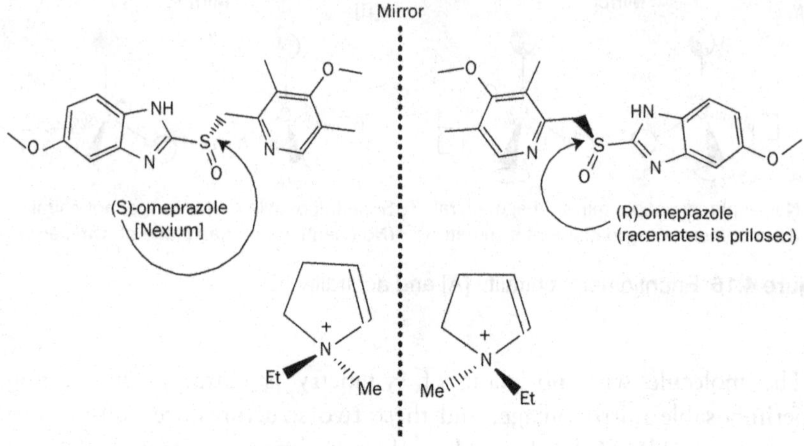

Figure 4.18 Stereoisomerism around sulfur and nitrogen atoms

When there are more pairs of enantiomers because of a greater number of chiral centers, another stereo term is used: diastereoisomers. The stereoisomers that are not mirror images of one another are called diastereoisomers. The enantiomers have identical properties aside from optical rotations, but diastereoisomers have different physical and chemical properties.

Stereoisomerism can occur in atoms other than carbon atoms. Sulfur atoms with three bond ($R^1R^2R^3S$), sulfonium salts ($R^1R^2R^3S^+A^-$), and sulfinyl compounds ($R^1R^2S = O$) exhibit chirality (R and S configuration). Similarly, N-containing compounds also show chirality around nitrogen atoms (Figure 4.18).

When a pair of enantiomers is present in equimolar amounts in a mixture, it is known as a racemate, or racemic mixture, and the optical rotation is cancelled to zero. In the synthesis of chiral organic compounds or chiral drugs, racemic mixtures are produced unless an asymmetric route is followed. Racemic mixtures can be separated into individual stereoisomers.

4.5.1 Chirality and pharmacological activity

The pharmacological activity of drugs depends on how the drugs interact with proteins, enzymes, receptors, nucleic acid, or biomembranes. Figure 4.19 illustrates the interaction between a stereoisomeric drug and biological receptors. The left structure fits well compared with the right one, so the left one is biologically active and the right one is biologically inactive because of the mismatch with biological receptors.

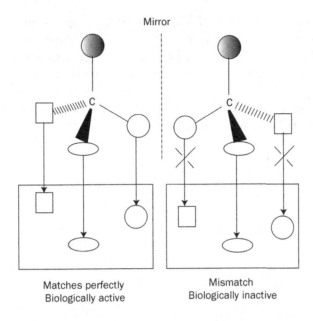

Figure 4.19 Matching interaction and biological activity

There are numerous examples of chirality and pharmacological activity. The most interesting examples are flavor-related: carvone and limonene. As shown in Figure 4.20, the (R) stereoisomer of carvone smells like caraway seeds, and the (S) stereoisomer of cavone smells like spearmint.

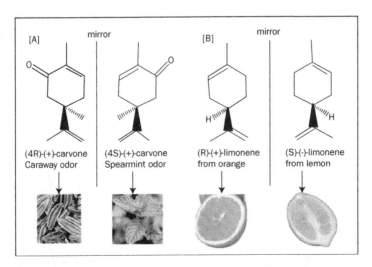

Figure 4.20 Flavor and tastes based on stereoisomers R and S

Published by Woodhead Publishing Limited

In other words, caraway seed contains the (R), and spearmint contains the (S) stereoisomer. Similarly, orange contains the (R)-(+)-limonene, and lemon contains the (S)-(–)-limonene. Most chiral drugs also show different pharmacological activity. In some cases, one enantiomer shows pharmacological activity and the other enantiomer (mirror image) does not, or it shows serious side effects. Some representative common drugs are listed in their (R) and (S) stereoisomer with pharmacological activity (Figure 4.21).

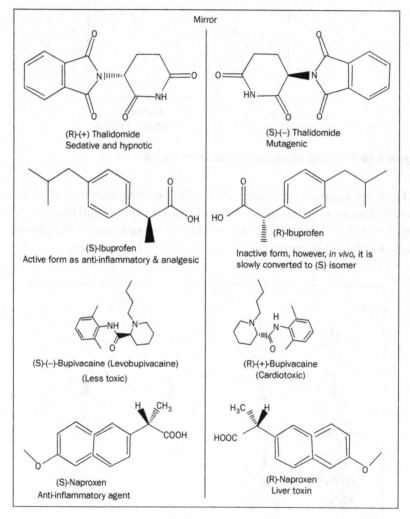

Figure 4.21 Pharmacological activity of certain drugs based on their configuration, R and S

Published by Woodhead Publishing Limited

The history of thalidomide and its disastrous effects led researchers to look more closely at the (R) and (S) enantiomers. Thalidomide was marketed in Europe in 1957 as a sedative-hypnotic drug, which pacified morning sickness in pregnant women. Soon the drug was discovered to cause deformities in newborns (teratogenic effect), and later studies revealed that the (S)-(–) thalidomide was responsible for fetal abnormalities. Recent studies, however, have shown that the (R)-(+) thalidomide undergoes epimerization to racemates *in-vivo*. In any case, stereochemistry, especially the enantiomerism, has taken a permanent place in the bulk drug industry. Figure 4.21 shows that (S) naproxen is an anti-inflammatory agent, but the (R)-naproxen is a liver toxin.

Two decades ago chiral drugs were marketed as racemates or racemic mixtures, but since 1992 the US FDA and European Committee for Proprietary Medicinal Products set the guidelines for pharmaceutical manufacturers to separate individual stereoisomers and characterize their pharmacological activity. Currently, most chiral drugs are marketed as a single stereoisomer with a better selectivity of drug action. The manufacturing of bulk, single-active stereoisomer chiral drugs is now an important concern for bulk drug production. Figure 4.22 lists drugs marketed as racemates and single enantiomers.

Currently there are also many drugs marketed as single enantiomers, including atorvastatin, simbastatin, pravastatin, and enalapril (Figure 4.23).

4.5.2 Resolution of racemic mixture

After the synthesis of chiral drug products, the individual stereoisomer is separated using the techniques shown in Figure 4.24.

AstraZeneca has used the technique of asymmetric synthesis to produce esomeprazole (brand name Nexium). The company launched the proton pump inhibitor omeprazole (brand name Prilosec) in 1988 as a racemic mixture. AstraZeneca then developed a method to produce the more active stereoisomer esomeprazole, which is the (S) stereoisomer of omeprazole. The company uses a pro-chiral sulfide intermediate to carry out asymmetric synthesis directly on (S)-omeprazole. In the conversion, cumene hydroperoxide is used as an oxidizing agent and titanium isopropoxide is used as a catalyst. The esomeprazole thus obtained is converted to magnesium salt, which is the active material for the brand name drug Nexium, which was launched in 2000 (Figure 4.25).

Published by Woodhead Publishing Limited

Drug marketed as racemate	Marketed as single enantiomer
1. Amphetamine Brand name: Benzedrine	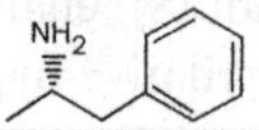 IUPAC name: (S)-1-phenylpropan-2-amine Generic name: dextroamphetamine Brand name: Dexedrine
2. Cetirizine Brand name: Zyrtec/Reactine	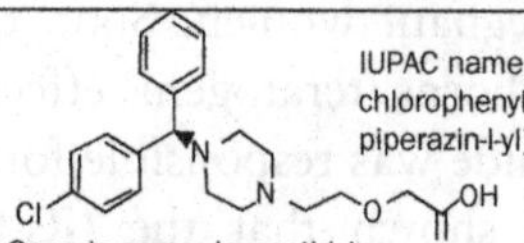 IUPAC name: 2-[2-[4-[(R)-(4-chlorophenyl)-phenyl-methyl] piperazin-l-yl]ethoxy]acetic acid Generic name: levocetirizine Brand name: Xyzal
3. Methylphenidate Brand name: Ritalin	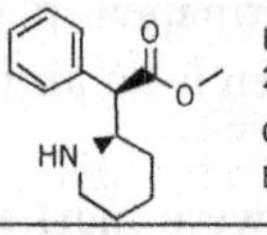 IUPAC name: (R,R)-(+)-methyl 2-phenyl-2-(2-piperidyl)acetate Generic name: dexmethylphenidate Brand name: Focalin
4. Omeprazole Brand name: Prilosec	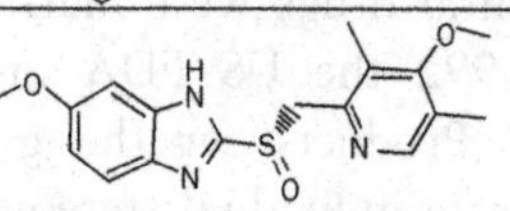 IUPAC name: (S)-5-methoxy-2-[(4-methoxy-3-5-dimethylpyridin-2-yl) methylsulfinyl]-3H-benzoimidazole Generic name: esomeprazole Brand name: Nexium
5. Salbutamol Brand name: Ventolin	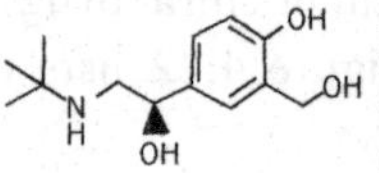 IUPAC name: 4-[(1R)-2-(tert-butylamino)-1-hydroxyethyl]-2-(hydroxymethyl)phenol Generic name: levalbuterol Brand name: Xopenex
6. Zoliclone Brand name: Imovane	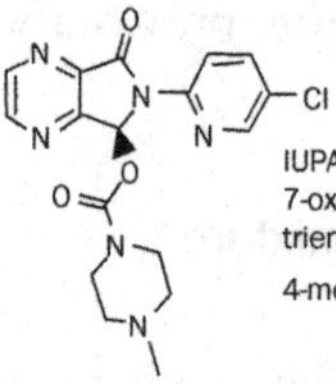 IUPAC name: (S)-[8-(5-chloropyridin-2-yl) 7-oxo-2,5,8-triazabicyclo [4.3.0]nona-1,3,5-trien-9-yl] 4-methylpiperazine-1-carboxylate Generic name: eszopiclone Brand name: Lunesta

Figure 4.22 Marketed drugs as racemates or single stereoisomers

The enzymes are stereospecific protein catalysts, which means the enzymes react or catalyze the reaction of one particular enantiomer, either (R) or (S). The active enantiomer of naproxen, the (S) stereoisomer, can be made using an enzyme catalyst. The racemic mixture of ester derivative of naproxen, when treated with an enzyme, esterase, in aqueous alkaline solution, only acts on the (S) stereoisomer of naproxen and not on the (R) ester. After the hydrolysis of the (S) ester of naproxen, it becomes a sodium salt, which is then acidified to produce naproxen (Figure 4.26).

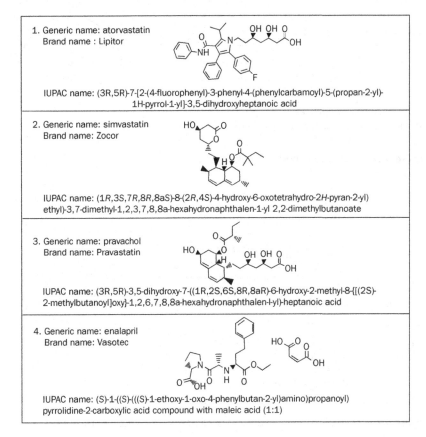

Figure 4.23 Marketed drugs with only one stereoisomer

Ibuprofen's racemic mixture can be separated by converting the racemates into disthererisomers using the resolving agent (S)-(+) α-phenylethylamine. The (S)-amine will form salt with the (R) acid form of ibuprofen and the (S) acid form of ibuprofen. Interestingly, the salt of (R, S) is aqueous soluble and the salt of (S, S) is aqueous insoluble. The (R, R) and (S, S) salts are diastereoisomers to each other and their physical and chemical properties are different.

The (S, S) salt can be isolated easily by filtration because of its insolubility in aqueous solutions. After its isolation, the (S) stereoisomer of ibuprofen can be made by acidification of the salt. Finally the (S)-ibuprofen can be extracted from the acidic solution using an immiscible organic solvent (Figure 4.27).

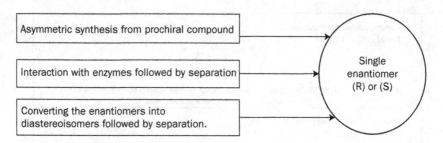

Figure 4.24 General methods of making single enantiomer

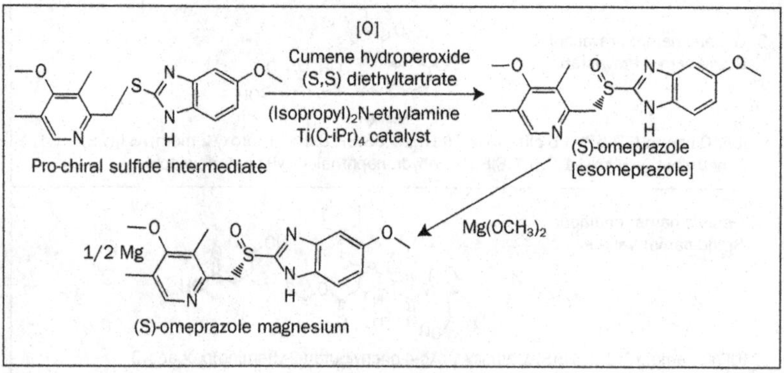

Figure 4.25 Production of single active enantiomer of omeprazole (Nexium)

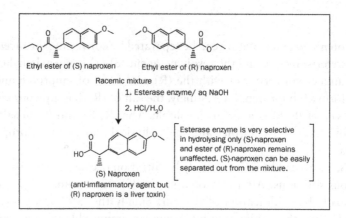

Figure 4.26 Production of (S) naproxen, an anti-inflammatory agent

Published by Woodhead Publishing Limited

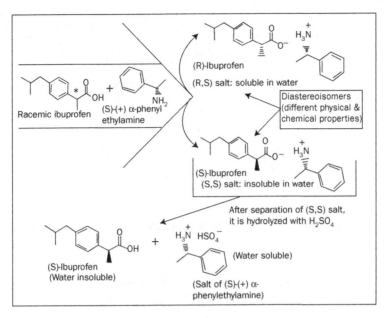

Figure 4.27 Separation of (S)-ibuprofen from its racemic mixture

4.6 Stability, degradation, and impurity profiles of bulk drugs

Instability, degradation, and impurity in drugs are closely connected and drugs with these characteristics may be sub-standard and not useable. The instability of drugs leads to degradation and degradation leads to impurity. There could be impurities from other sources too. Degradation of a drug is common, but what is important is whether the degraded impurity is within an acceptable limit or not. If a drug is stable, there will not be any degradation, nor any degradation related impurity (Figure 4.28).

Some environmental factors, such as moisture (water), air (oxygen), and light, can influence certain drugs to undergo degradation. Certain organic functional groups are sensitive to certain environmental conditions. Figure 4.29 gives a list of sensitive drugs and their types of degradation.

4.6.1 Impurity profile of bulk drugs[3]

Impurities in pharmaceuticals are the unwanted chemicals that remain with APIs. The presence of these unwanted chemicals, even in small amounts, may influence the efficacy and safety of the pharmaceutical products. The

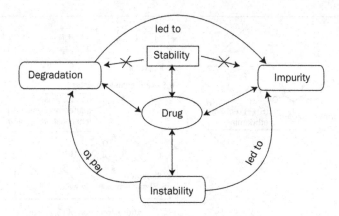

Figure 4.28 Relationship between stability, instability, degradation, and impurity in drugs

Functional groups		Drugs	Racemization
Hydrolysis		Drugs	Racemization
	Ester	Aspirin, Dexmethasne sodium phosphate, Nitroglycerin	(1)-Epineprine to (d)-Epineprine
	Lactone	Pilocarpine, Sapironolactone	Ionizing radiation
	Lactam	Penicillins, Cephalosporins	Atropine to degradation products
	Amide	Chloramphenicol	Ultrasound energy
	Imide	Glutethimide	Prednisolone acetate to degradation
	Carbamate	Barbiturates	
Oxidation			Photodegradation
	Catechols	Catecholamines (dopamine)	Piperzine ring in ciprofloxacin
	Thiols	Dimercaprol (BAL)	Ferrous ion in sodium nitroprusside
	Thioethers	Chlorpromazine	

Figure 4.29 Sensitive drugs and their types of degradation

different pharmacopoeias, such as the British Pharmacopoeia (BP) and the USP, are slowly incorporating limits for allowable levels of impurities present in the APIs. The ICH has published guidelines on impurities in new drug substances. In general, according to ICH guidelines on impurities in new drug products, identification of impurities below the 0.1% level is not considered to be necessary unless the potential impurities are expected to be unusually potent or toxic. In all cases, impurities should be qualified.

If data are not available to qualify the proposed specification level of an impurity, studies to obtain such data may be needed (when the usual qualification threshold limits given below are exceeded). According to the ICH, the maximum daily dose qualification threshold is:

$\leq$ 2g/day 0.1% or 1 mg per day intake (whichever is lower) $\geq$ 2g/day 0.05%

According to ICH guidelines, impurities associated with APIs are classified into the following categories:

- organic impurities (process and drug-related)
- inorganic impurities
- residual solvents.

4.6.1.1 Organic impurities

Organic impurities may arise during the manufacturing process and/or storage of the drug substance. They may be identified or unidentified, volatile or non-volatile, and include:

- starting materials or intermediates
- by-products
- degradation products
- enantiomeric impurities.

Starting materials or intermediates

These are the most common impurities found in APIs unless proper care is taken at every step of the multi-step synthesis. Although the end products are always washed with solvents, there is always the chance of having the residual unreacted starting materials remain unless the manufacturers are very careful about the impurities. In paracetamol bulk, there is a limit test for p-aminophenol, which could be a starting material for one manufacturer or be an intermediate for another.

By-products

In synthetic organic chemistry, getting a single end product with 100% yield is very rare; there is always a chance of having by-products. In the case of paracetamol bulk, diacetylated paracetamol (Figure 4.30) may form as a by-product.

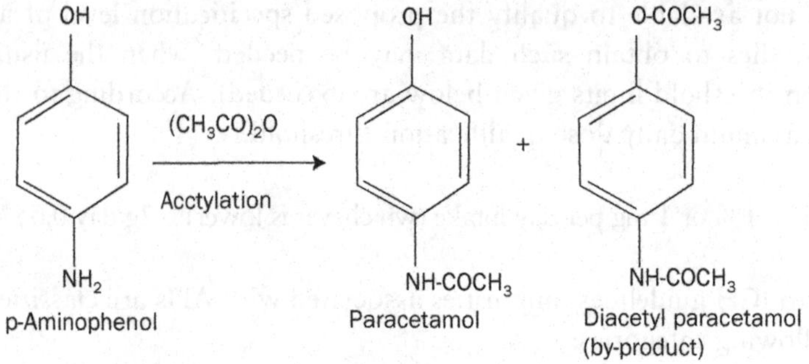

Figure 4.30 Production of paracetamol from the intermediate p-aminophenol

Degradation products

Impurities can also be formed by degradation of the end product during bulk drug manufacturing. However, degradation products resulting from storage, formulation to different dosage forms, or aging are common impurities in medicines. The degradations of penicillins and cephalosporins are well-known examples of degradation products (Figure 4.31). The presence of a ß-lactam ring as well as that of an a-amino group in the C6/C7 side chain plays a critical role in their degradation.

The manufacturers and different research groups performed a detailed investigation of impurities in semi-synthetic penicillin. Studies show the presence of traces of ampicillin polymers and hydrolyzed products in the API (Figure 4.32).

The presence of certain chemicals, such as triethylamine, has a degradative effect on the product. Ampicillin trihydrate samples with a triethylamine content of 2,000–4,000 ppm are found to be stable under accelerated stability testing, but the product showed appreciable degradation when the triethylamine content reached 7,000 ppm. Recent pharmacopoeia included the limit tests for the traces of impurities present in ampicillin and amoxycillin bulk raw materials. The residual solvents associated with these APIs have also been determined. As the organic impurities are the most

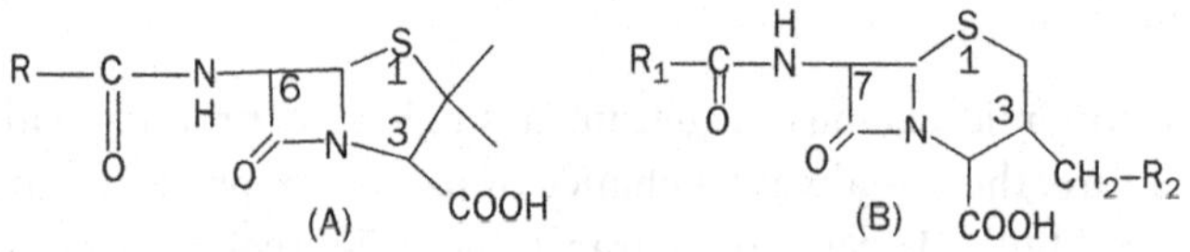

Figure 4.31 The general structure of penicillin (A) and cephalosporin (B)

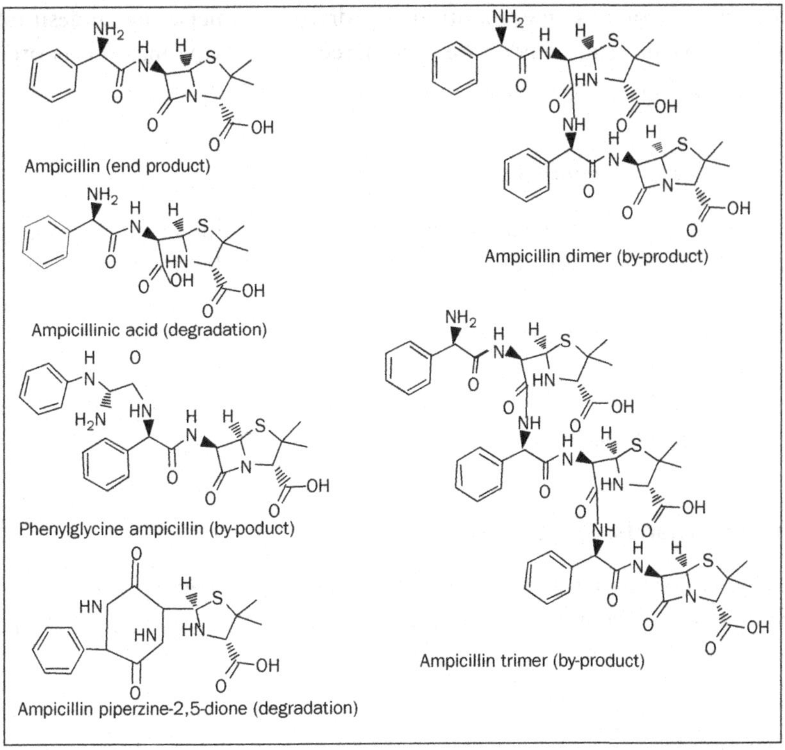

Figure 4.32 Structures of ampicillin and ampicillin-related products

common product- and process-related impurities, it is the responsibility of manufacturers of APIs and users (the formulators) to take care of these impurities according to ICH guidelines or compendia.

In addition, for an optically active single isomer drug, there could be enantiomeric impurities present in the API.

Enantiomeric impurities

The single enantiomeric form of a chiral drug is now considered an improved chemical entity that may offer a better pharmacological profile and an increased therapeutic index with a more favorable adverse reaction profile. However, the pharmacokinetic profile of levofloxacin (S-isomeric form) and ofloxacin (R-isomeric form) are comparable, suggesting a lack of advantages of the single isomer in this regard. In any case, cost benefits and a patient's compliance need to be considered when selecting drugs. For the manufacturers of a single enantiomeric drug (eutomer), the undesirable stereoisomers in drug control are considered in the same manner as other organic impurities.

4.6.1.2   Inorganic impurities

Inorganic impurities may also derive from the manufacturing processes used for bulk drugs. They are normally known and identified and include:

- reagents, ligands, and catalysts
- heavy metals
- other materials
- solvent residues.

Reagents, ligands, and catalysts

The chances of having these impurities are rare, but in some processes these impurities could create a problem unless the manufacturers take proper care during production.

Heavy metals

The main sources of heavy metals are the water used in the processes and the reactors (if stainless steel reactors are used) in which acidification or acid hydrolysis takes place. These impurities of heavy metals can easily be avoided by using demineralized water and glass-lined reactors.

Other materials

Filters or filtering aids, such as centrifuge bags, are routinely used in bulk drugs manufacturing plants, and in many cases activated carbon is also used. The regular monitoring of fibers and black particles in the bulk drugs is essential to avoid these contaminations.

Solvent residues

Residual solvents are organic volatile chemicals used during the manufacturing process or generated during production. It is very difficult to remove these solvents completely by the work-up process; however, efforts should be taken to meet the safety data. Some solvents that are known to cause toxicity should be avoided in the production of bulk drugs.

There are three classes of residual solvents:

- *class I* – solvents such as benzene (Class I, 2 ppm limit) and carbon tetrachloride (class I, 4 ppm limit); they should be avoided
- *class II* – the most commonly used solvents, such as methylene chloride (600 ppm), methanol (3,000 ppm), pyridine (200 ppm), toluene (890 ppm), N,N-dimethylformamide (880 ppm), and acetonitrile (410 ppm)
- *class III* – solvents such as acetic acid, acetone, isopropyl alcohol, butanol, ethanol, and ethyl acetate with permissible daily exposures of 50 mg or less per day.

ICH guidelines for limits should be strictly followed.

4.6.1.3 Environmental factors

The primary environmental factors that can reduce stability include:

- exposures to adverse temperatures
- light, especially UV light
- functional group-related typical degradation
- ester hydrolysis
- oxidative degradation
- photolytic cleavage
- decarboxylation.

Exposures to adverse temperatures

There are many APIs that are labile to heat or tropical temperatures. For example, vitamins as drug substances are very heat-sensitive, and degradation frequently leads to a loss of potency in vitamin products, especially in liquid formulations.

Light, especially UV light

Several studies have reported that ergometrine and methyl ergometrine injections are unstable under tropical conditions, such as light and heat, and found a very low level of active ingredient in many field samples. In only 50% of the marketed samples of ergometrine injections tested did the level of active ingredient comply with the BP/USP limit of 90–110% of the stated content. The custom-made injection of ergometrine (0.2 mg/mL) showed almost complete degradation when kept 42 hours in direct sunlight.

Ester hydrolysis

Aspirin, benzocaine, cefotaxime, cocaine echothiophate, ethyl paraben, and cefpodoxime proxetil are examples of ester hydrolysis (Figure 4.33).

Hydrolysis is also a common phenomenon for the ester type of drugs, especially in liquid dosage forms. Examples include benzylpenicillin, barbitol, chloramphenicol, chlordiazepoxide, lincomy-cin, and oxazepam.

Oxidative degradation

The hydrocortisone, methotrexate, adinazolam, and hydroxyl group directly bonded to an aromatic ring (e.g. phenol derivatives, such as catecholamines and morphine), conjugated dienes (e.g. vitamin A and unsaturated free fatty ac-ids), heterocyclic aromatic rings, nitroso and nitrite derivatives, and aldehydes (e.g. flavorings) are all susceptible to oxidative degradation.

Photolytic cleavage

Pharmaceutical products are exposed to light while being manufactured as solids or solutions, packaged, held in pharmacy shops or hospitals pending use, or held by the consumer pending use.

Ergometrine, nifedipine, nitroprusside, riboflavin, and phenothiazines are very labile to photo-oxidation. In susceptible compounds, photo-chemical energy creates free radical intermediates, which can perpetuate

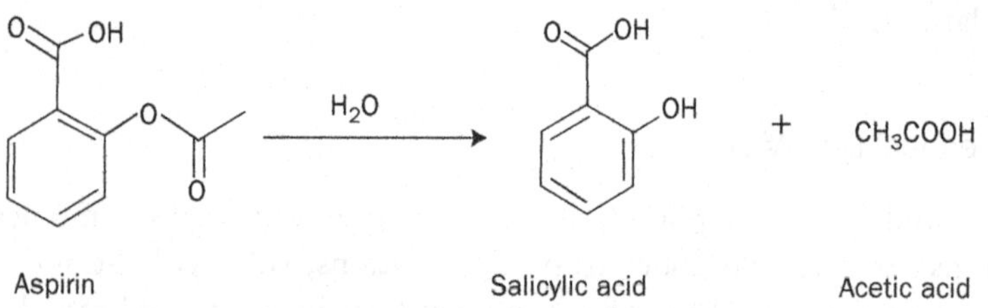

Aspirin   Salicylic acid   Acetic acid

Figure 4.33 Formation of salicylic acid impurity from aspirin

Published by Woodhead Publishing Limited

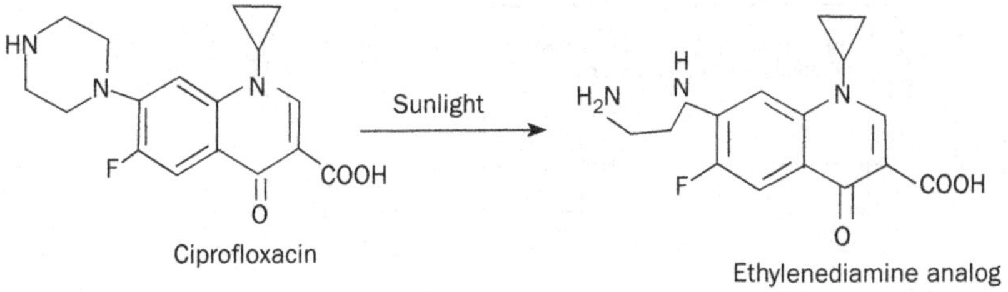

Figure 4.34 Photolytic cleavage of ciprofloxacin in eye drop preparation

chain reactions. Most compounds degrade as solutions when exposed to high energy UV exposure. Fluoroquinolone antibiotics are found to be susceptible to photolytic cleavage. In ciprofloxacin eye drop preparation (0.3%), sunlight induces photocleavage reactions, producing ethylenediamine analog of ciprofloxacin (Figure 4.34).

Decarboxylation

Some dissolved carboxylic acids, such as p-aminosalicylic acid, lose carbon dioxide from the carboxyl group when heated. Decarboxylation also occurs in the case of a photoreaction of rufloxacin.

4.6.2 Critical factors regarding bulk drug quality

4.6.2.1 During crystallization

The size of crystals sometimes determines the quality and stability of bulk drugs. Large crystals can entrap a minute amount of chemicals from the mother liquor, which ultimately causes the degradation of the drug (Figure 4.35). Thus, the manufacturers of bulk drugs should take care to produce finer crystals when isolating the products.

4.6.2.2 Washing the wet cake

Washing the wet cake or powder in the centrifuge should be thoroughly completed to remove unwanted chemicals, including residual solvents.

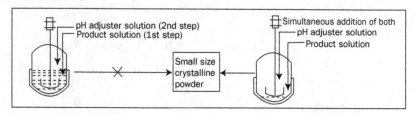

Figure 4.35 The process of crystallization leading to small size crystals

4.6.2.3 Drying

It is always preferable to use a vacuum dryer or fluid-bed dryer rather than a tray dryer in the pharmaceutical bulk drug industry. The high thermal efficiencies, reduction of drying time, and uniform drying are beneficial in drying sensitive drug substances. If a tray dryer is used, initial airflow at ambient conditions should be considered before exposing the materials to a relatively higher fixed temperature.

4.6.3 Forced degradation or stress testing

Bulk drug or API stability is the most important factor that determines the quality and safety of medicines. The ICH has comprehensive generalized guidelines for the quality of drugs and medicines, shown in Table 4.2.

Table 4.3 lists the ICH conditions for stress testing or forced degradation of API. This testing is also called accelerated stability testing. More severe conditions of humidity, heat, acidity, basicity, and photostability are used than in a normal accelerated testing. These tests help develop and validate the stability-indicating analytical methods. The degradation products, their

Table 4.2 ICH standards for some drug tests

Standard	Title
ICH Q1A(R2)	Stability Testing of New Drug Substances and Products (the parent guideline)
ICH Q1B	Photostability Testing of New Drug Substances and Products
ICH Q2B	Validation of Analytical Procedures: Methodology
ICH Q3A(R)	Impurities in New Drug Substances
ICH Q3B(R)	Impurities in New Drug Products

Table 4.3 ICH guidelines for stress or forced degradation of bulk drugs

Storage conditions	Testing period*
pH = 2, room temperature	2 weeks
pH = 7, room temperature	2 weeks
pH = 10–12, room temperature	2 weeks
H_2O_2 = 0.1–2% at neutral pH, room temp.	24 hours

* Storage time given or 5–15% degradation, whatever comes first

structures, and mechanisms of formation can be identified and established, and stability issues can be addressed and possible solutions presented.

The ICH has set regular or formal stability testing conditions (Table 4.4), which are universally used around the world.

An API is considered stable if it is within the defined/regulatory specifications when stored at 30±2 °C and 65±5% RH for two years and at 40±2 °C and 75±5%RH for six months.

4.7   Drug development, scale up, and analytical development

After the discovery of a new drug, from pre-clinical to submission of a new drug application (NDA), the scale up of a new bulk drug and the development of its analytical profile occurs simultaneously (Figure 4.36).

The development of an analytical profile is an integral part of the drug development processes. The NDA must contain a complete dossier of the drug's analytical profile. The generic companies also must develop their own analytical profile of the drug they are interested in bringing to the market. The documentation starts with the drug's nomenclature, such as the international non-proprietary name and chemical name. Its physical

Table 4.4 ICH regulatory or formal stability testing conditions

Storage temperature	Relative humidity	Minimum time period covered by data at submission
Accelerated: 40 ± 2 °C	75 ± 5%	6 months
Intermediate: 30 ± 2 °C	65 ± 5%	12 months
Long term: 25 ± 2 °C	60 ± 5%	12 (6) months

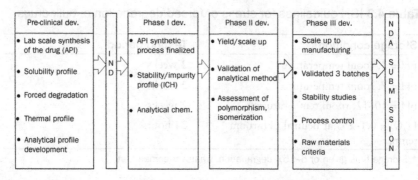

Figure 4.36 Scale up of a new drug and its analytical development

form, appearance, color, odor, chemical formula, structural formula, and molecular weight are also recorded.

The evidence of chemical structure or identification of the drug molecule by spectrometric measurements is one of the most important aspects of the analytical profile. As an example, celecoxib (brand name Celebrex) is discussed with a few spectral analyses. Its structure can be confirmed by the elemental analysis, infrared (IR), nuclear magenetic resonance (NMR), and mass spectrometry. The self-explanatory spectrum of IR (Figure 4.37), ^{1}H-NMR (Figure 4.38), ^{13}C-NMR (Figure 4.39) and mass (Figure 4.40) with identified peaks are provided.

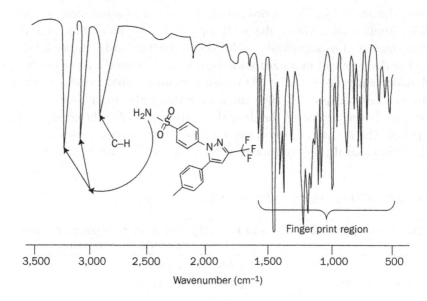

Figure 4.37 FTIR spectrum of celecoxib taken using KBr pellet

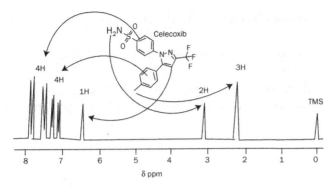

Figure 4.38 ^{1}H-NMR spectrum obtained on a 200 MHz machine using $CDCl_3$

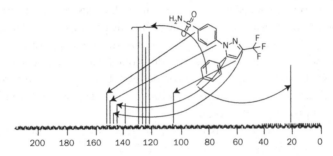

Figure 4.39 ^{13}C-decoupled NMR spectrum obtained on a 200 MHz machine using $CDCl_3$

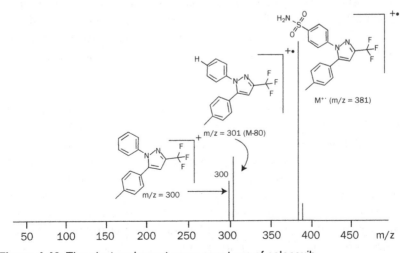

Figure 4.40 The electron impact mass spectrum of celecoxib

The other important features in the analytical profile dossier are:

- physico-chemical properties, such as solubility, pH, pKa values, and melting point
- analytical methodology – thin layer chromatography (TLC), high performance liquid chromatography (HPLC), and gas chromatography (GC)
- stability and degradation.

4.8 Green chemistry in bulk drug manufacturing

When producing a new molecular entity innovator pharmaceutical industries develop their own process of manufacturing bulk drugs. The manufacturing process before marketing a drug is somewhat different from the lab process used at an earlier stage in the drug's production. As more cost-effective or environmentally friendly processes are developed, earlier processes become obsolete. While providing medicine for people, it is important not to harm the environment, so pharmaceutical industries are getting involved in green chemistry to produce bulk drugs.

The concept of green chemistry has only recently begun to take shape. In 1991 the US Environmental Protection Agency established the Green Chemistry Program within the Office of Pollution, Prevention, and Toxics. According to the US Environmental Protection Agency:

> Green chemistry, also known as sustainable chemistry, is the design of chemical products and processes that reduce or eliminate the use or generation of hazardous substances. Green chemistry applies across the life cycle of a chemical product, including its design, manufacture, and use.[4]

Very simply, green chemistry is environmentally friendly chemistry.

In 1998, Anastas and Warner wrote *Green Chemistry*,[5] in which they put forward 12 principles of green chemistry (Figure 4.41). Slowly, different chemical societies, chemical organizations, government agencies, and non-government agencies started promoting the concept of green chemistry.

The 12 principles of green chemistry shown in Figure 4.41 are self-explanatory, but the atom economy may need explanation. The atom economy measures the environmental friendliness of chemical reactions in bulk drug production. Atom economy can be defined as:

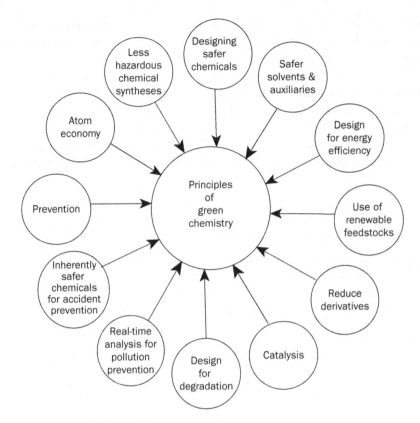

Figure 4.41 Twelve principles of green chemistry

$$\text{Atom economy} = \frac{\text{Total mass of atoms in desired product} + 100}{\text{Total mass of atoms in all the reactants}}$$

The better the percentage of atom economy, the greater the environmentally friendliness.

This is a simple example of a substitution reaction:

$$CH_3\text{-}CH_2\text{-}Cl + NaOH \rightarrow CH_3\text{-}CH_2\text{-}OH + NaCl$$

In this reaction, the desired product is ethanol, $CH_3CH_2\text{-}OH$, MW = 46 and total mass of reactants (64.5 for $CH_3CH_2\text{-}Cl$ and 40 for NaOH) = 104.5. Therefore, the percentage of the atom economy is (46/104.5 × 100) = 44%.

In bulk drug manufacturing, the production of ibuprofen can act as an example of green chemistry. Ibuprofen is an analgesic and anti-inflammatory drug discovered by Boots Company in the 1960s. The original production method by Boots included six steps (Figure 4.42). Its atom economy was only 40%.

After the patent expiration of ibuprofen in 1984, other companies started working on more efficient methods of production. Hoechst Celanese Corporation eventually developed a very efficient three-step method of producing ibuprofen with a 77% atom economy (Figure 4.43).

Boots and Hoechst Celanese jointly formed a company, BHC, and have been making ibuprofen since 1990. The first method by Boots produced

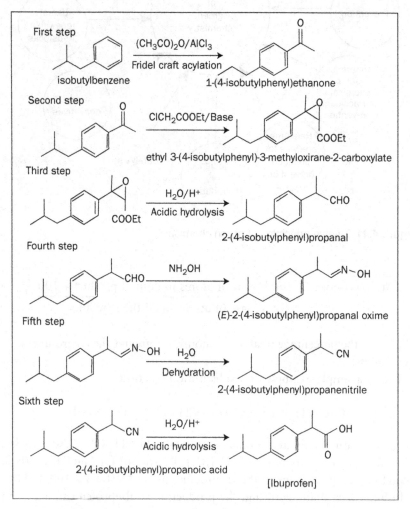

Figure 4.42 Original method of production of ibuprofen by Boots

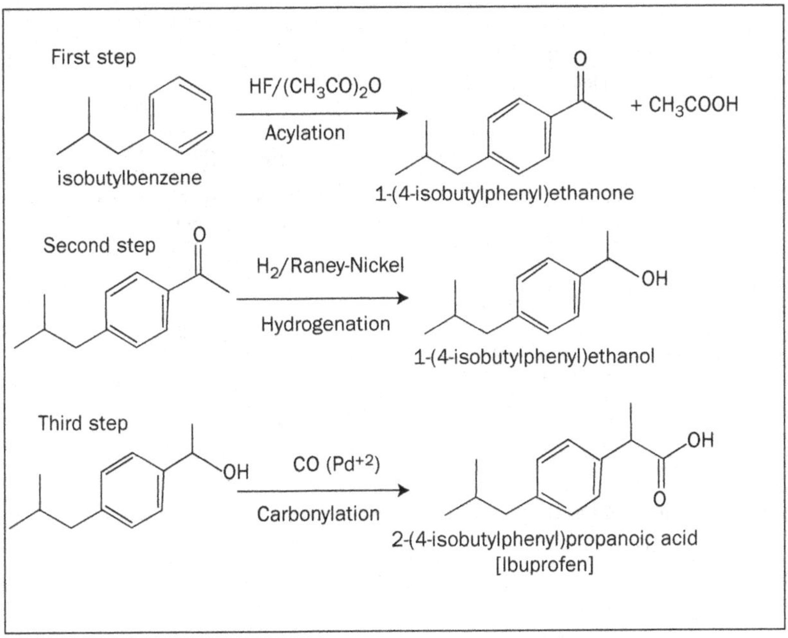

Figure 4.43 Improved method of production of ibuprofen by Hoechst Celanese Corporation

60% waste, and every year it was estimated to produce £40 million of waste against £30 million of ibuprofen. However, the second method produced only 1% waste with disposal costs.

Another important aspect of a green synthetic process is the production of by-products in addition to the desired product, rather than waste products. The second method produces a by-product, acetic acid, in the first step, which can be recycled, used to make acetic anhydride, or sold to other companies.

Pfizer initiated a green chemistry program in its bulk drug manufacturing and made a breakthrough in its implementation. The company received the 2003 UK Award for Green Chemical Technology for the sildenafil citrate process. According to an article published by Pfizer researchers, Pfizer has redesigned the commercial method for sildenafil citrate and cut down the waste production from 100% in the lab scale to 0.5% in the commercial scale (Figure 4.44).[6] The overall yield of sildenafil citrate increased from 9.8% during the lab scale to 75% during the commercial scale. The overall atom economy is around 54%. There are seven reactions with no isolation steps. The commercial synthetic processes are discussed in Chapter 11.

Published by Woodhead Publishing Limited

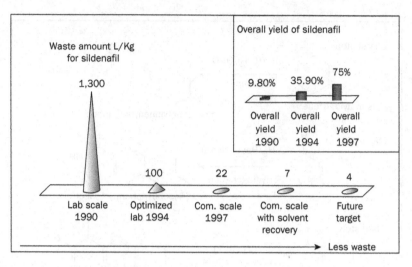

Figure 4.44 Generation of waste in the development of sildenafil citrate

Source: Dunn et al.[7]

Practice questions

1. What are bulk drugs? Are bulk drugs and APIs the same? What is the difference between bulk drugs and medicine?
2. Is there any difference between the bulk drug industry and the chemical industry? Compare the bulk drug industry for oral drugs with that for parenteral drugs.
3. In the industry for active pharmaceutical ingredients, reactors made of stainless steel and glass line are used. What types of reactions or processes take place in glass line reactors?
4. The API of a specific stereoisomer is costly compared with the racemate. Can you find any reason for this? Justify why in some cases racemic APIs cannot be used as a medicine.
5. What is green chemistry? Is there any role for green chemistry in the pharmaceutical industry?
6. Is there any therapeutic importance of the particle size of an API? Explain.
7. There are different steps involved in the manufacturing of bulk drugs, one of which is crystallization, and this step is considered very important. Explain why.

8. When we talk about drug solubility, what sort of solvent are we talking about for the drug? Why is drug solubility important? What method can be used to overcome the solubility problem of the drug?
9. Discuss the role of analytical chemistry in the identification of APIs. Name a few analytical methods used in the qualitative analysis of APIs.

Notes

1. International Conference on Harmonisation of Technical Requirements for Registration of Pharmaceuticals for Human Use, *Good Manufacturing Practice Guide for Active Pharmaceutical Ingredients Q7*, Current Step 4 version, ICH Harmonised Tripartite Guideline, November 2000, www.ich.org/fileadmin/Public_Web_Site/ICH_Products/Guidelines/Quality/Q7/Step4/Q7_Guideline.pdf (accessed February 15, 2011).
2. US Food and Drug Administration, 'Waiver of in vivo bioavailability and bioequivalence studies for immediate-release solid oral dosage forms based on a biopharmaceutics classification system', Guidance for Industry, August 2000, www.fda.gov/downloads/Drugs/GuidanceComplianceRegulatoryInformation/Guidances/ucm070246.pdf (accessed February 15, 2011).
3. Section based on Jiben Roy, 'Pharmaceutical impurities: a mini-review', *PharmSciTech Journal*, Vol. 3, No. 2, 2002, by permission of *AAPS PharmSciTech Journal*.
4. US Environmental Protection Agency, 'Green chemistry', www.epa.gov/gcc/ (accessed September 12, 2010).
5. Paul T. Anastas and John C. Warner, *Green Chemistry: Theory and Practice*, Oxford and New York: Oxford University Press, 1998.
6. Peter J. Dunn, Stephen Galvin, and Kevin Hettenbach, 'The development of an environmentally benign synthesis of sildenafil citrate (ViagraTM) and its assessment by green chemistry metrics', *Green Chem.*, Vol. 6, 2004, pp. 43–48.
7. Ibid.

Published by Woodhead Publishing Limited

5

Formulated drugs 1

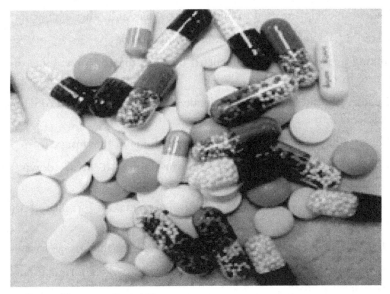

Source: Square Pharmaceuticals Ltd

Learning objective

This chapter is about medicines or formulated drugs. To make a medicine of a particular dosage form the active pharmaceutical ingredient (API) is mixed with non-APIs called excipients (Figure 5.1). The excipients play a very important role in formulating different dosage forms. This chapter explains why various types of dosage forms are required and how tablets, capsules, or solutions and suspension are manufactured. Though the process of manufacturing tablets and solutions has existed for many years it still evolves as new methods to enhance the safety, quality, and efficacy of medicines are found. The introduction of process analytical technology (PAT) – the current technique of in-line, on-line, at-line, or non-invasive process monitoring – will be discussed. Finally, there is a discussion of the very sensitive topic of pediatric dosage forms.

Key concept terms

Anti-oxidant: an expient used to prevent oxidation

API: active pharmaceutical ingredient

At-line: testing after isolating samples from the processing

Binder: an excipient used to bind API powders and other excipients

Blister: a packaging device for tablets and capsules

Bulking agent: a filler or diluent to increase the size or volume of a dosage form

Capsule: a solid dosage form, made up using powder of APIs and excipients into a gelatin shell

Diluent: filler to make a specific size or volume of the dosage form

Disintegrant: an exicipent used in the tablet to break down or disintegrate the tablet in the GIT

Exipient: substance other than an API used to make a formulated drug or medicine

Filler: a diluent to make specific size or volume of the dosage form

Flavoring agent: different flavored materials used in formulation to give a specific taste

Fluid bed dryer: a dryer used in drying wet APIs or wet granulated mixture of APIs and excipients

Formulated drug: a medicine made up of a drug (API) and excipients

FTIR: Fourier transform infrared

GIT: gastrointestinal tract

Granulator: a machine where granules of a mixture of APIs and excipients are made

Humectant: hygroscopic (absorbing moisture) excipient such as propylene glycol or glycerine

Published by Woodhead Publishing Limited

In-line: direct testing during formulation

LIBS: laser induced breakdown spectroscopy

LIF: light-induced fluorescence

Medicine: a formulated drug given to patients

NIR: near infrared

On-line: direct testing that bypasses processing steps using a loop

PAT: process analytical technology used in monitoring different formulation steps

Pediatric dosage form: form of medicines suitable for children

Sifter: a screener used in tablet manufacturing

Solution: a clear medicinal liquid

Strip: a packaging device for tablets and capsules

Suspension: an insoluble API suspended in liquid dosage form

Suspension agent: an excipient that helps in suspending insoluble APIs in liquid dosage form

Sweetening agent: an excipient used to sweeten dosage forms

Tablet: a solid dosage form made by compressing a mixture of APIs and excipients

TPS: terahertz-pulsed spectroscopy

XRF: X-ray fluorescence

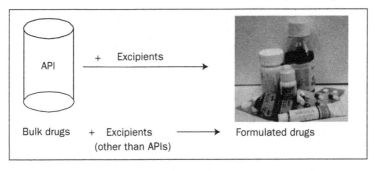

Figure 5.1 APIs + excipients = formulated drugs

Published by Woodhead Publishing Limited

5.1 Introduction

There is a saying that 'a doctor prescribes drugs, patients receive medicine'. Here drugs are defined as APIs, and more specifically pharmacologically active ingredients, and medicine is defined as a formulated API ready for administration. Thus a formulated drug is an API in its finished dosage form (Figure 5.1). A dosage form is a physical form of a final pharmaceutical preparation based on therapeutic intention, route of administration, and dosing. Figure 5.2 shows the major steps of getting APIs to patients.

Most APIs are in solid form, possibly crystalline or powder. We need small amounts of APIs, usually in the range of 5–500 mg, every time medicine is made. There are even drugs that need less than 1 mg of an API. We need dosage forms to ensure patients take the right amount of a drug in the correct form, depending on the requirements of the patient. For example, a patient in the emergency room of a hospital needs a drug immediately but is unable to take medicine orally. The parenteral (injectable) form is appropriate as it acts quickly. Some children cannot swallow pills, so they are given liquid dosage forms or chewable candy forms. There are dozens of reasons for having various dosage forms (Figure 5.3).

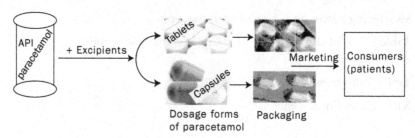

Figure 5.2 The major steps of getting APIs to patients

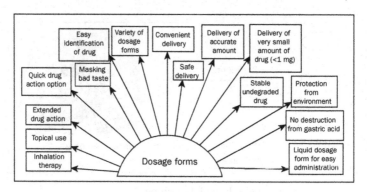

Figure 5.3 Reasons for having different dosage forms

Dosage forms, such as solid dosage forms (tablets or capsules) or liquid dosage forms (syrup or suspension), are made using the API and excipients, so they are convenient for patients and can be produced on a large scale. Excipients are indispensable in drug manufacture as without adding them to an API, no formulation of the drug is possible for mass scale production. Different excipients are used, depending on the dosage form.

5.2   The role of excipients

Excipients are an essential and integral part of medicine. They are so important there is a global organization that maintains quality in pharmaceutical excipients, the International Pharmaceutical Excipients Council Federation, which defines excipients as:

> substances, other than the active drug substance of finished dosage form, which have been appropriately evaluated for safety and are included in a drug delivery system to either aid the processing of the drug delivery system during its manufacture; protect; support; enhance stability, bioavailability, or patient acceptability; assist in product identification; or enhance any other attributes of the overall safety and effectiveness of the drug delivery system during storage or use.[1]

This is a comprehensive definition of excipients. The *US Pharmacopeia–National Formulary (USP–NF)* states that 'excipients are components of a finished drug product other than the API and are added during formulation for a specific purpose'.[2] Figure 5.4 shows the proportion of APIs (~25–30%) and excipients (~75–70%) in a drug.

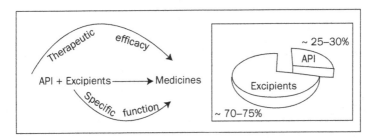

Figure 5.4 The proportion of APIs (~25–30%) and excipients (~75–70%) in a drug

The *USP–NF* classifies excipients according to their function, including for example disintegrants, coatings, binders, diluents, fillers, lubricants, glidants, emulsifying-solubilizing agents, sweetening agents, coating agents, antimicrobial preservatives, stabilizers, colorants, flavors, and buffering agents based on their functionalities (Figure 5.5).

The most common, convenient, and cheapest dosage form is the tablet form, which requires a number of excipients. Fewer excipients are used in injectable dosage forms. When making tablets, the oral solid dosage form, the objective is to have a balanced formulation so it undergoes immediate disintegration in the gastrointestinal tract (GIT) (Figure 5.6).

The primary objective of a drug therapy is to introduce the drug or API in an exact therapeutic dose (amount) at regular intervals, considering the patient's compliance. The direct use of an API is rare for three reasons:

- It is almost impossible to produce drugs using only APIs on a mass production scale while maintaining the accurate dose strength at the mg or µg level.

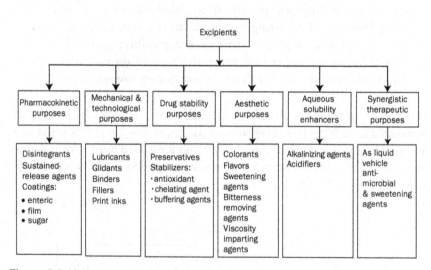

Figure 5.5 Various categories of excipients

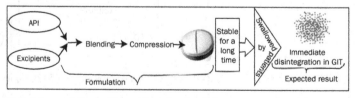

Figure 5.6 A formulation with an objective to disintegrate at the right place

Published by Woodhead Publishing Limited

- In the administration of drugs, the API powder is only feasible when taken orally, and in most cases has an unpleasant taste and smell.
- There is no choice over the route of administration, and it will not meet the therapeutic needs.

The use of excipients depends on the type of dosage form. For example, oral solid dosage forms, such as tablets, need diluents (fillers, bulking agents), disintegrants, binders, lubricants, and glidants; liquid dosage forms, such as solutions or suspension, do not need disintegrants, coatings, lubricants, glidants, or binders, but require solvents and/or co-solvents, buffering agents, preservatives, anti-oxidants, wetting agents, antifoaming agents, suspending agents, sweetening agents, or flavouring agents. There are several dozens of dosage forms based on the physical properties or route of administrations. Various dosage forms also exist for a particular API or drug.

5.2.1 Excipients for regular tablets

5.2.1.1 Fillers, diluents, or bulking agents

Filler is an inert substance used to fill up the bulk of the tablet to achieve the intended size, so the filler should have a good compressibility factor. Commonly used fillers are starch, lactose, microcrystalline cellulose, and mannitol. Fine grades of lactose are used in the wet granulation process and spray-dried lactose is used in the direct compression of tablets. Sometimes, to improve the flow properties of granules, microcrystalline cellulose are used in addition to lactose. In most cases, a small amount of an API in the range of 5–500 mg is used, which could make up 25–30% of the tablet.

5.2.1.2 Binders

Binders help to bind or hold all the substances used to make a tablet. They can be water insoluble (starch, microcrystalline cellulose), water soluble (methylcellulose, HPMC), or soluble in water and ethanol (povidone).

5.2.1.3 Disintegrants

Tablets are made by compression, so they become hard and solid, but once tablets are swallowed, they should disintegrate (break down immediately). Disintegrators help break up the compact tablet rapidly on exposure to moisture. The disintegration of tablets is a very important step in their functionality because the disintegration of a tablet is followed by the dissolution of a drug. Examples of disintegrants are crospovidone, croscarmellose sodium, carboxymethyl starch sodium, and sodium starch glycolate microcrystalline cellulose.

5.2.1.4 Lubricants

Tablets are made in a die punch under pressure; after compression, they should come out of the mold easily. This is a mechanical situation and the die punch requires some kind of lubrication. The inert lubricants magnesium or calcium stearate are widely used in the amount of 0.3–2%. Alternative lubricants are stearic acid, sodium stearyl fumarate, and sodium behenate. A high capacity, high-speed tablet compression machine can produce 6,000 tablets per minute (30 stations – three tablets per second per station) so effective lubrication plays a very important role in the tablet manufacturing process.

5.2.1.5 Glidants

The powders for tablets should have a smooth flowability and little inter-particle friction. Glidants such as colloidal silicon dioxide or talc in an amount of less than 0.1% are used to increase the flowability and reduce friction.

5.2.2 Excipients for coated tablets

Coated tablets require different excipients from those used in manufacturing regular tablets. Tablets are coated for various reasons: to protect the tablet from air or moisture, to mask bitter tastes, or to provide special characteristics of drug release, such as enteric release. The three most widely used coatings are sugar film enteric, film coating, and enteric-coated solid dosage forms.

5.2.2.1 Sugar film enteric coating

Sugar coating protects tablets from moisture, humidity, or air oxidation. The tablets are coated with shellac or cellulose acetate phthalate, and sugar syrup containing talc and acacia; then they are dried. Finally, a smooth coating with colorant is given. If imprinting and polishing are required, imprints may be embossed, engraved, or printed on the surface with ink. Polishing can be carried out by spraying the tablets with beeswax dissolved in non-aqueous solvents.

5.2.2.2 Film coating

Film coating of tablets has the same function as sugar film enteric coating: to protect them from moisture, humidity, and air oxidation. The components for non-aqueous film coating are film former-cellulose acetatae phthalate, alloying substances, such as polyethylene glycol, plasticizer such as castor oil, and opaquants, surfactants, sweeteners, glossants and volatile solvents such as alcohol-acetone mixture. Another method is aqueous coating, which can be applied provided the method is perfected over time.

5.2.2.3 Enteric coating

Enteric-coated solid dosage forms serve a special purpose. Enteric-coated tablets are supposed to pass through the stomach intact, disintegrate, and release the drug content for absorption in the intestines. The substances used in enteric coating are hydroxypropyl methylcellulose phthalate (HPMCP), polyvinyl acetate phthalate, diethyl phthalate, and cellulose acetate phthalate. In general, tablets can be coated using either a fluid-bed dryer or air suspension coating. Tablets can be sustained release or controlled release, which works for a longer period. A special type of excipient can be used to control the release of the API and excipients, such as polyvinyl acetate or glyceryl behenate.

5.2.3 Excipients for liquid oral dosage forms

5.2.3.1 Solvent and/or co-solvents

Water is the solvent most widely used in liquid oral dosage forms because it has a high solubility power, is physiologically compatible, and has no toxicity; however, water cannot be used as a vehicle if the drug is sensitive to hydrolysis, and it is prone to microbial growth. Propylene glycol, glycerol, or ethanols are used as co-solvents, which can provide better tastes and stable preparation, and prevent microbial growth.

5.2.3.2 Buffering agents

Maintaining the pH of the liquid dosage form is very important for a drug's chemical stability and the stability of other excipients, such as preservatives, flavors, and coloring materials. Commonly used buffers are citrate and gluconates.

5.2.3.3 Preservatives

The use of preservatives in liquid dosage forms, especially multi-use dosage forms, helps prevent the growth of microorganisms, including pathogens. The most common preservatives are sodium benzoate and parabens (methyl, propyl, or butyl paraben).

5.2.3.4 Anti-oxidants

To prevent the air oxidation of APIs, anti-oxidants such as butylated hydroxytoluene (BHT), butylated hydroxyanisole (BHA), or ascorbic acid (vitamin C) are used.

5.2.3.5 Sweetening agents

In general, most drugs do not taste good – some are bitter. To make the preparation palatable, sweetening agents are used. Among natural sweeteners, sucrose (sugar) and sorbitol (non-cariogenic) are used in a mixture with artificial sweeteners, such as saccharin, aspartame, or acesulfame.

5.2.3.6 Flavoring agents

Flavoring agents (natural, such as peppermints and lemon oils, or synthetic, such as tutti frutti, butterscotch, or any fruit flavors) compliment sweetening agents to enhance patient compliance.

5.2.3.7 Suspension agents

Suspension agents are not required for solution dosage forms, but for insoluble APIs in liquid vehicles, suspension agents such as methylcellulose, hydroxyethylcellulose, or microcrystalline cellulose are used to prevent settling or sedimentation of insoluble drug particles. There can be partial sedimentation, but shaking the liquid mixture produces a uniform composition for a dose.

5.2.3.8 Wetting agents

To aid the dispersion of insoluble API in liquid dosage forms, wetting agents such as polysorbates are used.

Published by Woodhead Publishing Limited

5.2.3.9 Antifoaming agents

To reduce foaming during the production of liquid formulation, an antifoaming agent, such as simethicone (polydimethylsiloxane-silicon dioxide), is used in the range of 1–50ppm.

5.2.3.10 Humectants

Humectants are hygroscopic (attracting moisture from the air) excipients such as propylene glycol or glycerine; they are also used as co-solvents. A small amount of a humectant can be used to prevent cap locking when they are not used as a co-solvent.

5.2.4 Drug and excipients interactions

5.2.4.1 Synergistic interaction (positive effect)

Excipients are usually thought to be biologically inert or inactive, which is not entirely true. Recently, some excipients contribute synergistically to the API's activity (see Figure 5.5). For example, recent research has confirmed that oleic acid – an excipient used with Herceptin to treat breast cancer – acts as a liquid vehicle for drugs and at the same time can inhibit the breast cancer gene. Similarly, gamma-linolenic acid and omega-3 fatty acids have some beneficial effects in antitumor activity and cardiovascular benefits, respectively. These excipients can be used as liquid vehicles for other drugs, but excipients can also destabilize APIs.

5.2.4.2 Counter interaction (negative effect)

Excipients can participate in physical and chemical interactions with the drug molecule, which can reduce the effectiveness of the drug. The physical interaction of excipients can affect the rate of dissolution of a solid dosage form. Some excipients can adsorb APIs, which ultimately leads to slower dissolution rates, resulting in less bioavailability of the drug. Colloidal silicon dioxide (glidant) can catalyze the degradation of nitrazepam through adsorption of the drug in the tablet dosage form.

The chemical interaction of excipients can lead to the degradation of an API. Soluble or ionizable excipients can produce counter ions that can interact with ionizable drugs. For example, sodium carboxymethylcellulose can interact with neomycine, producing a precipitate of drug-excipient

Published by Woodhead Publishing Limited

complex. Povidone can interact with the drug containing hydrogen-donating functional groups. Similarly, a drug molecule containing primary and secondary amines reacts with reducing sugars, such as excipients (namely lactose), resulting in a 'Maillard reaction' product. Lactose and fluoxetine or lactose and baclofen can produce Maillard reaction products in tablet dosage forms (Figures 5.7 and 5.8).

In some cases, the residue or impurities from the excipients can also degrade the drug. During the manufacturing of spray-dried lactose, there is a possibility of 5-hydroxyfurfural forming as an impurity. The presence of this impurity in lactose can react with the primary amine functional group of a drug, producing a Schiff base (Figure 5.9).

As an anti-oxidant, bisulphite is used in formulation, and this excipient is found to react with epinephrine, causing a sulfated product to form (Figure 5.10).

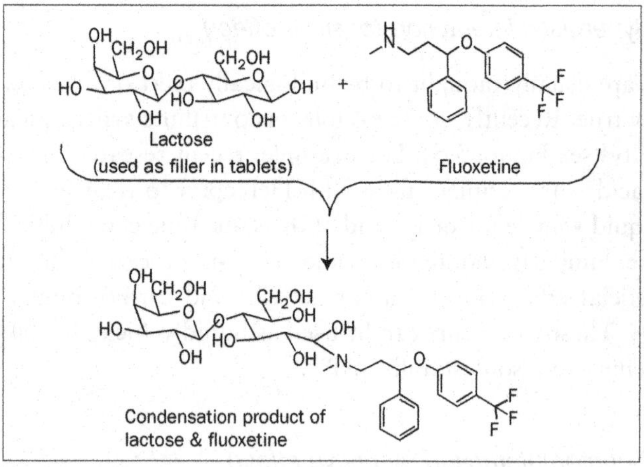

Figure 5.7 Maillard reaction between lactose and fluoxetine

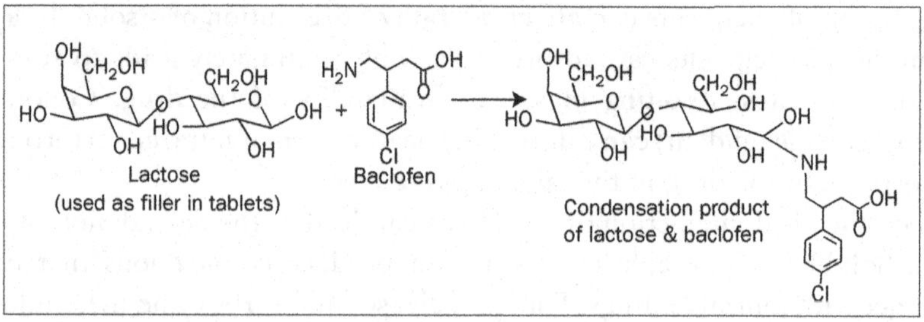

Figure 5.8 Maillard reaction between lactose and baclofen

Published by Woodhead Publishing Limited

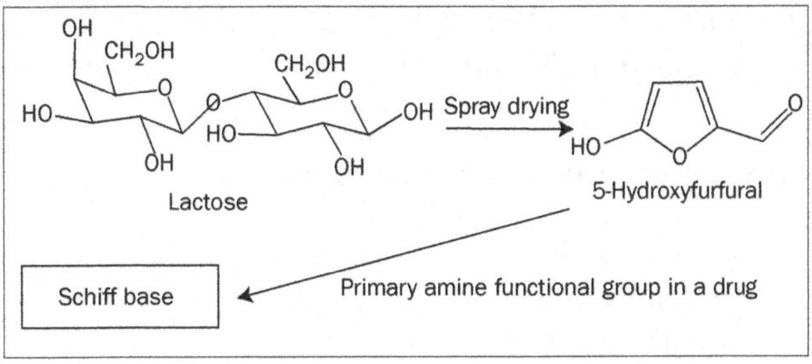

Figure 5.9 Interaction between the residue or impurity from a spray-dried lactose and drug

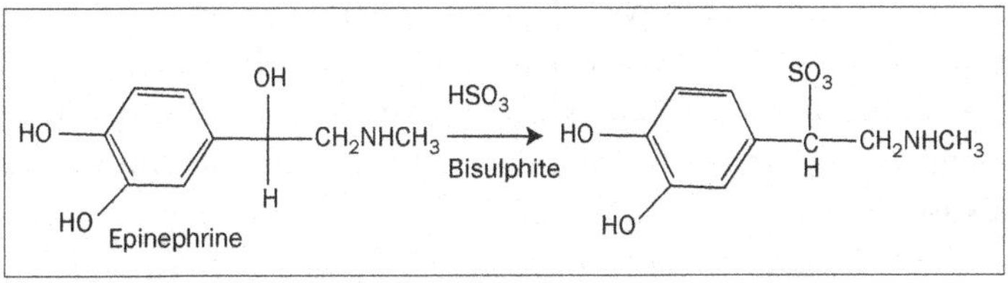

Figure 5.10 The reaction between bisulphite and epinephrine

An excipient's moisture, such as the high moisture content in polyvinyl pyrrolidone, can initiate hydrolysis of a certain drug molecule. Crowley and Martini of GSK found that the impurities found in common excipients can cause drug-excipient interaction.[3] Table 5.1 shows the residues in common

Table 5.1 Residues or impurities in common excipients

Excipient	Residue or impurity
Povidone, crosspovidone, polysorbates	Peroxides
Magnesium stearate	Antioxidants
Lactose	Aldehyde
Benzyl alcohol	Benzaldehyde
Polyethylene glycol	Aldehydes, peroxides, organic acids
Microcrystalline cellulose	Lignin, hemicelluloses, water
Starch	Formaldehyde
Talc	Heavy metals
Dibasic calcium phosphate dihydrate	Alkaline residue
Stearate lubricants	Alkaline residue
Hydroxymethyl/ethyl/propylcellulose	Glyoxal

Published by Woodhead Publishing Limited

excipients. Excipients should be tested and analyzed in the same way as APIs are tested and analyzed, including testing for the presence of impurities.

5.3   The classification of dosage forms

Dosage forms can be classified in two ways: by physical state of the drug or by route of administration (Figure 5.11). Dosage forms by route of administration are discussed in Chapter 6.

5.3.1 Dosage forms based on physical states

There are three different physical states – solid, liquid, and gas – and pharmaceutical dosage forms are available in these three forms. There are also semi-solid dosage forms and sterile and non-sterile dosage forms. Oral solid dosage forms, especially tablets and capsules, are the most commonly used because they:

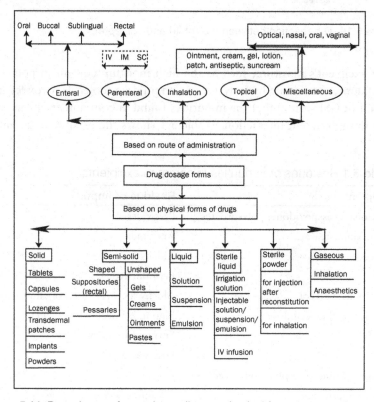

Figure 5.11 Drug dosage forms depending on physical form or route of administration

Published by Woodhead Publishing Limited

- are convenient to administer
- are convenient to store
- are a relatively stable form
- can be dosed with accuracy and reproducibility
- are comparatively cheap
- are simple to produce on a mass scale.

Tablets are solid dosage forms manufactured by compressing a mixture of APIs and excipients; a die punch is used to produce various size and shapes. Tablets used as medicines are called pills – the name originally given by the apothecary. All pills are tablets, but tablets are not necessarily pills. Although tablets are usually swallowed whole, some can be dissolved in water and then drunk; these are called effervescent tablets. Sometimes tablets are chewed or dissolved in the mouth. Figure 5.12 shows the various solid dosage forms, including different tablet forms.

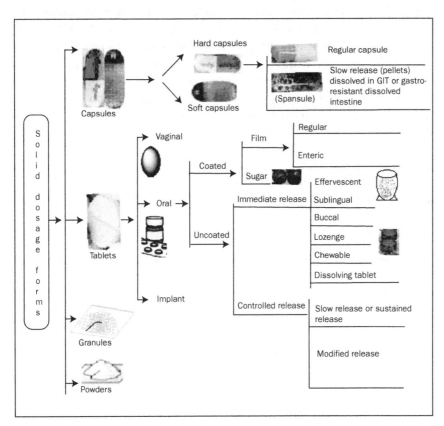

Figure 5.12 Various dosage forms depending on physical states

Published by Woodhead Publishing Limited

5.4   Formulation and manufacturing of tablets

There are certain general formulation criteria for producing tablet forms:

- formulation stability
- blend homogeneity
- flowability
- compressibility and compactibility
- lubricity
- tablet content uniformity
- hardness
- friability.

The most important formulation criterion for a tablet is that it should have the quickest possible disintegration time. Though there is no standardized disintegration time for tablets, a time of 5–30 minutes is considered acceptable as are 5-minute dissolutions of 40–60% and 45-minute dissolutions of > 90%. The quicker the disintegration time, the quicker the dissolution time, so the faster the physiological action. For immediate-release tablets, the dissolution step is the rate-limiting step for drug action. To achieve the above-mentioned formulation criteria for tablets, the following basic formulation materials in addition to the API are needed:

- a compressible diluent
- a disintegrant
- a glidant
- a lubricant.

When making tablets the following machinery is needed:

- a sifter
- a planetary mixer or high-speed granulator
- a fluid bed dryer
- a mill or granulator
- a double-cone blender
- a steam-jacketed pan
- a tablet compression machine
- blister, strip, or container packing.

Figures 5.13 shows the three different processes involved in producing tablets or capsules:

- direct compression or capsule filing via sieving or milling and blending
- dry granulation followed by compression or capsule filing
- wet granulation followed by compression or capsule filing.

Figure 5.14 illustrates the manufacturing process of tablets.

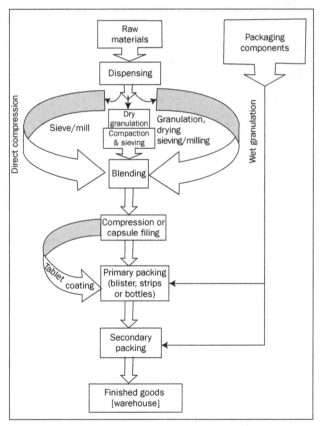

Figure 5.13 Flow diagram of production of tablets and capsules via direct compression, dry granulation, and wet granulation followed by compression

Published by Woodhead Publishing Limited

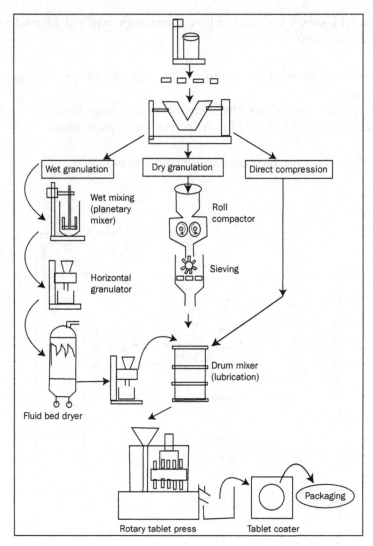

Figure 5.14 Flow diagram of the manufacturing process of tablets

5.5   Problems with tablet manufacturing and the use of process analytical technology

The most common problems encountered in tablet manufacturing include capping, cracking, chipping, lamination, picking, sticking, orange peel, color variation, mottling, black spots, hardness variation, thickness variation, and double impression. Figure 5.15 illustrates some of the problems.

These problems have different sources and can be machinery related, raw materials related, or manufacturing process related. Problems can be caused by:

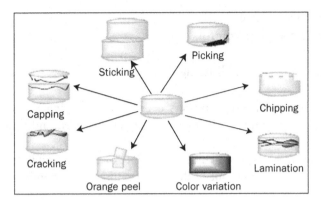

Figure 5.15 Problems in tablets caused by manufacturing processes

- compressibility and ejection properties or the quality of die-punches of tablet presses
- the poor quality of raw materials, such as pharmaceutical active ingredients and various excipients used in making tablets
- the important tablet manufacturing processes blending, granulating, drying, and milling of total ingredients.

5.5.1 Conventional in-process controls

To obtain good tablet products it is necessary to carry out the following control checks.

During preparation of the tableting mixture check:

- conformity of ingredients
- exactness of ingredient weights
- screen size control
- mixing time control
- drying temperature control.

During tablet compression check:

- conformity of ingredients
- exactness of ingredient weights
- screen size control

Published by Woodhead Publishing Limited

- mixing time control
- drying temperature control.

During packaging, when blistering check:

- sealing and tightness of blisters every hour, plugging in a methylene blue under vacuum at 50 mm Hg for ten minutes, and that no blue spots appear
- the printing of date of manufacture, date of expiry, and batch number
- that the tablet comes out of the blister with simple thumb pressure.

5.5.2 Process analytical technology

Current manufacturing processes of tablets involve a stepwise route where product or in-process qualities are checked. If the optimum quality is not obtained in the first instance, the materials need to be reprocessed. The reprocessing may produce a quality product in the end, but if the quality is built in or quality by design (QbD) is established, most of the problems can be avoided. QbD can be implemented by using process analytical technology (PAT) in tablet manufacturing channels. PAT is an on-line technique that can ensure the quality of tablets by monitoring every step of manufacturing, from raw materials to the end product. The US Food and Drug Administration (FDA) has guidelines for using PAT, which it defines as:

> a system for designing, analyzing, and controlling manufacturing through timely measurements (i.e., during processing) of critical quality and performance attributes of raw and in-process materials and processes with the goal of ensuring final product quality.[4]

The main objective of using PAT is 'to understand and control the manufacturing process, which is consistent with our current drug quality system: quality cannot be tested in products; it should be built-in or should be by design'.[5] A number of technologies are available, including near infrared (NIR), laser induced breakdown spectroscopy (LIBS), X-ray fluorescence (XRF), Fourier transform infrared (FTIR) spectroscopy, air coupled acoustic techniques, light-induced fluorescence (LIF), and terahertz-pulsed spectroscopy (TPS). Figure 5.16 compares the conventional tablet manufacturing process with the use of PAT.

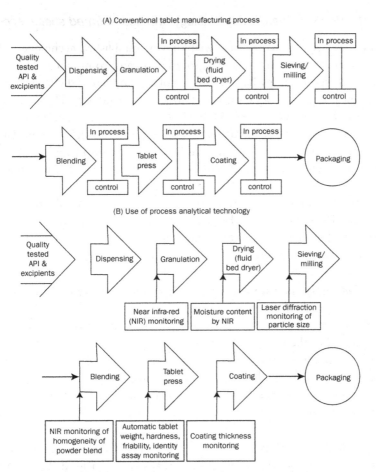

Figure 5.16 The conventional tablet manufacturing process compared with using process analytical technology

Though the initial investment for implementing PAT is high, the technology has many advantages. It:

- is a non-destructive process
- requires no sample preparation
- can control content uniformity better
- can control moisture content better
- can control particle size
- can control flow characteristics and bulk density
- ensures better batch-to-batch consistency
- ensures better product quality
- does not require reprocessing or rejection of batches.

Published by Woodhead Publishing Limited

5.5.2.1 Process analytical technology and near-infrared spectroscopy

Infrared (IR) spectroscopy is a well-known, established technique, which provides information on functional groups of organic compounds. The closely related NIR spectroscopy has recently become a popular and effective on-line and at-line process technology in the pharmaceutical industry. The IR radiation covers the wave number range 4,000–400 cm⁻¹ (0.25–2.5 μm), whereas NIR covers the range 12,820–3,959 cm⁻¹ (wavelength 780–2,526 nm). The IR radiation makes molecules vibrate, and these vibrations of molecular bonds lead to IR spectra. The case of NIR is similar, but it is less sensitive than IR. This lack of sensitivity makes NIR advantageous in performing measurements without any sample preparation or pretreatments. Chemical and physical characteristics of samples can be predicted from a single spectrum.

NIR can be used for at-line, on-line, in-line, or non-invasive analysis of manufacturing processes:

- *at-line analysis* – sample is isolated and analyzed in close proximity to the manufacturing process stream
- *on-line analysis* – sample is diverted from the process, tested, and returned to the process stream
- *in-line analysis* – direct testing where sample is not removed from the process stream; can be invasive or non-invasive
- *non-invasive analysis* – when there is no need to isolate or come into contact with the sample.

Using real-time analysis of different in-process materials, manufacturing risks can be minimized and product quality can be ensured (Figure 5.17). Though NIR technology is much ahead of PAT instruments, other analytical

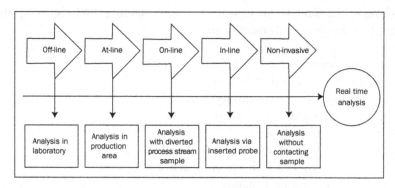

Figure 5.17 Real-time analysis of a production process

Published by Woodhead Publishing Limited

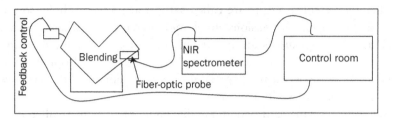

Figure 5.18 In-line monitoring of blending operation in table production

instruments are also used, including IR, Raman spectroscopy, light induced fluorescence, chemical imaging, reflective UV, fast HPLC, and acoustic methods. Uniformity in blending is a critical step in tablet manufacturing; it can be monitored in-line using fiber-optic probes (Figure 5.18).

5.6 Liquid dosage forms

There are many different liquid dosage forms, including oral and parenteral forms (Figure 5.19). Oral liquid dosage forms are easier to swallow and thus suitable for children and elderly patients. The solution form is homogenous and dosing accuracy can easily be maintained. The therapeutic action of the solution form is relatively quicker than that of solid dosage forms.

Solutions are clear homogenous liquid preparations containing one or more APIs dissolved in suitable solvents. Aqueous solutions with sugar or

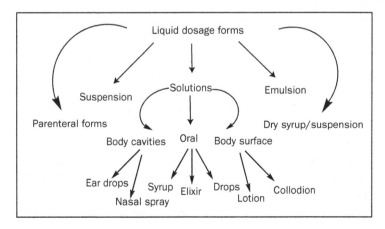

Figure 5.19 Liquid dosage forms

Published by Woodhead Publishing Limited

artificial sweetening agents are called syrups; aqueous alcoholic solutions are called elixirs. Suspensions are liquid preparations where the active ingredient or ingredients are not readily soluble and are dispersed in the liquid vehicle. Suspending agents or thickening agents – hydrophilic colloids such as cellulose derivatives, acacia, or xanthan gum – are used to prevent sedimentation and agglomeration.

Emulsions are made of two immiscible liquid phases; the smaller amount is dispersed into the larger amount. To prevent the separation of phases, emulsifying agents such as sodium lauryl sulfate, triethanolamine stearate, sodium oleate, or glyceryl monostearate are used. There are two types of emulsions depending on whether oil or water is dispersed: the oil in water (o/w) type when oil is dispersed and the water in oil (w/o) type when water is dispersed.

Dry syrups or suspensions are medicines supplied as dry powders; a measured amount of water is added to them to reconstitute the medicine before consumption. A few aqueous unstable antibiotics are supplied as dry suspensions or syrups.

5.6.1 Critical factors in liquid dosage forms

To make liquid dosage forms, the drugs or APIs must be sufficiently stable in an aqueous solution to maintain the required potency until the expiry date. Whatever degradation takes place, the degradants must not be toxic at all. An option to avoid hydrolysis of APIs is to use a formulation of dry syrup (in dry powder form). In the formulation, certain measures are taken to protect the dosage form from the growth of molds, yeast, and other microorganisms to maintain the correct viscosity, flowability, and dosage uniformity to make the dosage form palatable, with a pleasant taste and agreeable appearance. In order to achieve the above-mentioned objectives, a number of excipients are added to the API, and the excipients play an important role in the formulation.

These excipients are used in liquid dosage forms:

- buffering agents such as dibasic sodium phosphate and citric acid; these act as buffers to keep the required pH range for the stability of the solution
- antimicrobial preservatives such as methyl/propyl-p-hydroxybezoate (paraben), the main preservative of the preparation
- solvents as preservatives such as alcohol; these are solubilizing agents for paraben and contribute to the preservation and taste of the solution

Published by Woodhead Publishing Limited

- flavoring agents such as fruit flavor, to flavor the syrup
- sweetening agents such as sorbitol, which is also effective in preventing microbial growth in the solution, and glycerine, which reinforces the sweet and fresh taste given to syrup by sorbitol and acts as a preservative
- viscosity imparting agents
- chelating agents
- anti-oxidants
- bitterness removing agents
- solubilizing agents
- water in a quantity sufficient to make specific volume.

5.7   Production of oral solution and suspension dosage forms

The manufacturing processes of oral solutions and suspensions are relatively simple and basic (Figure 5.20), but contamination can occur easily during the manufacturing process and batch-to-batch manufacturing systems. Thus the equipment, including pumps, valves, flow meters, and pipelines, should be of sanitary design to be easily cleaned and sanitized.

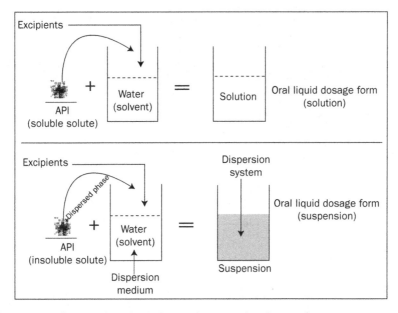

Figure 5.20 Schematics of solution and suspension dosage forms

Published by Woodhead Publishing Limited

For suspension, the API has to be a finely divided powder of particle size less than 25 micron (colloidal suspension = 1 nm to 0.5 μm and coarse suspension = 1–100 μm). The particles should settle slowly, and once settled should be easily redispersed with shaking. The dispersed phase should never settle permanently, which would ultimately form a cake. The process of aggregation or caking of dispersed particles is a common phenomenon in oral suspension, resulting from:

- adsorption of surface active agents
- minor changes in the surface of the dispersed particles
- the presence of electrolytes.

Oral suspension formulations are generally used for antacid, antibiotics, analgesics, anthelmintics, and antifungal and anticonvulsant drugs. They are particularly useful for children and elderly patients. Figure 5.21 summarises the process of making oral solutions and suspensions.

Figure 5.22 illustrates the process in more detail.

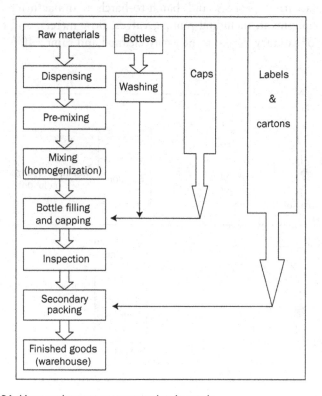

Figure 5.21 How oral syrup or suspension is made

Published by Woodhead Publishing Limited

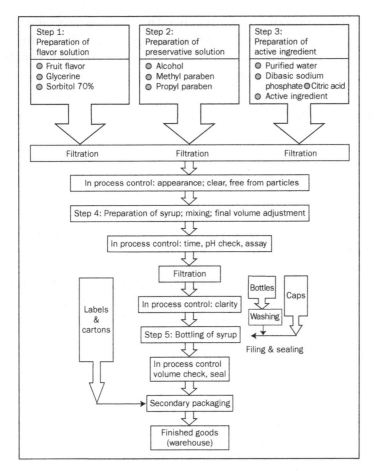

Figure 5.22 Typical production processes for making syrup

5.8 Dosage forms in pediatrics

The pediatric population comprises 20–25% of the total world's population and is very susceptible to various diseases. When giving medicine to children they cannot be treated as 'little adults' and simply be given the same drugs used for adults but in smaller quantities. Medicines do not work in this way; there are variations in the absorption rate of medicines in pediatric patients, especially premature newborn and infants.

Clinical trials are not usually carried out on children while a drug is marketed, so pharmacokinetic and pharmacodynamic (see Chapter 9) data on children is usually unavailable. The US FDA and the European Medicine Evaluation Agency (EMEA) have guidelines for the purposes of clinical trials and licensing medicines for children. The International Conference on Harmonization of Technical Requirements for Registration of Pharmaceuticals for Human Use (ICH) categorizes the pediatric population into the following age groups:

- preterm newborn infants
- term newborn infants (0–27 days)
- infants and toddlers (1–23 months)
- children (2–11 years)
- adolescents (12–16 or 12–18 years).

Although many adult dosage forms are not suitable for infants and children, there are plenty of suitable dosage forms for this population: solutions, syrups, suspensions, scored tablets, chewing tablets, effervescent tablets, orally disintegrating tablets, sublingual strips, lozenges, lollipop formats, wafers, sachets, powder for reconstitution, suppositories, and transdermal patches. The most commonly used ones are solution and suspension forms because of their rate of drug bioavailability (explained in Chapter 3) in oral dosage forms:

> Rate of bioavailability of dosage forms: solution > suspension > capsule > tablet

Figure 5.23 shows how the rate of dissolution of a drug affects its absorption into the blood stream. After swallowing, the tablet has to disintegrate, dissolve, and finally be absorbed into the blood stream.

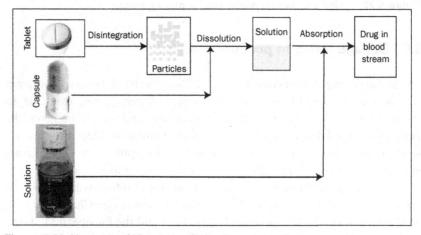

Figure 5.23 How rate of dissolution limits drug absorption

Published by Woodhead Publishing Limited

Liquid dosage forms are already in dissolution form, so are absorbed into the blood stream more quickly than a tablet would be and therefore act faster. In general, the liquid dosage form, also known as the pediatric dosage form, is used in pediatrics. It is convenient, but taste is very important and the use of alcohol and sugar in the formulation should be avoided.

It is very important to measure liquid medicine accurately to get the right dose. Measuring devices include dosing cups, syringes, droppers, and dosing spoons that come with medicine bottles (Figure 5.24). Teaspoons and tablespoons are usually available at home. When measuring liquid medicine into a teaspoon (tsp) or tablespoon (tblsp) the following conversion measurements apply:

1 ml = 1 cc

2.5 ml = 1/2 tsp

5 ml = 1 tsp

15 ml = 3 tsp = 1 tblsp

30 ml = 2 tblsp = 1 fluid ounce

The dose volume for pediatric liquid formulation is usually a maximum 5 ml (one teaspoon) per dose for children under 5 years old and a maximum 10 ml per dose for children above 5 years old.

Solid dosage forms, or odispersible tablets, lyophilized wafers, and thin films, are in great demand because they melt on the tongue and no water is required. Chewable tablets are also valuable pediatric dosage forms. Chewable tablets include antacids, antibiotics, anticonvulsants, analgesics, ant-asthmatics, vitamins, and cold preparations. Suppositories are sometimes used for infants.

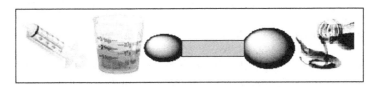

Figure 5.24 Measuring devices for liquid dosage forms

Published by Woodhead Publishing Limited

Practice questions

1. Define medicine. What is meant by 'formulated drugs'? What is an API?
2. What does 'excipient' mean? Do you think excipients are totally inactive? Discuss the role of excipients in the formulation of drugs.
3. Do you think excipients used for manufacturing solid dosage forms can also be used in manufacturing liquid dosage forms? What excipients are used in solid and liquid dosage forms?
4. Which solid dosage form, tablet or capsule has the fastest therapeutic action in our body? Explain.
5. Distinguish between solution and suspension dosage forms.
6. What is PAT? How does this technology help in perfecting the formulation processes of manufacturing tablets?
7. Describe the functions of the following excipients: binders, disintegrants, lubricants, glidants, preservatives, humectants, and enteric coating.
8. Which analytical tool is currently used to monitor the manufacturing processes of tablets directly? What other PATs are available?
9. What is the function of tablet compression machine? How are different shapes and sizes of tablets obtained?
10. What is the difference between the disintegration and dissolution of tablets? Which is the limiting step of drug action of tablets?
11. Explain the following statement: 'The rate of bioavailability of dosage forms is: solution > suspension > capsule > tablet.'

Notes

1. International Pharmaceutical Excipients Council, 'The IPEC Excipient Composition Guide, 2009', p. 2, www.ipec-europe.org/UPLOADS/IPEC CompositionGuidefinal.pdf (accessed February 15, 2011).
2. 'Excipients', USP Guideline, 2007, www.usp.org/pdf/EN/USPNF/chapter3.pdf (accessed February 15, 2011).
3. Patrick Crowley and Luigi G. Martini, 'Drug–excipient interactions', *Pharmaceutical Technology Europe*, Vol. 13, No. 3, 2001, pp. 26–34, www.callumconsultancy.com/articles/DrugExcipientInteractions.pdf (accessed February 15, 2011).
4. US Food and Drug Administration, 'Guidance for industry, PAT – a framework for innovative pharmaceutical development, manufacturing, and quality assurance', September 2004, www.fda.gov/downloads/Drugs/guidancecompliance regulatory information/guidances/ucm070305.pdf (accessed February 15, 2011).
5. Ibid.

6

Formulated drugs 2

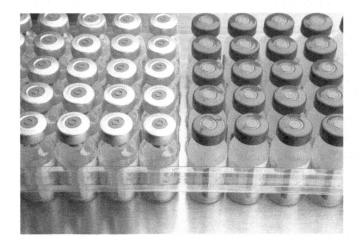

Learning objective

In this chapter there is a discussion of a couple of advanced routes of administration. The parenteral route of administration and the pulmonary route of administration seem simple but are very delicate, and very good current good manufacturing practice (cGMP), quality control (QC), and quality assurance (QA) are required. Parenteral routes require the dosage forms to be sterile; aerosol dosage forms do not need to be sterile unless in aqueous-based inhalers. This chapter will show how water for injection (WFI) is made and kept sterile during storage. Other subjects covered in this chapter are lyophilization, an important technology for biotechnology based drugs; aerosol dosage forms; and metered dose inhalers (MDIs).

Published by Woodhead Publishing Limited

Key concept terms

Aerosol: suspension of colloidal solid particles in air; a dosage form for the pulmonary route of administration

Biologic: therapeutic or prophylactic product made from a living system

Biopharmaceutical: biologic

cGMP: current good manufacturing practice, e.g. to avoid any contaminations and other unusual environmental conditions

DPI: dry powder inhaler

First-pass metabolism: a drug absorbed through the GIT has to pass through the liver, where a certain amount of the drug is metabolized

Freeze drying: at low temperature icy water is removed by being converted directly to vapor

GIT: gastrointestinal tract

GMP: good manufacturing practice

IM route: intramuscular route

IV route: intravenous route

Lyophilized: freeze dried

MDI: metered dose inhaler

Ocular: through the eye

Otic: through the ear

Parenteral route: when a drug enters the body directly through the blood stream (rather than the GIT)

pMDI: pressurized metered dose inhaler

Potable water: drinkable water

Pulmonary route: when a drug is absorbed through the lungs after being inhaled nasally or orally

Pyrogen: bacterial endotoxin

QA: quality assurance

QC: quality control

Rapid onset: quick absorption of drug to obtain therapeutic blood concentration

SC route: subcutaneous route

Sterile: free from microorganisms

WFI: water for injection, free from microorganisms and endotoxins

Published by Woodhead Publishing Limited

6.1 Dosage forms according to route of administration

Route of administration refers to the method of getting drugs into the body. Dosage forms depend on the route of administration and vice versa. There are a number of routes of administration (Figure 6.1).

When determining the route of administration of a drug these are the factors to consider:

- Does the patient need local action or systemic action?
- Is it an emergency? Is rapid onset of action needed?
- What is the site of therapeutic action?
- How easy is it to administer the drug?
- What is the patient's condition and age?
- What are the characteristics of available drugs' dosage forms (biologics are only available in injectable form)?

6.2 The parenteral route of administration

The word parenteral comes from the Greek where 'para' means outside and 'enteron' means intestine, so the parenteral route of a drug involves a drug entering the body (blood stream) not via the intestine but directly. Alternative terms are injection, infusion, and shots. The parenteral route has advantages:

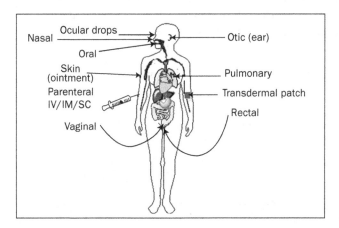

Figure 6.1 Routes of administration of drugs

Published by Woodhead Publishing Limited

- as it brings rapid onset of action
- as it bypasses 'first-pass' metabolism
- as it is the preferred route in emergencies
- as it allows the blood level concentration of the drug to be easily maintained
- during surgery, when the use of infusion saline or anesthesia is a common practice

and disadvantages:

- as needles are painful for some people, especially children
- if there are any serious side effects, the drug must be washed from the blood stream
- as there are some discomforts or complications from injection or infusion
- as self-medication is not possible; professional or hospital settings are required for the use of some parenteral medications.

There are different types of sub-route of administration in parenteral dosage forms (Figure 6.2):

- *the intravenous (IV) route* – needle is directly inserted into the vein and medication directly mixed with the blood stream; certain drugs, such as antibiotics, anesthesia, or life saving drugs, are given intravenously in emergencies, and nutritional fluid and electrolytic fluids are given through infusion for a longer time
- *the intramuscular (IM) route* – needle is inserted into muscles, usually a shoulder or buttock; used for administering antibiotics, vitamins, and iron
- *the subcutaneous (SC) route* – needle is inserted under the skin into the subcutaneous layer; used for giving insulin, adrenaline, heparin, and vaccines

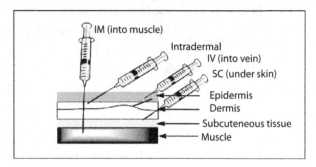

Figure 6.2 Sub-routes of parenteral dosage forms

Published by Woodhead Publishing Limited

- *intradermal (ID) route* – needle is inserted right below the epidermis; used for local anesthesia and immunization shots, and some diagnostic tests such as for TB.

Other sub-routes of parenteral dosage forms include intra-arterial, intrathecal, and intraperitoneal routes.

6.2.1 The production process of parenteral dosage forms

It is simple to manufacture parenteral dosage forms, but not easy to keep them in their required state:

- free of microorganisms (sterile)
- free of pyrogen
- free of particles (clear).

Figure 6.3 illustrates the dress code required in the manufacture of these dosage forms. See Section 8.4 for more information about GMP in sterile production manufacturing.

6.2.2 Water for injection

Water for injection is water used to dilute or dissolve drugs for parenteral administration. This water is sterile and free of pyrogen and dust particles, as are parenteral drugs. According to the US Pharmacopoeia (USP), there are several different types of water, including:

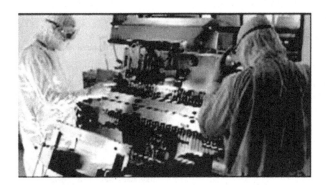

Figure 6.3 Parenteral production (filling section) in an aseptic area

Source: Square Pharmaceuticals Ltd

Published by Woodhead Publishing Limited

- potable water (drinkable water)
- purified water (microbial count < 10,000 cfu/100ml, pathogen free, and endotoxin not specified)
- WFI (microbial count < 10 cfu/ml, pathogen free, and endotoxin < 0.25)
- sterile WFI (free of microorganisms and endotoxin < 0.25).

The British Pharmacopoeia (BP) states that WFI must be a sterile preparation.

Sterilization of WFI can be achieved using ion exchange filtration followed by distillation, reverse osmosis, or both. The use of reverse osmosis to prepare WFI is acceptable to the USP but not the BP. A combination of double pass reverse osmosis/electrodeionization systems with built-in, pump-less, closed loop recirculation makes high quality WFI. Figure 6.4 illustrates the process for making WFI.

6.2.3 Lyophilization or freeze drying of biologics

Lyophilization, or freeze drying, is a process for manufacturing parenteral dosage forms. Biologics are available in the parenteral form, and

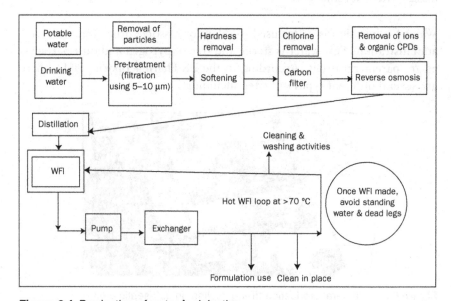

Figure 6.4 Production of water for injection

lyophilization is the best-suited technique to make dry powder vial forms of biologics. According to the US FDA:

> Lyophilization or freeze drying is a process in which water is removed from a product after it is frozen and placed under a vacuum, allowing the ice to change directly from solid to vapor without passing through a liquid phase.[1]

The key process is sublimation, by which liquid is converted to solid.
  The process includes the following steps:

- The active biopharmaceutical ingredient, excipients, and WFI are mixed in a tank to make a solution.
- The solution is sterilized by being filtered through a 0.22 micron filter.
- The sterile solution thus formed is used to fill individual sterile container (vial) with a stopper partially fixed.
- The filled vials are placed in a freeze dryer and frozen by lowering the temperature.
- The frozen solvent (water) is removed by converting ice to water vapor without passing through liquid water, done under strong vacuum.
- Once the medicine inside the vial is dried, the vials are fully stoppered.

Figure 6.5 illustrates the lypholization or freeze drying process.

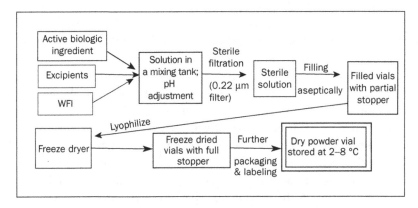

Figure 6.5 The lyophilization or freeze drying process

Published by Woodhead Publishing Limited

There are many biologics (biotechnology products), and many pharmaceutical parenteral products, especially antibiotics, such as some semi-synthetic penicillins, cephalosporins, and some salts of erythromycin, doxycycline, and chloramphenicol, are produced using this freeze drying technology. Table 6.1 lists some examples of marketed biologics made in this way.

Table 6.1 Marketed biologics made through freeze drying technology

Generic	Indication	Company
Advate	Hemophilia	Baxter
Avonex	Multiple sclerosis	Biogen Idec
Betaferon	Multiple sclerosis	Berlex, Bayer and Merck
Enbrel	Arthritis	Amgen
Herceptin	Breast cancer	Genentech
Remicade	Arthritis, Crohn's	J&J

6.3   The pulmonary route of administration

The pulmonary route of administration is the name for the route used when drugs are administered directly to the lungs through the mouth or nose. The commonly used preparation of drugs for this route of administration is aerosol, and this technique is also called an aerosol drug delivery system.

The pulmonary route of administration is not new. Thousands of years ago Indians used to smoke *Atropa belladonna* leaves to suppress coughing, and the smoking of tobacco, cigarettes, marijuana, and hashish (psychotropic drugs or hallucinogens) has been well documented throughout history. Pharmaceutical scientists used this smoking technique to deliver drugs to the blood stream via the lungs as they recognized that this technique is fast; the drug is systemically absorbed quickly, bypassing first-pass metabolism. It is convenient to use, non-invasive and has few side effects.

Engineers are critical for the successful use of parenteral dosage forms because the delivery vehicle device (e.g. syringes) is very important. There are different delivery platforms to introduce drugs to the lungs; the most common one is a pressurized metered-dose inhaler (pMDI or MDI). Others include pMDIs with spacers (especially for children), dry-powder inhalers (DPIs) and nebulizers, and breath actuated inhalers. Figure 6.6 shows an MDI, and its schematic drawing. In the pressurized MDI, an inert propellant in the form of liquefied gas is used to force out the micronized drug particles.

Published by Woodhead Publishing Limited

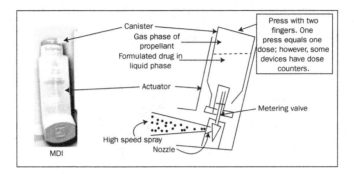

Figure 6.6 A metered-dose inhaler and its mechanism of action

Source: Square Pharmaceuticals Ltd

The most common and widely used propellant in the past was chlorofluorocarbon (CFC), but it has not been used since the mid-1990s because of its ozone depleting reaction at the stratospheric level in the atmosphere. Hydrofluroalkane types of compounds are now used as propellants.

The MDI formulations include:

- a propellant (liquefied gas, hydrofluoroalkanes)
- a micronized active pharmaceutical ingredient (API) (sizes are 0.001–100μm)
- surfactants or dispersing agents (e.g. oleic acid to stabilize suspension formulation; the micronized API is suspended or kept as a solution in the liquefied propellant)
- co-solvents (sometimes volatile solvents are used as a formulation aid; e.g. ethanol)
- a flavoring agent (e.g. menthol).

When the canister is pushed down by the finger (hand–mouth–breathing coordination is very important when using pMDI), the formulated drug comes out through the actuator nozzle in a high-speed spray. Almost instantaneously, the drug substance passes through the trachea and bronchioles to alveoli (Figure 6.7). The liquefied gas vaporizes, leaving the deposit of drugs around the alveolis, where the absorption into the blood stream takes place.

Aerosol dosage forms are mainly used for the treatment of respiratory diseases with local effects, such as asthma. However, the drugs administered through this pulmonary route easily undergo systemic circulation, so this

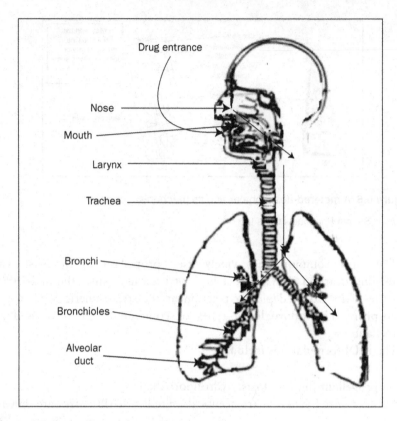

Figure 6.7 Aerosols and the respiratory system

route is being used increasingly to treat non-respiratory diseases, such as diabetes and analgesics, and genetic diseases (Table 6.2).

The technology of the pulmonary route of administration is gradually advancing. There was an aerosol form of insulin on the market, but it was withdrawn for lack of market demand. A development in aerosol inhalation allows very rapid systemic absorption, even within a few minutes. The process known as the 'Staccato system' is the rapid vaporization of a drug as it passes through the pulmonary route.

6.3.1 Production of metered dose inhalers

There are two important aspects of the production of MDIs. One is the valve–actuator assembly house – where the drug container is placed.

Table 6.2 Marketed metered-dose inhaler drugs

API generic name	Brand name	Amount of drug per actuation	Company
Albuterol sulfate	Ventolin	90 µg	GSK
Beclomethasone dipropionate	Qvar	40 or 80 µg	Teva
Fluticasone propionate	Flovent	44, 110, or 220 µg	GSK
Fluticasone propionate and salmeterol xinafoate	Advair	45, 115, or 230/21 µg	GSK
Ipratropium bromide	Atrovent	17 µg	Boehringer Ingelheim
Ipratropium bromide and albuterol sulfate	Combivent	18/90 µg	Boehringer Ingelheim
Levalbuterol tartrate	Xopenex	45 µg	Sunovion Pharmaceuticals

Usually other companies manufacture and supply valve–actuator assembly houses. The second is the formulation part – where a homogenous mixture of APIs and excipients (usually called a concentrate), other than propellant, is made and put into the container (canister). Then the propellant is fed into the canister and sealed. The filling of propellant in the right proportion is important and there are two methods for this, the cold filling method and the pressure filling method.

6.3.1.1 The cold filling method

In the cold filling process, the concentrate, propellant, and drug container are chilled below 0 °C. The valve and actuator assembly are then fixed on the drug container and the container is filled with the chilled propellant.

6.3.1.2 The pressure filling method

This method is carried out at room temperature, and the propellant is forced under pressure into the container through the valve orifice. The trapped air has to be forced out of the container.

Practice questions

1. Name five important routes for the administration of drugs.
2. Under what circumstances are injectables the preferred route of the administration of drugs? Why is IV a faster acting route than the IM or SC routes?
3. What are the criteria of parenteral products? What types of products are produced by the lyophilization method?
4. Solid drug powders are used in the pulmonary route of administration, but the absorption of the drug takes place very fast. Explain why.
5. The aerosol drug delivery system is based on high technology. Discuss this unique delivery technology.

Note

1. US Food and Drug Adminstration, 'Lyophilization of parenterals: guide to inspections of lyophilization of parenterals', April 2009, www.fda.gov/ICECI/Inspections/InspectionGuides/ucm074909.htm (accessed February 15, 2011).

7

The stability of medicines

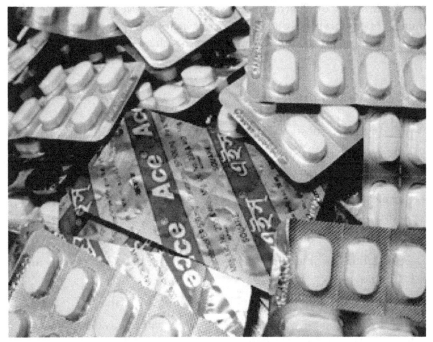

Source: Square Pharmaceuticals Ltd

Learning objective

All medicines have certain life-times. The appropriate term for this life-time is 'shelf-life' or expiration date, which is when aging medicines deteriorate. Whether made chemically or biologically, medicines deteriorate because of environmental factors and dosage form-related degradations. The stability of medicines is thus an important aspect for consumers and the pharmaceutical industry. This chapter begins by discussing different categories of stability (physical, chemical, microbiological, therapeutical, toxicological, and genotoxic), using specific marketed medicines to exemplify them. The following stability related issues are addressed:

- how to store medicines at home
- how to stabilize the dosage forms
- how instability can be studied before marketing medicines
- the chemistry of kinetics and its application in medicines
- packaging.

The International Conference on Harmonization of Technical Requirements for Registration of Pharmaceuticals for Human Use (ICH) is one of a number of organizations and regulatory agencies that set stability guidelines, and its stability protocol is introduced in this chapter.

Key concept terms

Anti-oxidant: a substance that prevents oxidation

API: active pharmaceutical ingredient

cGMP: current good manufacturing practice

Chemical stability: when there is no degradation as a result of chemical reaction

Decarboxylation: loss of CO_2 from carboxylic acid functional group

Degradation: break down of medicines, which can lead to toxicity and loss of potency

Expiration date: last date on which medicines are usable

Genotoxic stability: when there is no DNA damage leading to cancer from medicine or its metabolite

Half-life: the time required for a drug to undergo degradation by 50%

Hydrolysis: breakdown of molecule by water

ICH: International Conference on Harmonization of Technical Requirements for Registration of Pharmaceuticals for Human Use

Microbiological stability: when there is no microbial growth in a drug

Oxidation: change of molecule because of influence of oxygen

Published by Woodhead Publishing Limited

Photo-oxidation: light induced oxidation

Physical stability: when there is no change in physical appearance in a drug

Preservative: something that helps to prevent the growth of a microorganism

Racemization: change of configuration of the molecule

Shelf-life: period of storage

Stability kinetics: studies on the rate of degradation of medicines

Stability: when a medicine retains its integrity and quality within specified limits during its shelf-life

Therapeutical stability: when there is no change in therapeutic action of a drug as a result of disintegration or dissolution

Toxicological stability: when there is no development of toxic impurity in a drug

7.1 Stability – an essential criterion of medicines

The US Pharmacopoeia (USP) defines the stability of medicines as:

> the extent to which a product retains, within specified limits, and throughout its period of storage and use, i.e., its shelf life, the same properties and characteristics that it possessed at the time of manufacture.[1]

There is a mandatory expiration date on all manufactured medicines and until this date the medicines should retain their integrity and quality in all respects. In general, there are six categories of stability recognized in the pharmaceutical sciences:

- physical
- chemical
- microbiological
- therapeutic
- toxicological
- genotoxic.

Throughout the shelf-life of medicines, there should be no change in physical appearance, palatability, dissolution and suspendability (physical stability); no loss of leveled potency beyond specified limits (chemical stability); no microbial growth or loss of sterility (microbial stability); no change in therapeutic effects (therapeutic stability); no toxicity (toxicological stability); and no genotoxicity from the medicine or its metabolite (genotoxic stability). The types of stability are shown in Figure 7.1.

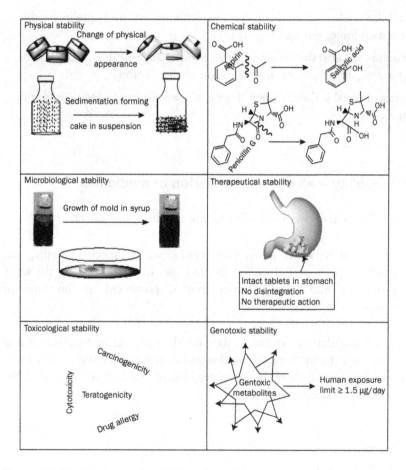

Figure 7.1 Various types of stabilities of medicines

Published by Woodhead Publishing Limited

7.1.1   Physical stability

The physical stability of drugs is the ability of drugs to retain physical characteristics including drug content uniformity, pharmaceutical elegance (color, odor, and so on), dissolution, and palatability. This stability is more prominent in liquid dosage forms. Liquid solutions can lose flavor and color or can form precipitate. Similar situations can occur in parenteral solutions too. The suspension liquid dosage form has different stability problems, including cake formation and the growth of crystals. The solid dosage form, such as tablets and capsules, can have instability problems: in tablets, there could be changes in disintegration, dissolution, hardness, friability, and appearance. Capsules may have appearance and dissolution problems. These are some examples of physical instability:

- aspirin tablet color becomes pink in storage
- adrenaline color becomes red on exposure to air
- calcium gluconate (solution for injection) precipitate and crystallization
- ranitidine tablets melt in humid environments.

7.1.2   Chemical stability

The chemical instability of drugs may cause reduced efficacy, formation of toxic degradation products, or physical instability. The most common chemical reactions involved in the degradation of drugs include hydrolysis, oxidation, photolysis, racemization, and decarboxylation. These reactions and rates of degradation are affected by the presence of metals, moisture, air, light, heat, and pH of solutions.

7.1.2.1   Hydrolysis

Drugs susceptible to hydrolysis are mostly the derivatives of carboxylic acid, such as lactam, ester, amide, lactone, and carbamates. Some examples of hydrolytic instability of medicines are shown in Figure 7.2.

The drug substance or active pharmaceutical ingredient (API) sensitive to water cannot be formulated in liquid aqueous form, but a dry powder form is made and reconstituted with pure water to form what is known as dry syrup.

Published by Woodhead Publishing Limited

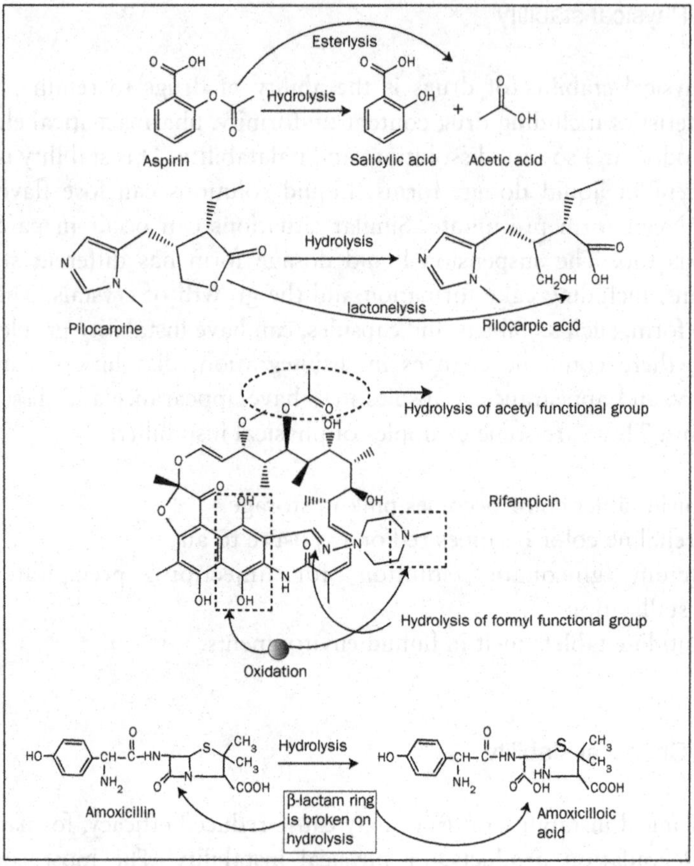

Figure 7.2 Examples of medicines susceptible to hydrolysis

7.1.2.2 Oxidation

The structures in the drug molecule likely to undergo oxidation are phenolic derivatives, such as catecholamine, aldehydes, conjugated dienes, and so on. Figure 7.3 shows the oxidative degradation of methyldopa.

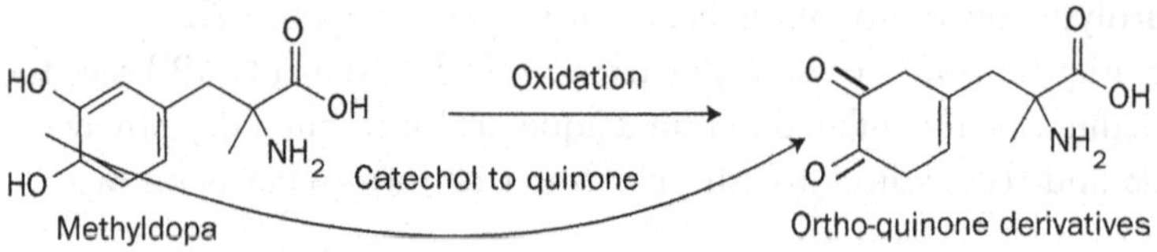

Figure 7.3 The oxidative degradation of methyldopa

Published by Woodhead Publishing Limited

7.1.2.3 Photo-degradation

Light, especially UV light, can induce degradation in medicines. Photo-oxidation or photolysis of medicines, such as nifedipine, riboflavin, chlorpromazine, ergosterol, ciprofloxacin, and vitamin K, is common. Light-protected packaging, such as strips, opaque blisters, amber bottles, or opaque plastic containers, can override this stability concern. Figure 7.4 gives some examples.

7.1.2.4 Racemization

For chiral drugs, racemization is a problem, especially when the other enantiomer is inactive or toxic. Figure 7.5 illustrates the racemization of oxazepam.

7.1.2.5 Decarboxylation

Some drug molecules containing a carboxylic functional group can lose carbon dioxide when heated to a relatively high temperature. An example of this is 4-aminosalicylic acid produce 2-aminophenol after decarboxylation (Figure 7.6).

7.1.2.6 Epimerization and dehydration

Epimerization is a process in stereochemistry in which there is a change in the configuration of only one chiral center. As a result, a diastereomer is

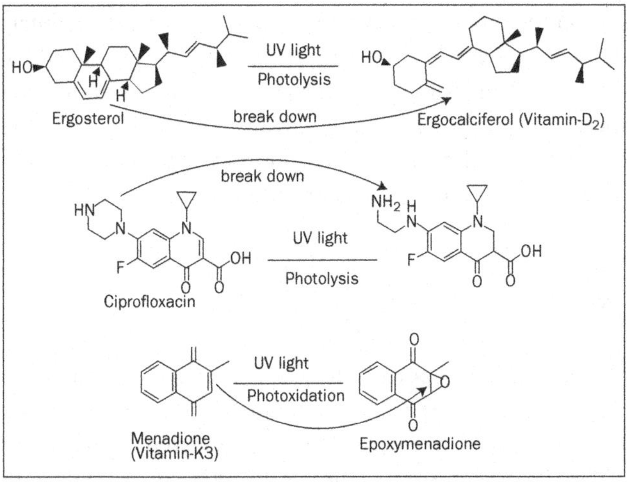

Figure 7.4 Photo-degradation of three drug substances

Published by Woodhead Publishing Limited

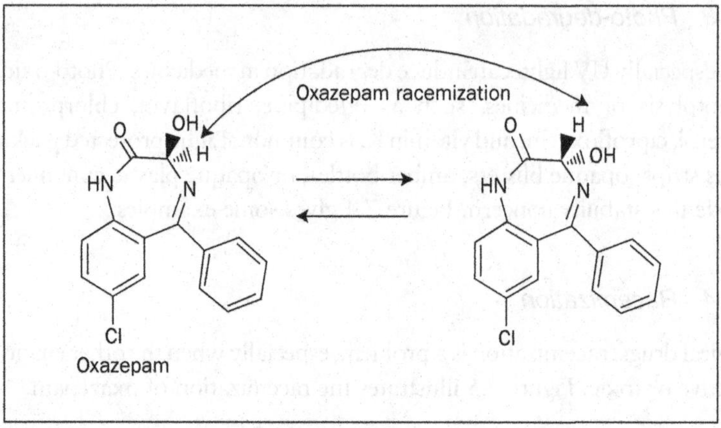

Figure 7.5 The racemization of oxazepam

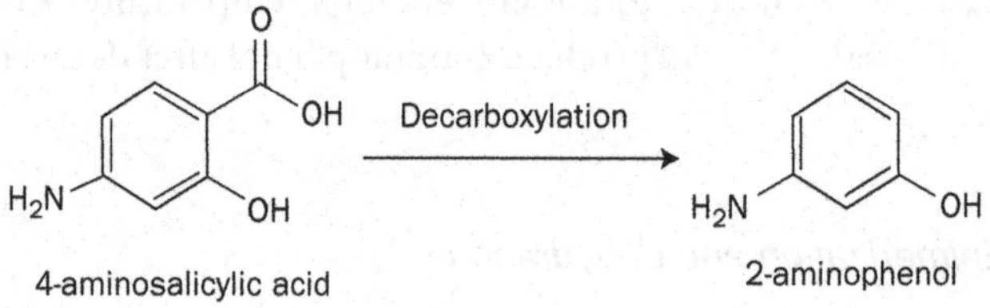

Figure 7.6 The decarboxylation of 4-aminosalicylic acid

formed. The classical example of this in medicine is tetracycline. In acidic conditions around pH 4, tetracycline readily undergoes epimerization at position 4, and an inactive 4-epitetracycline is produced, which on dehydration forms 4-epianhydrotetracyline, a highly toxic product. This toxic compound can also be formed from acid catalyzed (at lower pH) dehydration of tetracycline via anhydrotetracycline. Figure 7.7 shows the process of epimerization and dehydration.

7.1.3 Microbiological stability

A medicine has microbiological stability if it has no microbial growth during its life-time. The formulations or medicines containing water are at risk of contamination from microorganisms. Current good manufacturing practice (cGMP) has an important role in preventing microbial contamination as antimicrobial agents or preservatives are added to the formulation to

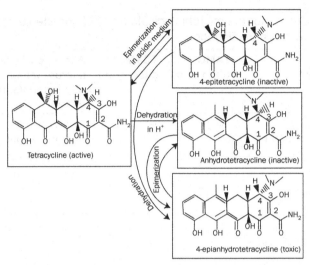

Figure 7.7 The epimerization and dehydration of tetracycline

prevent the growth of microorganisms. Possible sources of microbial growth, other than water and air, include some pharmaceutical raw materials, such as starch, gum, antacid ingredients, personnel, packaging, and so on. Microbiological control is essential (Figure 7.8).

Sterile medicines are free from all microorganisms. In non-sterile dosage forms there is an acceptable limit of non-pathogens, but there should be no pathogens. Table 7.1 lists the microbiological quality criteria of non-sterile medicines by route of administration.

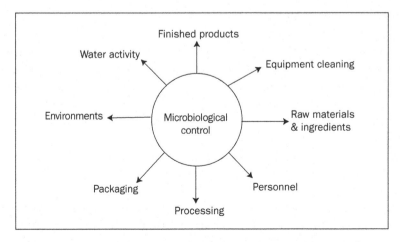

Figure 7.8 The microbiological control required in all pharmaceutical operations

Published by Woodhead Publishing Limited

Table 7.1 Criteria for the microbiological quality of non-sterile dosage forms by route of administration

Route of administration	TAMC* cfu/g or ml	TCYMC** cfu/g or ml	Absence of specific microorganism requirements in 1 g or 1 ml
Non-aqueous preparation of oral use	10^3	10^2	Escherichia coli, Salmonella spp.
Aqueous preparation of oral use	10^2	10^1	Escherichia coli
Rectal products	10^3	10^2	–
Oromucosal use, gingival use, cuteneous use, nasal use, auricular use	10^2	10^1	Staphylococcus aureus, Pseudomona. aeruginosa
Vaginal use	10^2	10^1	S. aureus, P. aeruginosa, Candida albicans
Transdermal patches	10^2	10^1	S. aureus (1 patch), P. aeruginosa (1 patch)
Inhalents	10^2	10^1	S. aureus, P. aeruginosa, bile-tolerant gram-negative bacteria (1 g or 1 ml)

*TAMC = total aerobic microbial counts; **TCYMC = total combined yeasts/molds counts

7.1.4 Therapeutic stability

Therapeutic stability is the most important factor influencing the efficacy of medicines. It is the process by which non-expired medicine, after being taken (through any route of administration), should start functioning via absorption, distribution, metabolism, and elimination. There is thus an art in manufacturing medicines by which therapeutic functions remain unabated throughout their shelf-life.

If a drug does not function therapeutically there is a problem. For example, a patient was prescribed a painkiller to take twice a day. After taking it for almost a week, the pain intensified rather than improved. Finally, the patient underwent surgery, and all the intact tablets were found in the patient's stomach. This was clearly a formulation problem. The tablets did not disintegrate at all, so there was no dissolution, thus no action.

Published by Woodhead Publishing Limited

Disintegration followed by dissolution is the absolute minimum action required of drugs in tablet form. Depending on storage conditions, some medicines, such as nifedipine andcarbamazepine, can change from the amorphous to the crystalline phase, resulting in a change in dissolution. The validated (proven and documented) stability study plays an important role in determining a drug's performance until expiry.

7.1.5 Toxicological stability

Some drugs may produce toxic impurities when they degrade. Tetracycline, on dehydration, produces 4-epianhydrotetracycline, which is nephrotoxic. Figure 7.7 shows the epimerization and dehydration of tetracyclin.

7.1.6 Genotoxic stability

Genotoxic impurities (GTIs) are known to damage DNA and can cause cancer. Certain functional groups and organic structures can cause genotoxicity alerts. The synthesis of bulk drugs includes starting materials, intermediates, reagents, catalysts, and solvents, which ultimately produce the desired end-product along with by-products and impurities. Researchers now scrutinize possible GTIs before designing and planning bulk drug synthesis. If GTIs are unavoidable, the threshold level of toxicological concern must be below 1.5 μg/day. DNA damage can be caused by genotoxic organic structures in several mechanisms, such as strand breaks, cross-linking, or oxidative reaction (Figure 7.9).

Certain functional groups (Figure 7.10) in the drug molecule can lead to the formation of degradants and metabolites as genotoxic impurities.

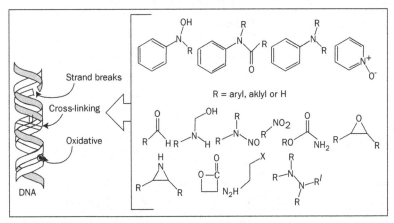

Figure 7.9 DNA damage caused by organic compound of genotoxic alerts

Published by Woodhead Publishing Limited

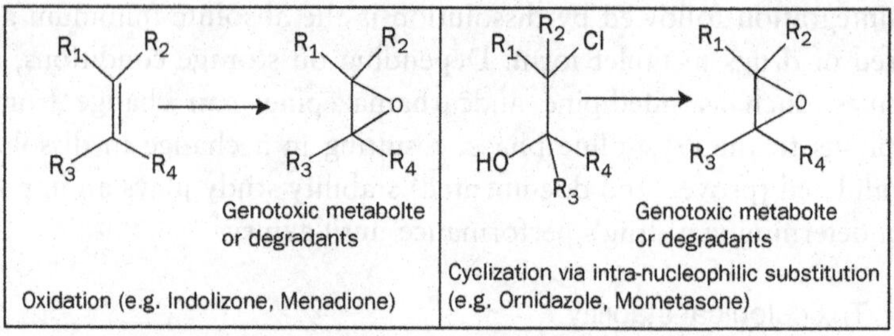

Figure 7.10 Formation of compounds genotoxic alerts from different functional groups

7.2 Label instructions and stability of medicines at home

It is now clear why there is a universal instruction on medicine labels to 'keep medicines in a cool, dry place away from heat and light sources', to encourage people to store medicines correctly so they do not undergo degradation. Table 7.2 lists the USP's definitions of different storage conditions and the temperatures required for them.

Everyone must be careful when storing medicines at home. Under no circumstances should medicines be stored in bathroom cabinets (because of the moisture in bathrooms, which makes most medicines unstable), on windowsills, or near heat sources. Before taking medicines, it is very important to read the drug facts label. Another common instruction is 'keep medicines out of reach of children' as accidental ingestion of medicines by children can lead to serious problems. The other important instructions are:

Table 7.2 USP definitions of different storage conditions

Storage condition	Definition
Freezer	Any temperature between −25 °C and −10 °C (−13 to 14 °F)
Cold	Any temperature not exceeding 8 °C (46.4 °F); a refrigerator's range of 2–8 °C (35.6–46.4 °F) is acceptable
Cool	Any temperature 8–15 °C (46.4–59 °F)
Room temperature	Temperature of working areas; the comfortable range of temperature is 20–25 °C (68–77 °F)
Warm	Any temperature 30–40 °C (86–104 °F)
Excessive heat	Any temperature above 40 °C (104 °F)
Dry place	Average relative humidity should not exceed 40%

- keep medicines in original containers
- do not use medicines after they are past the labeled expiration date.

7.3 Drug stability kinetics

Medicines change over time, depending on dosage forms. Medicines in liquid dosage form change faster than those in solid dosage form. Tablets are the most stable of the solid dosage forms. Drug kinetics can show the rate of degradation (how fast or slowly the medicine degrades) and allow scientists to predict the expiration date of medicines. The regulatory agency requires that the expiration date be placed on most prescription and over-the-counter medicines, but most medicines retain their potency beyond the manufacturer's expiration date. A US Food and Drug Administration (FDA) study conducted on a stockpile of medicines bought by the US military showed that most drugs were safe and effective years after expiration. Bayer's cipro (ciprofloxacin) tablets were found to be good more than nine and half years after the expiration date. Later, the US FDA approved two-year extensions to the expiration date of cipro tablets.

Drug stability kinetics provides information on three important aspects of drug stability:

- *half-life of the drug* – $t_{1/2}$, the time required for the drug to undergo degradation by 50%
- *shelf-life of the drug* – $t_{0.1}$, the time required for 10% deterioration, determined by extrapolation
- *expiration date* – ± 5% beyond the labeled potency is considered acceptable in most countries.

Basic mathematics can provide a straight-line equation or linear equation such as

$$y = mx + b$$

where y = dependent variable (ordinate), m = slope, x = independent variable (abscissa), and b = intercept. The graph of this equation is shown in Figure 7.11.

When the order of reaction (some power of concentration of reactants, such as 0, 1, 2, and so on) is known, then the rate of decomposition of drug can be written as

Published by Woodhead Publishing Limited

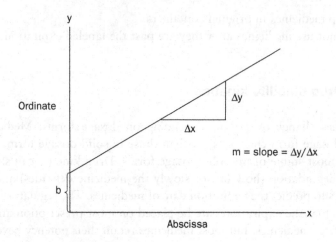

Figure 7.11 The equation y = mx + b in graph form

$$\text{Rate} = -dC/dt = kC^n$$

where C = concentration of reacting substance, t = time, k = proportionality constant, and n= order of reaction. In drug chemistry, the degradation of a drug is mostly a first order or pseudo first order reaction, and zero order is rare.

For a zero order reaction, n = 0 and rate becomes

$$-dC/dt = kC^0 = k$$

$$dC = -kdt \text{ on integration}$$

$$\int_C^C dC = -K\int_0^t dt \qquad \begin{array}{l} C_0 = \text{initial concentration} \\ C_t = \text{concentration at time, t} \end{array}$$

$$C_t = C_0 - kt$$

$$\text{At } t_{1/2} \ kt_{1/2} = C_0 - C_0/2 = 0.5C_0$$

See Figure 7.12.

$$t_{1/2} = 0.5C_0/k; \text{ same way, } t_{0.1} = 0.9C_0/k$$

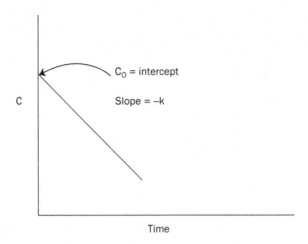

Figure 7.12 Concentration vs time for a zero order reaction

For a zero order reaction, the rate is independent of drug concentration. The oxidation of vitamin A in an oily solution is a zero order reaction.

In the case of first order reaction, the rate is directly proportional to concentration of drug:

Rate = $-dC/dt = kC^1 = kC$

or $dC/C = -kdt$ on integration,

$lnC_t - lnC_0 = -kt$

$log\ Ct = logCo - kt/2.303$

See Figure 7.13.

$t_{1/2} = ln\ 2/k = 0.693/k$

If we plot log C_t against t, a straight line will be obtained for a first order rate of degradation, for which the slope will be $-k/2.303$ and intercept at time 0 will be log C_0 (Figure 7.13).

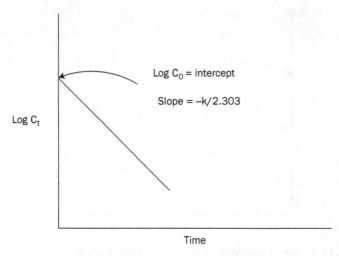

Log C_0 = intercept

Slope = $-k/2.303$

Log C_t

Time

Figure 7.13 Log concentration vs time for a first order reaction

A real-time stability study at different storage conditions takes time, but studies at higher temperatures can be used to predict the stability of a drug and an expiration date. The effect of temperature on the rate constant, k, is given by the famous Arrhenious equation: $k = Ae^{-Ea/RT}$ where A is constant, Ea = activation energy, R = the gas constant and T = temperature in °K. The equation can be rearranged substituting the logarithm, $\log k = \log A - Ea/2.303 R (1/T)$. On plotting 1/T against log k, a straight line will be obtained from which the energy of activation, Ea, can be calculated from slope = $-Ea/2.303R$. The intercept will be equal to log A. To find out the shelf-life within 10% of the deterioration of a drug, stability studies at different temperatures, such as 40–80 °C, are performed to plot 10% deterioration time against 1/T.

The graph in Figure 7.14 shows the degradation of a hypothetical drug at temperatures of 40–80 °C. Using the data from degradation studies at different temperatures, a graph can be plotted using a log of the number of weeks needed for 10% deterioration vs 1/T (Figure 7.15). By extrapolating the straight line to the room temperature or refrigeration temperature, the maximum storage time can be found.

This study shows the preliminary drug behavior at different temperatures and the shelf-life at room temperature and refrigeration temperature. This methodology is also useful in setting up a preliminary expiration date for a new drug or new formulation, but later it should be replaced by real-time stability studies.

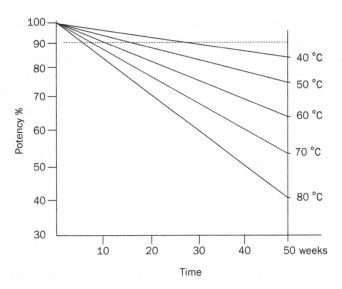

Figure 7.14 Potency vs time at different temperatures of a drug's degradation (%)

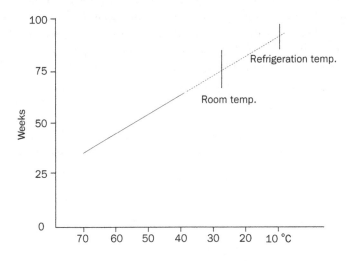

Figure 7.15 Determination of shelf-life at different temperatures by extrapolation

7.4 Stabilization of pharmaceutical products

All medicines are somewhat sensitive to environmental conditions and show some extent of instability, and some dosage forms (e.g. aqueous liquid dosage forms) are more unstable than others. Dosage forms are based on the properties of the drug substances. There is always an alternative dosage form. If the liquid dosage form is unstable for a longer period, a dry powder form is made and reconstituted to liquid form during dispensing time. Stability studies suggest that 10–15 days is fine for this form, if kept in the refrigerator. This is how some antibiotic 'dry syrup' dosage forms are marketed. For some stability problems, such as microbiological stability, it is hard to get the certain dosage form completely free of non-pathogenic microorganisms, but it is possible to suppress them from proliferating. Some measures taken to stabilize dosage forms are discussed below.

7.4.1   Use of antimicrobial preservatives

Antimicrobial preservatives are parts of excipients added to dosage forms to reduce initial microbial loads, suppress their proliferation, or prevent new microbial contamination in a preparation of multiple doses. The concentration of preservatives in the final dosage form cannot exceed the level that is toxic to humans. Figure 7.16 shows the structure of various antimicrobial preservatives used in pharmaceutical formulations.

Most of the compounds are organic aromatics in nature. They interfere with microbial growth and multiplication using different cellular level mechanisms. Phenols and chlorinated phenols work by denaturing cytoplasmic membranes. Benzoic acid and parabens work by denaturing protein.

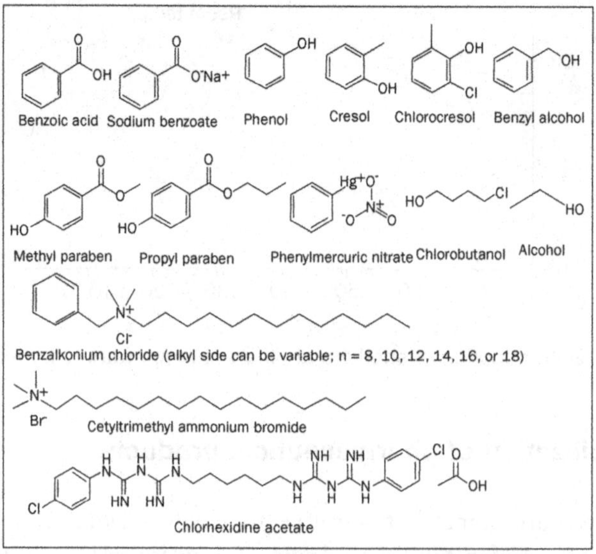

Figure 7.16 Structures of various antimicrobial preservatives

Published by Woodhead Publishing Limited

Alcohols and quaternary salts act by breaking down membranes. The selection of preservatives based on the properties, dosage forms, solubility, and amounts depend on accurate and precise consideration. Preservatives should be compatible with the other ingredients of the formulation. Table 7.3 lists the concentration limits of some antimicrobial preservatives.

7.4.2 Stabilization against oxidation

Containers can be filled up with nitrogen gas by replacing air (oxygen in air) after the drug products are inside. The oxidation reaction can also be slowed down by using anti-oxidants, several of which are commonly used in the formulation. These are mostly organic compounds such as butylated hydroxytoluene (BHT), butylated hydroxyanisole (BHA), tocopherols, ascorbic acid, and propyl gallate. They work as radical scavengers. Inorganic salts (e.g. sodium sulphite or sodium metabisulphite) are also much used in different formulations. Metals can catalyze oxidation reaction, so chelating agents such as EDTA can be used.

7.4.3 Stabilization against hydrolysis

Solid dosage forms, especially tablets and capsules, should be packaged in tightly closed containers, or moisture-proof blisters or strips. Tablets can be coated with waterproof coating materials. Nonaqueous solvents such as glycerol, propylene glycol, or alcohol can be used for liquid preparations. Sometimes certain pHs can stabilize drugs better in liquid formulations.

Table 7.3 The concentration limits of some preservatives

Antimicrobial preservative	Concentration limit (%)
Benzoic acid	0.1–0.2
Sodium bezoate	0.1–0.2
Phenol	0.1–0.5
Cresol	0.1–0.5
Alcohol	15–20
Chlorbutanol	0.5
Benzalkonium chloride	0.002–0.01
Combined mixture of methyl and propyl paraben	0.1–0.2

Published by Woodhead Publishing Limited

7.5   The International Conference on Harmonization

The International Conference on Harmonization of Technical Requirements for Registration of Pharmaceuticals for Human Use (ICH) is a joint initiative of regulators and research-based industry representatives of the European Union, Japan, and the USA that ensures safe, effective, and high quality medicines are developed and registered in the most efficient and cost-effective manner (Figure 7.17).

Table 7.4 shows the different storage conditions required for drugs in different climatic zones.

The ICH lists on its website (www.ich.org) its guidelines in the following stability-related areas:

- *Q1A(R2)* – Stability Testing of New Drug Substances and Products
- *Q1B* – Stability Testing: Photostability Testing of New Drug Substances and Products
- *Q1C* – Stability Testing for New Dosage Forms
- *Q1D* – Bracketing and Matrixing Design for Stability Testing of New Substances and Products
- *Q1E* – Evaluation of Stability Data
- *Q1F* – Stability Data Package for Registration Applications in Climatic Zones III and IV.

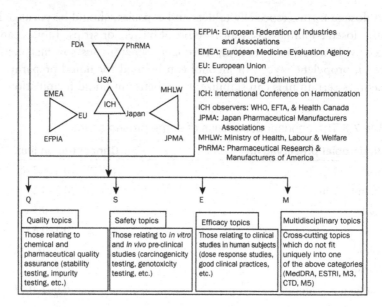

Figure 7.17 The ICH framework and functionality

Published by Woodhead Publishing Limited

Table 7.4 Storage conditions for drugs in different climatic zones

Climatic zone	Definition	Storage condition	Region or countries
I	Temperate climate (cool summer)	21 °C/45% RH	Great Britain, Northern Europe, Canada, Russia
II	Subtropical and Mediterranean climates (semi-arid)	25 °C/60% RH	The USA, Japan, southern Europe, Mediterranean region
III	Hot, dry climate (arid)	30 °C/35% RH	Iran, Iraq, Sudan
IVa	Hot, humid (tropical dry)	30 °C/65% RH	Brazil, Ghana, Nicaragua
IVb	Hot with higher humidity (tropical wet)	30 °C/75% RH	Bangladesh, Cambodia, Indonesia, Laos, Malaysia, Myanmar, Thailand, Philippines, Singapore, Vietnam

RH relative humidity

7.6   Product stability protocol

Stability protocols can be developed following the guidelines of the ICH listed in Table 7.5. The purpose of stability testing is to provide evidence for how the quality of a drug substance or drug product varies with time and under the influence of various environmental stress factors, such as temperature, humidity, and light. The testing protocol will help show the most stable formulation in the shortest possible period (within six months),

Table 7.5 The ICH stability protocol for drugs

Study	Storage condition	Minimum time covered by data at submission
Long term*	25 °C ± 2 °C/60% RH ± 5% RH or 30 °C ± 2 °C/65% RH ± 5% RH	12 months
Intermediate**	30 °C ± 2 °C/65% RH ± 5% RH	6 months
Accelerated	40 °C ± 2 °C/75% RH ± 5% RH	6 months

RH relative humidity

* It is up to the applicant to decide whether long-term stability studies are performed at 25 °C ± 2 °C/60% RH ± 5% RH or 30 °C ± 2 °C/65% RH ± 5% RH.

** If 30 °C ± 2 °C/65% RH ± 5% RH is the long-term condition, there is no intermediate condition.

Published by Woodhead Publishing Limited

so an accelerated condition should be used. The rationale behind this protocol is that storage at elevated temperatures should quickly show less stable formulations, ideally within six months.

In general, 'significant change' for a drug product is defined as:

- a 5% change in assay from its initial value, or failure to meet the acceptance criteria for potency when using biological or immunological procedures
- any degradation of the product exceeding its acceptance criterion
- failure to meet the acceptance criteria for appearance, physical attributes, and functionality tests (e.g. color, phase separation, resuspendibility, caking, hardness, dose delivery per actuation); some changes in physical attributes (e.g. softening of suppositories and melting of creams) may be expected under accelerated conditions and are appropriate for the dosage form
- failure to meet the acceptance criterion for pH
- failure to meet the acceptance criteria for dissolution for 12 dosage units.

Initial feasibility studies will produce data to give confidence in selecting a formulation for registration and other purposes. A minimum shelf-life of 12 months, preferably 24 months, is desirable for this purpose. The latter can be predicated if the product shows good stability for six months at 40 °C ± 2 °C and 75% ± 5% RH. At this stage, a potential primary container will be selected for evaluation. Routine or long-term stability studies should be carried out, preferably on three batches, as discussed below.

7.6.1   Routine or long-term stability studies

Routine stability studies are long-term studies carried out on already-marketed products, based on a time-to-time analysis of the retention sample. The objective is to generate real-time data on the marketed product in order to confirm and extend (if required) the shelf-life predicted from earlier studies.

Materials are subject to ambient or 'room temperature' conditions (30 °C ± 2 °C/65% RH ± 5% RH). The sample is preserved in retention storage whose temperature and humidity complies with ambient, uncontrolled room temperature and is monitored regularly.

The batches tested are produced on equipment and a scale that can be equated with normal production batches. They comply with the analytical specification and are stored in marketing packs. The study protocol is similar to that shown in Table 7.6.

Based on the dosage forms, test parameters are determined. Table 7.7 presents some common dosage forms and their test parameters.

Table 7.8 presents typical data from an accelerated stability study of a 500 mg tablet.

Table 7.6 Study protocol for long-term stability of marketed products

Storage condition	Time (months)						
	0	6	12	18	24	30	36
Ambient condition	*				*		*
	✓	✓	✓	✓	✓	✓	✓

* Microbial test as appropriate

✓ Examine for physical or chemical test

Table 7.7 Common dosage forms and their stability test parameters

Dosage form	Test parameters	Comment
Tablet	Appearance, color and odor disintegration, dissolution test assay, and degradation analysis	Assay: two approaches may be used, which are equally acceptable: ● Use of a stability indicating assay, suitably validated to show that degradation products are separated or do not interfere. HPLC or GLC is the most likely technique. ● Use of a non-specific assay, supported by a test to show the absence of degradation products. UV assay is a typical example, with a TLC screen (suitably validated and shown to separate degradation products, with a known limit of detection) as a supporting test.
Capsule	Appearance, color and odor, disintegration and dissolution test	Assay (see notes under tablets) and impurities
Emulsion	Appearance, color and odor, microscopic examination pH, viscosity, and assay	● The stability protocol should also include a short cyclic storage study, e.g. 4–40 °C at daily intervals for 1–2 weeks.

Table 7.7 Common dosage forms and their stability test parameter (Cont'd)

Dosage form	Test parameters	Comment
		• If the product is preserved, there should also be an assay for preservative content. A challenge test should be conducted initially, after one year and at the end of the proposed shelf-life.
Oral solution and suspension	Appearance, color, odor and clarity, redispersability, and microscopical examination (suspensions) pH and assay	• Samples at 25 °C should also be stored inverted in order to detect any reaction with the closure system. • Preservative assay if preservative is present in the formulation. • Challenge test initially, after one year and at the end of shelf-life.
Metered dose inhalation-aerosol	Appearance of product in can and inside of can; assay per actuation, dispersion spray pattern, weight per actuation, detection of degradation products in residue in can after evaporation of propellants	• A separate test of ten numbered aerosols to monitor loss in weight due to leakage of propellant at 25 °C should be carried out in parallel to the main study. • Initial test should include (as part of manufacturing specification) absence of pathogens and total microbial count.
Topical products (cream or ointment)	Appearance (esp. through length of tubes) pH, consistency assay sterility or microbial count (if appropriate) preservative (if present)	Samples should be taken from the top, middle, and bottom of container (separately examined) and the area around a tube crimp examined carefully.
Eye drops and Nasal sprays	Appearance, pH, viscosity (if appropriate) assay, preservative (if present) sterility or microbial challenge test (0, 1 year and end of shelf-life)	
Small volume parenteral	Appearance (including particulates) pH, assay, preservative (if present)	Samples should also be stored inverted at 25 °C, for products with rubber closures, and examination made for reactions with closure (e.g. extractives)

Published by Woodhead Publishing Limited

Table 7.7 Common dosage forms and their stability test parameter (Cont'd)

Dosage form	Test parameters	Comment
Large volume parenteral	Appearance (including particulates) pH, assay, preservative (if appropriate) sterility (0, 1 year, and end of shelf-life)	Also store samples at 25 °C inverted and examine for reactions with closures.

Table 7.8 A typical accelerated stability study of a blistered tablet

1. Name of product	Product X 500 tablet
2. Description of container	4 tablets in a blister having aluminum film on one side and PVC film on other side.
3. a) Batch no.	PD10E41
b) Mfg date	May 2010
c) Date tested	May 3, 2010; August 8, 2010; and November 6, 2010
4. Test parameters	a) Appearance b) Hardness c) Disintegration time d) Potency

Storage time	Storage condition		Product specification	Result		
	Temperature	Relative humidity		Initial	After 3 months	After 6 months
Up to 6 months and 3 months interval	40 °C ± 2 °C	75% ± 5%	Appearance: a creamish oval caplet shaped tablet embossed logo on one side and breakline on other sides	Complies	Complies	Complies
			Hardness: not less than 7 kg	9.6 kg	9 kg	8.9 kg
			Disintegration time: not more than 30 minutes at 37 °C	9 min. & 45 sec	9 min. & 50 sec	8 min.
			Potency: content of secnidazole/ tablet: 450– 550 mg	500.15 mg	500.02 mg	498.99 mg

Tested by: _____   Checked by: _____

Approved by: _____

Published by Woodhead Publishing Limited

7.7 Packaging and stability of medicines

Medicines can become unusable because of packaging-related degradation even though everything else, from API to dosage formulation, may work perfectly. Thus the packaging of medicines is very important, and packaging stability should be evaluated before medicines are used. Medicines inside packaging should be protected from moisture, air, light, and temperature. The most common containers and closures for medicines are glass, plastic, rubber, and metal, as illustrated in Figure 7.18.

Tablets and capsules are packaged in blisters or strips, made of plastic or aluminum foil, or plastic containers. Injectables are usually packaged in glass vials with rubber septums or glass ampoules. Oral liquid dosage forms are packed in glass bottles or plastic containers. Figure 7.19 lists the characteristics that packaging materials should and should not have.

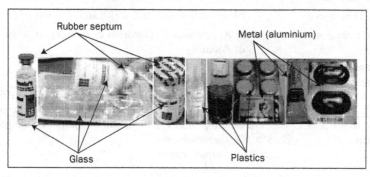

Figure 7.18 Packaging of some dosage forms

Source: Square Pharmaceuticals Ltd

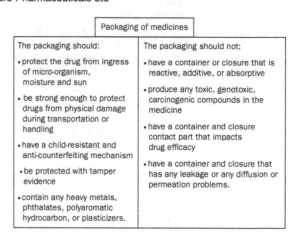

Packaging of medicines	
The packaging should:	The packaging should not:
• protect the drug from ingress of micro-organism, moisture and sun • be strong enough to protect drugs from physical damage during transportation or handling • have a child-resistant and anti-counterfeiting mechanism • be protected with tamper evidence • contain any heavy metals, phthalates, polyaromatic hydrocarbon, or plasticizers.	• have a container or closure that is reactive, additive, or absorptive • produce any toxic, genotoxic, carcinogenic compounds in the medicine • have a container and closure contact part that impacts drug efficacy • have a container and closure that has any leakage or any diffusion or permeation problems.

Figure 7.19 Characteristics of medicine packaging

Published by Woodhead Publishing Limited

Glass is the most commonly used packaging material, as it is resistant to physical and chemical changes. The selection of glass is important because the alkalinity of glass surfaces may change the pH of drugs; borosilicate glass is the best, though amber-colored glass is used for photosensitive drugs. A buffer can be used to prevent any interaction between ions from the drugs and glass. The USP classifies glass bottles into four types:

- *type I glass* – made of borosilicate, the least reactive glass, used for all applications including ampoules of water for injection; can be used without any surface treatment
- *type II glass* – made of de-alkalized soda lime glass, which has a higher percentage of sodium hydroxide and calcium hydroxide; good for products with pHs below 7
- *type III glass* – made of soda lime glass and suitable for liquid formulations insensitive to alkali
- *type NP soda lime glass* – for non-parenteral products, usually used for tablets and capsules.

There is a wide variety of plastics, which all incur potential problems. There could be two-way migrations of drugs through plastics, moisture, and oxygen from the environment to the drugs (Figure 7.20).

There is also a possibility of leaching of plastic ingredients into drugs or absorption of medicinal materials by the plastics, which will contaminate the medicines. The plastic manufacturers are aware of these concerns and

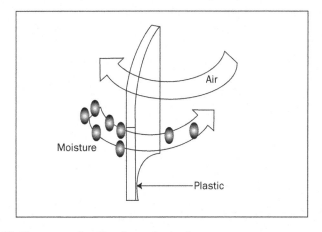

Figure 7.20 Two-way migration through plastics

Published by Woodhead Publishing Limited

produce lacquered plastics for pharmaceutical use, but the pharmaceutical industry should carry out stability testing on the leaching of plastics.

Metals, especially aluminum tubes, are used for packing medication such as ointment, creams, and pastes. Interaction between medicines and aluminum can occur, so polymer-coated aluminum tubes are used to avoid this. Rubbers are used inside stoppers and as septums in injection vials and come in direct contact with the medicines. Interaction and leaching of rubber into the drugs is also possible. Pretreatment with water and steam can improve the leaching problem, and teflon coatings can be used to avoid direct interaction with the drug.

For solid dosage forms, especially tablets and capsules, packaging is very important for acceptability in the market. In the USA bottles are preferred; in Europe and most other countries blister packs are more common. The pharmaceutical industry in the USA uses clear blisters, peel-push, and tear notch blister packs with secondary child resistant packs; in the EU, opaque and push-through blisters are used. For the blister packaging of tablets or capsules various plastic and aluminum packaging materials act as moisture barriers for stability. Figure 7.21 illustrates the relationship between the moisture barrier performance of a drug and its cost.

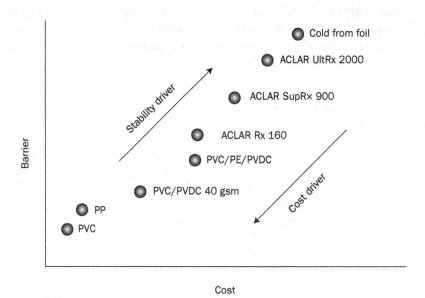

Figure 7.21 Pharmaceutical blister packaging: moisture barrier versus cost

Source: Elder and Mills[2]

Published by Woodhead Publishing Limited

Practice questions

1. Drug molecules are synthesized through bond formation and similarly the bonding of a drug molecule can be broken on aging. What environmental factors are responsible for breaking down the bonding of drug molecules?
2. Degradation of some drug molecules can lead to a toxic fragmented molecule or in some cases the breakdown product is non-toxic, which can lead to loss of potency of medicine. Give examples of drug molecules showing both situations.
3. How can you determine the rate of degradation of medicine? How can you determine the expiry date of a drug? Is there any role for the ICH on these stability studies? Discuss.
4. Discuss the influence of heat or temperature and humidity on the stability of medicines.
5. Discuss the role of different types of packaging in the stability of medicines.

Notes

1. US Pharmacopeia, 'Stability considerations in dispensing practice', USP29/NF24, p. 3029.
2. See Dave Elder and Simon Mills, 'Packaging', workshop held in Cape Town, South Africa, April 2007, http://apps.who.int/prequal/trainingresources/pq_pres/TrainingZA-April07/Packaging.ppt (accessed February 15, 2011). Aclar® film is a polychlorotrifluoroethylene material developed by Honeywell.

8

Quality assurance in medicines

$$QA_{medicine} = \int_{Start}^{Patient} df\,(GMP+QC)$$

Learning objective

The objective and function of the pharmaceutical industry is to produce (and discover, for some industries) and market safe, high-quality, and efficacious medicines. Many organizations have formulated guidelines for producing quality medicines, including the US Food and Drug Administration (FDA), the Medicines and Healthcare Products Regulatory Agency (MHRA), the European Medicine Evaluation Agency (EMEA), the International Conference on Harmonization of Technical Requirements for Registration of Pharmaceuticals for Human Use (ICH), the World Health Organization (WHO), the Pharmaceutical Inspection Co-operation Scheme (PIC/S), and the International Organization for Standard (ISO). These criteria are met through quality management systems that ensure quality assurance (QA), current good manufacturing practice (cGMP), and quality control (QC). This chapter will introduce these systems and GMP regulations by exploring different aspects of the production and quality of medicines.

Key concept terms

API: active pharmaceutical ingredient

Aseptic filtration: heat sensitive injectables sterilized by filtration through a 0.22-micron size filter

cGMP: current good manufacturing practice

Cross contamination: when products mix, especially penicillin and non-penicillin

EMEA: European Medicines Evaluation Agency

FDA: Food and Drug Administration

GMP: good manufacturing practice

ICH: International Conference on Harmonization of Technical Requirements for Registration of Pharmaceuticals for Human Use

ISO: International Organization for Standardization

MHRA: Medicines and Healthcare Products Regulatory Agency

Paracetamol tragedy: when many children died after being given diethylene glycol in paracetamol syrup

PIC: Pharmaceutical Inspection Convention

PIC/S: Pharmaceutical Inspection Co-operation Scheme

QA: quality assurance

QbD: quality by design

QC: quality control

Sterile production: when strict enforcement of cGMPs is required

Terminal sterilization: when injectable products are sterilized at the end of a process

Thalidomide tragedy: teratogenic (malformation of fetus) effects observed after pregnant women took this medicine

Validation: documented records that the process works as expected

WHO: World Health Organization

8.1 The concept of quality assurance

The main purpose of manufacturing and marketing medicine in an environment using a quality assurance system is to make sure that the medicines reaching patients are safe, effective, and of the highest possible quality. The MHRA's Orange Guide defines quality assurance in the following way:

> Quality Assurance is a wide ranging concept which covers all matters which individually or collectively influence the quality of a product. It is the sum total of the organized arrangements made with the object of ensuring that medicinal products are of the quality required for their intended use.[1]

Thus the concept of QA is embedded in the life of a medicine, and that life ends when the medicine is consumed by a patient. GMP is required in the production and marketing of medicines to ensure consistency of products. QC is a criterion when medicines are tested for compliance. Thus QA in medicines is a function of GMP and QC, which begins when medicines are manufactured and continues until they are consumed by patients. Figure 8.1 illustrates the integral relationship between QA, GMP, and QC in the manufacturing and marketing of medicines.

Regulatory agencies, such as the US FDA, the EMEA, the MHRA, the WHO, the ICH, the Pharmaceutical and Medicinal Devices Agency (PMDA), and the Central Drugs Standard Control Organization (CDSCO),

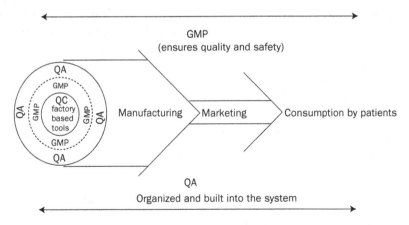

Figure 8.1 QA, GMP, and QC in the manufacturing and marketing of medicines

have GMP guidelines of their own. Overall, they are similar, but cGMP regulations evolve, so there are some differences from country to country.

In the last two decades there have been several incidents around the world in which people died because of negligence in maintaining proper GMP or following QA and QC systems. Dozens of children died in Nigeria, India, Bangladesh, and Haiti because they consumed a toxic syrupy medication. When syrup is manufactured for medication, glycerin and/or propylene glycol are used to dissolve the active pharmaceutical ingredient (API), but when the syrups responsible for these deaths were manufactured there was clearly inadequate QA, GMP, and QC. There are two possible reasons for this. First, the pharmaceutical companies responsible for manufacturing and marketing the syrupy medication, using toxic diethylene glycol, manufactured and marketed the toxic syrup intentionally (possibly because it was cheap to produce), knowing that diethylene glycol was a toxic solvent not to be used in any pharmaceutical preparation of syrup. These companies should not have been given a license. Second, the companies used diethylene glycol unintentionally, in which case they were in violation of GMP, QA, and QC because there was:

- no validated vendor as a supplier of excipients
- unauthorized buying of excipients from a local vendor
- no testing on the excipients before use
- no validated methods
- no quality control
- no record keeping
- no recall system.

Medicines exist for the wellbeing of sick people, which is why the system of manufacturing and marketing medicines is gradually improving. Figure 8.2 illustrates the attributes of quality medicines.

Quality by design (QbD) is used to ensure and maintain the quality of medicines. The ICH defines QbD as a 'systematic approach to development that begins with predefined objectives and emphasizes product and process understanding and process control, based on sound science and quality risk management'.[2] To implement QbD, design experiments are required, as well as process analytical technology and risk assessment (Figure 8.3).

8.2 Evolution of quality testing and safety of medicine

Testing the efficacy, safety, and regulation compliance of a medicine has developed gradually over many years. Sometimes the occurrence of

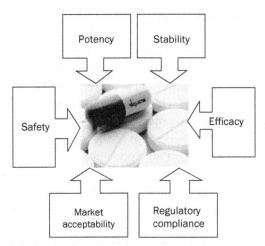

Figure 8.2 Attributes of quality medicines

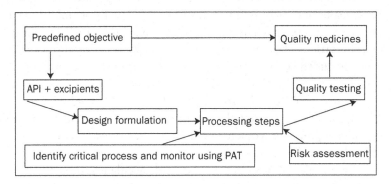

Figure 8.3 Elements involved in quality by design

accidents caused by negligence leads to stricter control over the use and sale of medicines. Historical records show that the testing of medicines for their efficacy goes back to 120 BC when the King of Pontus, Mithridates, made a 'Mithridatium', a mixture of 41 ingredients ranging from natural herbs to venoms such as panacea. He tested each ingredient individually on condemned criminals. He also prepared another mixture of 55 ingredients, called 'Galene'. Mithridatium and Galene found their way into apothecary shops in England.

In England, in 1540, the Royal College of Physicians formulated a Drug and Stuffs Act to control drugs by inspecting apothecaries' wares. Animal testing began in 1847 as a result of human fatalities from the use of chloroform as an anesthesia.

In the USA, testing, quality, and safety evolved in the following way:

- *1848, importation of drugs* – The Drug Importation Act prohibited the importation of unsafe or adulterated drugs to the USA.
- *1902, biological therapeutics* – There were regular inspections of the production facilities of vaccines, sera, antitoxins, and similar products and testing for purity and potency.
- *1906, labeling of drugs* – Because of the availability of adulterated or misbranded drugs in interstate commerce, the US FDA implemented the Pure Food and Drug Act for labeling selected dangerous or addicting substances, such as alcohol, morphine, heroin, and cocaine. The US Pharmacopoeia (USP) and National Formulary became the official standards for drugs.
- *1938, drug safety* – In 1937 elixir sulfanilamide, manufactured and marketed by S. E. Massengill Company, killed 107 people, including many children. The company used a poisonous antifreeze solvent, diethylene glycol. It became a priority to prove that a medicine was safe before marketing it.
- *1951, prescriptions* – The US FDA recognized that a number of drugs or drug groups should be sold only with physician prescriptions. The drugs included sulfas, barbiturates, amphetamines, and thyroids. This was the beginning of prescription-only drugs.
- *1962, the thalidomide tragedy and stronger drug regulation* – Thalidomide was marketed in western Europe as a pill for morning sickness in pregnant women, and it dominated the market instantly, but the pills caused birth defects in thousands of babies. The drug was not marketed in the USA, but the thalidomide accident caused the US FDA to strengthen drug regulation. Since then, manufacturers have had to prove that their drugs were effective and safe before marketing them.
- *1962, drug amendment* – After several tragic events with food and medicines, the US Congress instructed the FDA to implement GMP in the production of medicines. The word 'current' was later added to GMP; cGMP includes technological advancements.

In the twenty-first century can QA, GMP, and QC prevent the sometimes serious side effects from drugs that are withdrawn from the market? These can occur even after a drug has been withdrawn from the market for ten or more years. Drugs are not customized to individuals and are marketed without investigating their long-term side effects. However, although drugs can have harmful side effects these have to be placed in the context of the benefits drugs provide – the benefit–risk ratio of drugs is important. Table 8.1 lists drugs withdrawn from the market since 1967 and the reason for their withdrawal.

Published by Woodhead Publishing Limited

Table 8.1 Drugs withdrawn from the market since 1967

Year	Drug	Reason for being withdrawn from market
1967	Phenytoin, anti-epileptic drug	Decalcification of bones
1982	Benoxaprofen, NSAID	Liver damage
1984	Fenclofenac, NSAID	Liver damage
1990	Pemoline, for attention deficit hyperactivity disorder	Liver damage
1998	Terfenadine, anti-histamine	Risk of cardiac arrhythmia
1998	Mibefradil, for hypertension	Serious heart arrhythmias
1999	Astemizole, anti-histamine	Serious cardiac arrhythmias
2000	Cisapride, for night-time heartburn	Serious cardiac arrhythmias
2000	Alosteron, for irritable bowel syndrome	Serious life-threatening gastrointestinal adverse effects
2000	Troglitazone, anti-diabetic and anti-inflammatory drug	Adverse liver effects
2001	Cerivastatin, cholesterol reducing drug	Kidney damage
2004	Rofecoxib, Cox-2 NSAID	Miocardial infarction
2005	Valdecoxib, Cox-2 NSAID	Serious cardiovascular problems
2010	Rosiglitazone, anti-diabetic drug	Increased risk of heart attack and death, so withdrawn from European market; the FDA has not found enough evidence for it to be withdrawn from the US market

8.3 Quality management systems

A quality management system is an integral part of a pharmaceutical company at the highest level of management, providing leadership in implementing QA, GMP, and QC. Top managers of pharmaceutical companies must direct and be closely involved in all quality activities. Unless they are sincere and believe in the core values inherent in the quality system, there will not be continuous improvement in the functionalities of manufacturing and marketing quality medicines. For example, if managers in the pharmaceutical industry want to market a rejected product or insist

Published by Woodhead Publishing Limited

that a factory manufactures a penicillin product in a facility with equipment used to produce other products, QA, GMP, and QC are useless.

There are plenty of examples of inexperienced and unqualified people being in top management and leadership roles in pharmaceutical companies in developing countries; these managers are unlikely to make quality decisions. There have been several fatalities in Nigeria, Haiti, India, and Bangladesh resulting from inadequate checking of paracetemol. All quality managers should understand the key issues of QA, GMP, and QC, illustrated in Figure 8.4.

Quality management systems evolved out of cGMPs. Until 1970 GMPs included only QC to ensure quality medicine, based mainly on laboratory testing. QA has been introduced since then and GMP is now embedded in it, to maintain quality until medicines are consumed by patients.

The world's top pharmaceutical industries have implemented quality management systems, the most important features of which are to implement quality by design (QbD), process analytical technology (PAT), and risk management and assessment (Figure 8.5). These system measures are not regulations set by the the US FDA or the EMEA – they are called the guidance of continuous improvement.

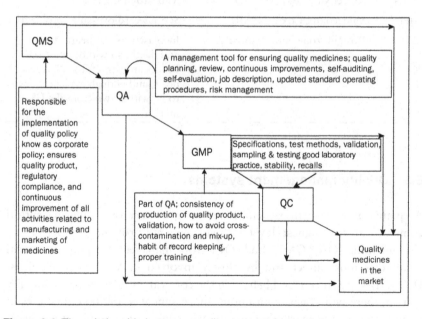

Figure 8.4 The relationship between quality systems for medicines

Published by Woodhead Publishing Limited

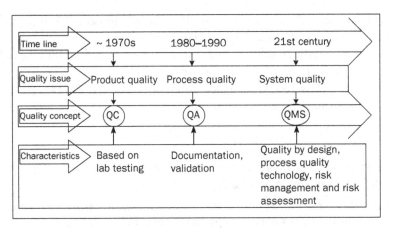

Figure 8.5 The evolution of GMPs at the US FDA

8.4 Good manufacturing practice in sterile production

Sterile means free of viable microorganisms, and sterile pharmaceutical products must in particular be free of:

- particulates
- microorganisms
- pyrogens.

Sterile pharmaceutical products are used for parenteral products, eye preparations, and wound dressings. The US FDA, the EMEA, the ICH, and the WHO specify that it is cGMP to produce sterile products in clean rooms, where workers and raw materials enter through air-lock systems. The Federal Standard 209 E describes a clean room as 'a room in which the concentration of airborne particles is controlled and which contains one or more clean zones'.[3] The clean room classification is based on particle limits at rest and in operation and microbiological limits in operation. The WHO's clean room classification is shown in Table 8.2.

The US FDA has a similar air classification with different category names and units based on a maximum number of particles in the air, listed in US Federal Standards 209E.[4] There are four grades:

Published by Woodhead Publishing Limited

- *grades A and B* – class 100 (particle count not to exceed 100 particles per cubic foot of a size 0.5µ and larger)
- *grade C* – class 10,000 (particle count not to exceed 10,000 particles per cubic foot of a size 0.5µ and larger)
- *grade D* – class 100,000 (particle count not to exceed 100,000 particles per cubic foot of a size 0.5µ and larger).

Table 8.2 WHO guidelines for an air classification system for the manufacture of sterile products

Grade	Maximum number of particles permitted per m^3 (at rest)		Maximum number of particles permitted per m^3 (at operation)		Maximum number of viable microorganisms per m^3
	0.5–5 µm	> 5 µm	0.5–5 µm	> 5 µm	
A	3,500	None	3,500	None	Less than 1
B	3,500	None	350,000	2,000	5
C	350,000	2,000	3,500,000	20,000	100
D	3,500,000	20,000	Not defined	Not defined	500

8.4.1 Clean room environments

Operations of sterile preparations include handling of raw materials, preparation of solution (suspension, powder, or ointment), filling of solution, and sterilization, and these operations should be performed in separate clean room facilities. The manufacturing operations are divided into two categories: terminally sterilized (preparation, filling, and sterilization) and aseptic preparation (some or all stages). In general, the Grade A room category is used for high-risk operations, such as filling and making aseptic connections; Grade B is used for the background environment of Grade A in aseptic preparation and filling; and Grade C and D clean rooms are used for less critical operations. Figure 8.6 shows the steps in preparing sterile parenteral solutions.

The Pharmaceutical Inspection Convention (PIC) is an international organization working for harmonized GMP standards and quality systems. The PIC Scheme (PIC/S) specifies that clean rooms facilities are required for terminally sterilized and aseptic preparations (Table 8.3).

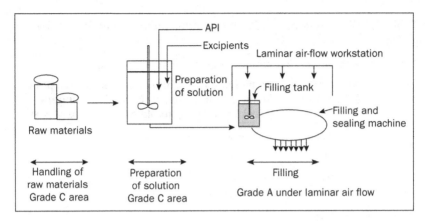

Figure 8.6 Sterile solution preparation with grade areas

Table 8.3 PIC/S guidelines on clean room grades and manufacturing operations by grade

Grade	Operations for terminally sterilized products
A	Filling of products, when unusually at risk
C	Preparation of solutions, when unusually at risk; filling of products
D	Preparation of solutions and components of subsequent filling

Grade	Operations for aseptic preparation
A/B	Aseptic preparation and filling with a Grade B background environment
C	Preparation of solutions to be filtered
D	Handling of components after washing

Table 8.4 lists PIC/S recommended limits of microbiological monitoring of cleaning areas during operations.

8.4.2 Sterilization methods

Sterile production takes place in clean room environments, but a clean room alone is not sufficient. The ultimate sterilization is performed by either aseptic filtration or by terminally sterilizing the drug. Worldwide, it

Published by Woodhead Publishing Limited

Table 8.4 PIC/S recommended limits of microbial contamination by grade

Grade	Recommended limits of microbial contamination[a]			
	Air sample (cfu/m³)	Settle plates (diam. 90 mm) (cfu/4 hours[b])	Contact plates (diam. 55 mm) (cfu/plate)	Glove print 5 fingers (cfu/glove)
A	<1	<1	<1	<1
B	10	5	5	5
C	100	50	25	–
D	200	100	50	–

[a] These are average values
[b] Individual settle plates may be exposed for less than 4 hours

is only acceptable worldwide for sterile drugs to be manufactured by aseptic processing when terminal sterilization processing is not feasible. Sterilization methods include:

- moist (steam) heat using autoclave
- dry heat
- ionizing radiation
- sterilizing gaseous agents (e.g. ethylene oxide)
- the filtration method (using 0.22 micron size).

The moist (steam) heat method is universally used for the terminal sterilization of pharmaceutical products, provided there is no degradation in the components of the medicines and packaging materials. Figure 8.7 illustrates commonly used sterilization methods in the pharmaceutical industry.

There is one more thing to consider when deciding whether a product is pyrogen free or pyrogens are within established limits. Pyrogen is the lipopolysaccharide endotoxin produced by gram negative microorganisms, and it is difficult to remove it once present in a product. The presence of pyrogen in an injectable product can induce fever, which is unacceptable. There are tests to detect pyrogen, but no easy method to destroy or remove it from medicines. Tests include:

- the limulus amebocyte lysate test; if this test is found incompatible with the product, the pyrogen test is conducted by injecting the product into rabbits and checking the increase in body temperature
- the turbidimetric method

Published by Woodhead Publishing Limited

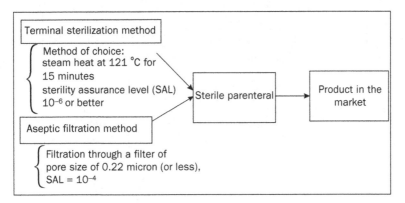

Figure 8.7 Commonly used sterilization methods in the pharmaceutical industry

- the colorimetric method
- the gel clot test
- the chromogenic assay method.

There are different sources of pyrogens, including water used as a solvent or in processing and raw materials or equipment used in manufacturing the medicines. It is thus very important to keep or use materials and resources free from endotoxins. If pyrogen is detected in water, the most common source of the endotoxin, it can be purified by distillation.

8.4.3 Clean room dress

Researchers have shown that every person emits 100,000 particles (particle size ≥ 0.5 µm) per minute while standing and sitting without moving, and 5,000,000 particles per minute when walking slowly at the rate of approximately 3.5 km/h. Humans are also a source of microorganisms. Microbes are dispersed from our skin cells every 24 hours.

Clean room air quality is maintained by wearing clean room clothing. Clean room dress can function as a barrier to the particles emitted by the human body and to the particles and fibers emitted by undergarments, and one piece of clean room dress can reduce the number of particles by 15 times. Different clean room categories require clothing of different qualities. The dress code for employees moving from an uncontrolled environment to a controlled environment in the pharmaceutical industry are shown in Figure 8.8.

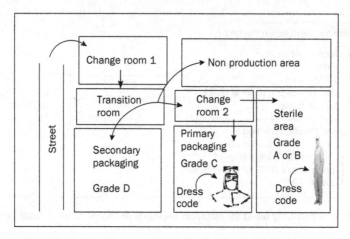

Figure 8.8 Change room dress code in the pharmaceutical industry

8.5 Validation

The US FDA defines the objective of validation as to 'establish documented evidence which provides a high degree of assurance that a specific process will consistently produce a product meeting its predetermined specifications and quality attributes'.[5] The equipment used in pharmaceutical manufacturing has an important role in maintaining medicine quality. Thus the validation considered a prerequisite for quality starts with installation qualification (IQ), followed by operation qualification (OQ), and then performance qualification (PQ) (Figure 8.9).

The first step of validation is to check that the installation and calibration of equipment meets the manufacturer's specifications. It includes checking wiring, utilities, preventative maintenance, safety features, spare lists and supplier documentation, drawings, and manuals. The critical parameters are evaluated in the OQ step, which includes process control parameters,

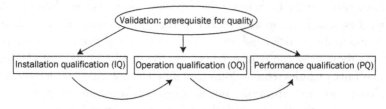

Figure 8.9 The relationship between validation qualifications

Published by Woodhead Publishing Limited

operating procedures, and change control. Finally manufacturing process performance is tested (PQ) and process repeatability is evaluated.

The pharmaceutical industry is built on three different technologies: utility, production, and quality control. Some systems and equipment from these technologies and their validations are shown in Table 8.5. Validation of technologies and processes helps reduce:

- rejection and reprocess
- testing
- process failure
- equipment failure
- overall cost.

The industry should have a validation team comprising staff in engineering, production, quality assurance, and quality control.

Table 8.5 Systems, equipment, and machinery for different technologies in the pharmaceutical industry with necessary validation

Technology	Systems, equipment, and machineries
Utilities	Air (heating, ventilating, and air conditioning), compressed air, vacuum system, boiler, potable water, water for injection
Production	Tablet compression machine, capsule filling machine, blister machine, liquid filling machine, fluid bed dryer, blender, lyophilizer, oven, autoclave etc.
Quality control	pH meter, incubator, centrifuge, dissolution tester, disintegrator, friability tester, freezer, refrigerator, HPLC, UV-VIS, FTIR, NIR, GC, GC-MS

8.6 Contamination control in formulation factory

The presence of anything undesirable in medicine is called contamination, and contamination of any kind in medicines is not acceptable. Contamination of pharmaceuticals from pathogens such as *Pseudomonas aeruginosa*, Salmonella, or *E. coli* is extremely harmful and health hazardous. Even the presence of non-pathogens makes medicines inconsumable. Non-pathogens in any dosage forms can produce bad odors, color changes, and texture

Published by Woodhead Publishing Limited

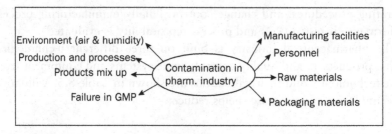

Figure 8.10 Origins of contamination in the pharmaceutical industry

changes, and they can destroy the elegance of dosage forms, especially liquid dosage forms. The contamination arises from product mix-ups, particularly penicillins with non-penicillin products, which is considered one of the worst health hazards in the pharmaceutical industry. Any dirt or dust particles or pieces of metals, glass, or even hairs can ruin certain dosage forms such as injectables. Potential sources of contamination are shown in Figure 8.10.

Contamination can be broadly categorized into:

- microbial contamination
- particle contamination
- chemical contamination.

According to cGMP, the production environment must have microbiological, cross contamination, and dust controls.

8.6.1   Microbiological control

In a manufacturing environment it is essential that the colony forming unit, a measure of viable bacterial or fungal numbers, is low. Identified sources of bacteria are:

- raw materials
- water
- equipment – tanks, containers, and other vessels
- manufacturing equipment – machines and filters
- facilities – walls, floors, ceiling, built-in furnishings, and work areas; these must be easy to clean and disinfect; there should be smooth, durable surfaces and no crevices or cracks

Published by Woodhead Publishing Limited

- air
- packaging materials
- personnel hygiene – humans are always critical factors in clean rooms; their skin, hair, clothing, and nasal passages harbor microbes that are continuously released into the environment, so there should be adequate facilities for changing clothes, sufficient facilities for washing hands, physical examination on employment, and periodic check-ups, depending on the degree of health of those involved.

Potential sources of microbial contamination and the actions to be taken to reduce the contamination are presented in Figure 8.11.

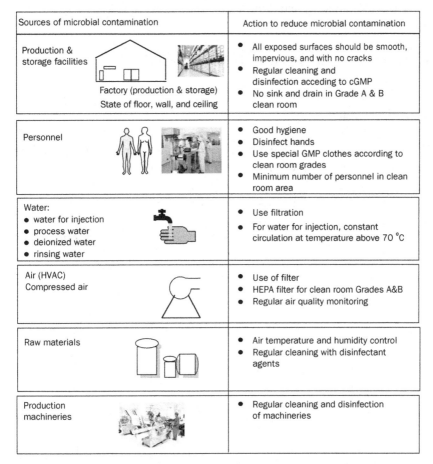

Sources of microbial contamination	Action to reduce microbial contamination
Production & storage facilities Factory (production & storage) State of floor, wall, and ceiling	• All exposed surfaces should be smooth, impervious, and with no cracks • Regular cleaning and disinfection acceding to cGMP • No sink and drain in Grade A & B clean room
Personnel	• Good hygiene • Disinfect hands • Use special GMP clothes according to clean room grades • Minimum number of personnel in clean room area
Water: • water for injection • process water • deionized water • rinsing water	• Use filtration • For water for injection, constant circulation at temperature above 70 °C
Air (HVAC) Compressed air	• Use of filter • HEPA filter for clean room Grades A&B • Regular air quality monitoring
Raw materials	• Air temperature and humidity control • Regular cleaning with disinfectant agents
Production machineries	• Regular cleaning and disinfection of machineries

Figure 8.11 Sources of microbial contamination and how they can be reduced

8.6.2 Cross contamination control

Cross contamination may occur through the mixing of dust particles from one product with another. Cross contamination caused by penicillin, cephalosporins, steroids, hormones, and anticancer drugs is harmful to patients and employees.

Apart from safety concerns, there can be financial losses for a company and damage to its image when there is cross contamination. Figure 8.12 illustrates how this can be minimized, for example using:

- a dedicated air handling system
- once-through air systems that do not recycle
- appropriately designed airlocks, pressure differentials
- air filtration
- dust control
- better housekeeping and validated cleanliness.

8.6.3 Dust control

Dust generation is a common phenomenon in the pharmaceutical industry, and needs to be controlled. This can be achieved using:

- pressure zones and air locking systems
- proper dust extraction processes
- an automation system and avoiding manual handling of products.

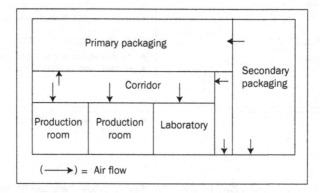

Figure 8.12 An air flow system to reduce cross contamination

Published by Woodhead Publishing Limited

8.7   Limits of good quality

All dosage forms of medicines are manufactured with a certain strength API, which is shown on the label. For example, paracetamol tablets are made with a strength of 500 mg; this is the amount of the API: each tablet contains 500 mg of paracetamol. It is very difficult to maintain a consistency of exactly 500 mg in each tablet when thousands of tablets are made in one batch. The regulatory authority or the pharmacopeia has specification limits for the tablets of 500 mg strength (± 5%). While manufacturing this tablet, the industry should set its own acceptable limits and work to make the product meet them (Figure 8.13).

A company wants value added activities in manufacturing, so its productivity must reflect the value of accountancy. In manufacturing, there could be other situations, such as those shown in Figure 8.14.

Both situations shown in Figure 8.14 are unacceptable. If the situation B remains within the upper specification limit, it will be acceptable to release for marketing, but this is not value added production. The manufacturing process thus has to be finalized at the beginning and validated with proper documents for at least three consecutive batches.

8.7.1   Analytical quality control

The API and excipients required for tablet manufacturing have to be analyzed and stored. The API should be analyzed for:

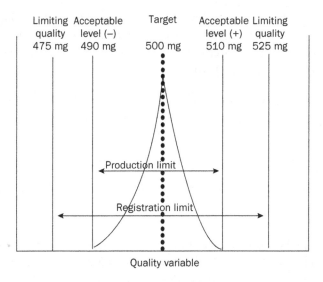

Figure 8.13 Quality variable: limits of good quality

Published by Woodhead Publishing Limited

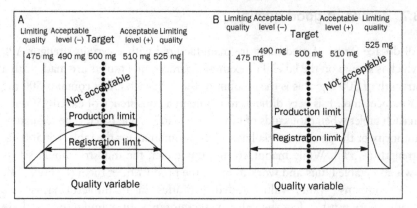

Figure 8.14 Quality variable: extended to lower and upper specification limits [A]; extended at upper specification limit [B]

- appearance
- purity
- impurities
- residual solvents
- heavy metals
- particle size
- bacterial endotoxins
- microbial limits.

The manufacturing process (direct compression, dry granulation, or wet granulation) and the critical steps involved in the process must be reviewed. The control of critical steps should be monitored according to the pharmacopeia's specifications for:

- loss on drying
- bulk density
- particle size
- blend uniformity
- weight variability
- hardness
- friability.

Finally the quality control department should evaluate the batch of tablets before giving approval. In the final analysis, the following characteristics should be checked using a validated methodology:

- appearance (visual)
- label claim analysis preferably using high-performance liquid chromatography
- degradants
- content uniformity
- disintegration
- dissolution
- hardness
- friability
- moisture
- residual solvents.

After successfully maintaining QA, GMPs, and QC, there should not be any problems in the marketed medicines. However, no system is 100% problem free. The following problems have been associated with recent drug recalls:

- sterile products found to be non-sterile
- sub-standard medicines (less potency than label claims)
- microbial contamination
- chemical contamination
- penicillin cross-contamination in another marketed product
- impurities or degradants found in higher amounts than the specific limits
- drug solubility problems
- foreign materials found in the product
- disintegration and dissolution problems.

Practice questions

1. Explain the relationship between quality management systems, quality assurance, quality control, and current good manufacturing practice regulations, and describe their objectives.
2. Discuss the role of validation in ensuring the quality and safety of medicines.
3. How are sterile products produced? Compare terminal sterilization and aseptic filtration.
4. How is cross contamination prevented in the pharmaceutical industry?
5. What is QbD? Briefly discuss this concept.
6. What was the thalidomide disaster?

Answers to some practice questions

6. When thousands of deformed babies were born because their pregnant mothers had taken the thalidomide sleeping pill. This was an example of a drug having a teratogenic effect, resulting in growth deficiency and/or mental retardation.

Notes

1. Medicines and Healthcare Products Regulatory Agency, *Rules and Guidance for Pharmaceutical Manufacturers and Distributors*, [the Orange Guide], London: Pharmaceutical Press, 2007.
2. FDA, 'Policies and procedures' in *Manual of Policies and Procedures*, 2011, www.fda.gov/downloads/AboutFDA/CentersOffices/CDER/ManualofPolicies Procedures/UCM242665.pdf (accessed December 5, 2010).
3. *Federal Standard 209E: Airborne Particulate Cleanliness Classes in Cleanrooms and Clean Zones*, 1992, www.lascoservices.com/Federal_Standard_209.pdf (accessed September 10, 2010).
4. The Engineering ToolBox, 'Clean rooms – Federal Standard 209', [n.d.], www.engineeringtoolbox.com/clean-rooms-d_932.html (accessed September 10, 2010).
5. Validation and Compliance Institute, 'What is validation?', 2010, www.vcillc.com/what_is.html (accessed July 5, 2010).

Published by Woodhead Publishing Limited

9

Pharmacological concepts and drugs

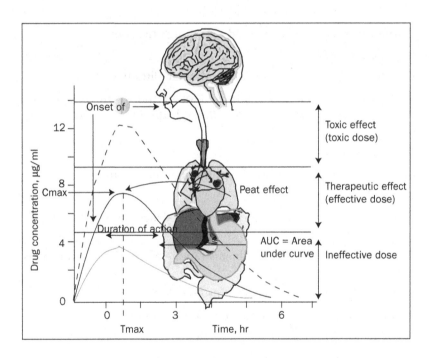

Learning objective

This chapter deals with pharmacology – how medicine works in the body. Once the body ingests a drug, the drug substances interact with the body's internal systems. The interactions lead to therapeutic effects, and sometimes side effects.

Key concept terms

Absorption: the diffusion of drugs through cell membrane

ADME: absorption, distribution, metabolism, excretion

API: active pharmaceutical ingredient

AUC: area under curve; quantitative estimation of drug concentration in the blood stream

Bid: twice a day

Bioavailability: drug availability in the blood stream

Bioequivalence: when there is a similar drug profile (pharmacokinetic) between brand name and generic drugs

Distribution: the spreading of a drug through the body

ED: effective dose

Excretion: the elimination of drugs or metabolites from the body

First-pass effect: the effect of a fraction of an orally administered drug being metabolized when it passes through the liver; it is considered wastage

GIT: gastrointestinal tract

Inhaler: aerosol breathed into lungs through the mouth

LD: lethal dose

Metabolism: the biotransformation of drugs into other forms (metabolites)

Parenteral: route of drug administration where GIT pathway is bypassed

Pharmacodynamics: interaction of drug with the organs of the body

Pharmacokinetics: rate of movement of drugs in the body

Pharmacology: the science of drug action and drug efficacy

Phase I reaction: a metabolic reaction that changes a drug by generating a new functional group for phase II reaction

Phase II reaction: conjugation reaction (joining together) of mostly phase I products

Qid: four times a day

Therapeutic effect: result of an effective dose

Tid: three times a day

9.1 Drug action

Drugs have different effects depending on the way in which they are taken (orally, intravenously, intramuscularly, subcutaneously, through inhalation, or topically). For example, if a patient has an infection in his or her leg, and the doctor has prescribed an orally administered antibiotic, it is not immediately clear how the antibiotic will work in the leg since the patient is taking the medicine orally. Antibiotics taken orally are first absorbed into the blood stream, then distributed all over the body through blood circulation. Then the drug starts working to fight the infection.

To find out how drugs work it is necessary to understand pharmacology, and more specifically the pharmacokinetics and pharmacodynamics of the drugs. Pharmacology is the science of drugs, their action, and efficacy in the body. It includes all the aspects of drug action, including absorption (A), distribution (D), metabolism (M), and excretion (E), also known as ADME; thus it covers the mechanism of drug action, drug interaction, and toxicity.

Pharmacokinetics is a specialized branch of pharmacology that explains the processes by which the body's organs handle drugs, especially the rate of movement of drugs in the body and the ultimate end of the drugs. Pharmacodynamics explains how drugs act or interact with different organs in the body. Figure 9.1 shows the relationship between pharmacokinetics and pharmacodynamics.

Once someone takes a drug it starts interacting with his or her body as it passes through the system, regardless of how it was administered. The most important action is absorption of the drug in the blood serum. The faster this absorption occurs, the faster the drug will act. For example, if the drug is taken orally, it has to pass through different organ systems and

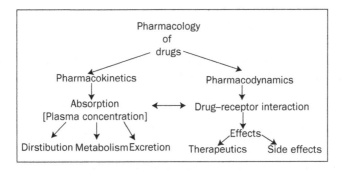

Figure 9.1 The relationship between pharmacokinetics and pharmacodynamics

undergo different steps of transformations before absorption. When a drug is administered parenterally (using an injection syringe), it enters the blood stream immediately and is distributed; this is called systemic circulation. The drug quickly reaches the target site to have a therapeutic effect, so the drug action happens more quickly. Figure 9.2 illustrates how drugs enter the body through oral and parenteral administration.

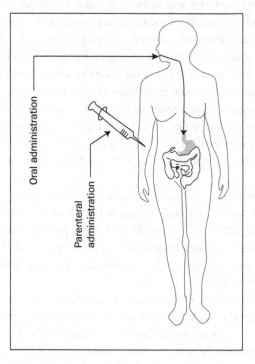

Figure 9.2 Oral and parenteral administration of drugs

9.2 Routes of drug administration

Drugs can be administered by many different routes (Figure 9.3), each of which has its own specificity and advantages.

9.2.1 The enteral route

The enteral route is the alimentary canal, digestive tract, or gastrointestinal tract (GIT). Drugs entering the system through this route are taken orally

Published by Woodhead Publishing Limited

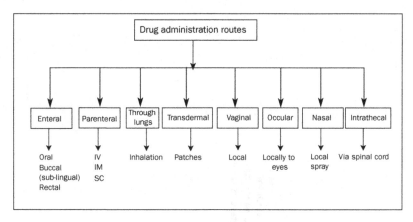

Figure 9.3 Drug administration routes

(through the mouth), sub-lingually (placed under the tongue), or rectally (inserted into the rectum). It takes time for drugs to be absorbed into the bloodstream when they enter the body through the enteral route. The oral route is the most widely used method of ingestion; it is convenient and inexpensive compared with other routes.

The absorption of drugs into the bloodstream from oral dosage forms depends on many factors, including:

- the dosage form, e.g. tablet, capsule, syrup, or suspension
- interaction with foods
- other drugs in the body
- gastrointestinal discomforts.

9.2.2 The parenteral route

The parenteral routes include intravenous (IV), intramuscular (IM), subcutaneous (SC), and intrathecal routes, all of which deliver drugs to the bloodstream more quickly than the enteral route (Figure 9.4). The most direct route to get drugs into the blood circulation system is to inject them intravenously. Drugs may be injected into the muscles of the upper arm, thigh, and buttock using the IM route. This is easier than IV injection because finding a vein can sometimes be difficult. For the SC route the needle is inserted right under the skin. Insulin injections are usually given subcutaneously. The intrathecal route is a specialized route for rapid action of anesthetic and analgesics drugs and is given in the spinal canal by needle injection.

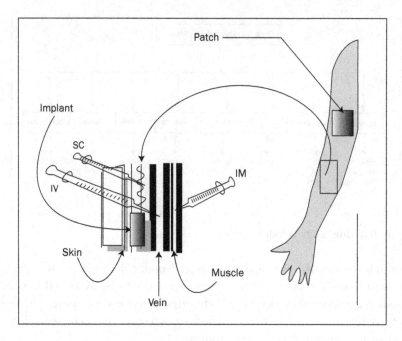

Figure 9.4 How parenteral drugs are administered

9.2.3 The inhalation route

Drugs administered using an aerosol can be breathed into the lungs through the mouth, which is known as inhalation (Figure 9.5). This is the best route of administration of drugs for asthma patients to achieve rapid drug action. Other routes, including vaginal, ocular, and nasal spray, are for localized use.

9.3 Mechanism of oral medication

Once oral medication is swallowed the drug passes to the stomach through the esophagus and small intestine where absorption takes place. It then moves to the liver and undergoes first-pass metabolism, and becomes active through biotransformation by liver enzymes. If the drug is extensively metabolized, higher doses are required for drug action. Drugs can be

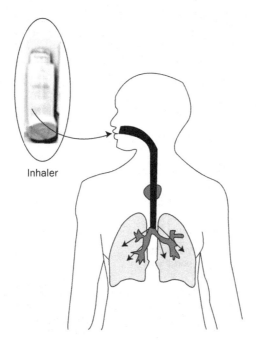

Inhaler

Figure 9.5 How drugs are inhaled

designed as prodrugs, which are inactive forms that are converted to active forms while passing through the liver.

After passing through the liver, the drug in the bloodstream is rapidly circulated throughout the body. Fat-soluble drugs pass through the blood brain barrier and affect the central nervous system. Water-soluble drugs such as penicillin do not cross the blood brain barrier. On recirculation, drugs from the bloodstream begin moving out of the bloodstream into tissues, which is how drugs taken orally can cure infections in the leg.

Figure 9.6 illustrates the movement of orally administered drugs in the body.

The ultimate end of drugs in the body occurs during excretion or elimination. Before elimination, the drugs or metabolites are converted to more water-soluble products so they can easily leave the body in urine via the kidneys. A fraction of the drug is also eliminated as it is. In some cases, small fractions of drugs are eliminated as sweat, saliva, or breast milk.

The mechanism of oral drug action consists of four steps:

- *absorption* – the diffusion of drugs through cell membranes
- *distribution* – spreading throughout the body

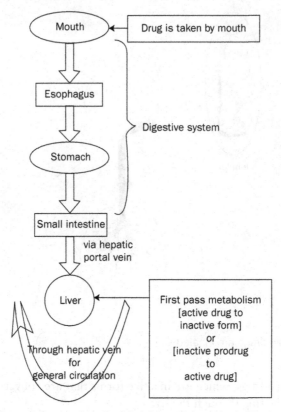

Figure 9.6 The movement of orally administered drugs in the body

- *metabolism* – the bioconversion of drugs into other forms (metabolites)
- *excretion* – the elimination of drugs or metabolites from the body.

This process is called ADME (Figure 9.7).

All dosage forms of the enteral route follow the same process of ADME. The parenteral drugs, especially the intravenous (IV) route, do not go through the first step of absorption because the drugs are introduced directly into the bloodstream. Orally administered drugs, in general, are absorbed through the membrane of the GIT and have to pass through the liver before reaching systemic circulation. While passing through the liver, drugs undergo metabolism by liver enzymes, the cytochrome P450 family, which is called first-pass metabolism (Figure 9.8). Unless the administered drugs are prodrugs, some fractions of the drugs become inactive because of

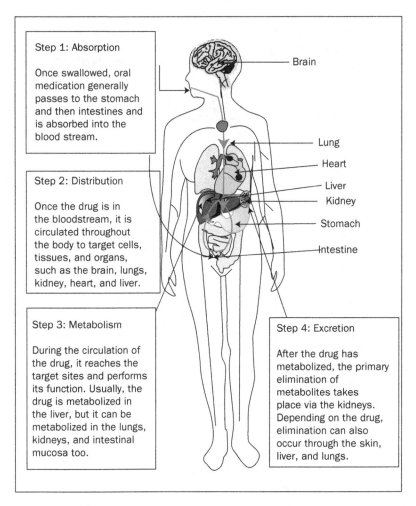

Step 1: Absorption

Once swallowed, oral medication generally passes to the stomach and then intestines and is absorbed into the blood stream.

Step 2: Distribution

Once the drug is in the bloodstream, it is circulated throughout the body to target cells, tissues, and organs, such as the brain, lungs, kidney, heart, and liver.

Step 3: Metabolism

During the circulation of the drug, it reaches the target sites and performs its function. Usually, the drug is metabolized in the liver, but it can be metabolized in the lungs, kidneys, and intestinal mucosa too.

Step 4: Excretion

After the drug has metabolized, the primary elimination of metabolites takes place via the kidneys. Depending on the drug, elimination can also occur through the skin, liver, and lungs.

Brain

Lung

Heart

Liver

Kidney

Stomach

Intestine

Figure 9.7 Absorption, distribution, metabolism, and excretion of oral medication

metabolism. This metabolism explains why oral dosage forms contain larger amounts of drugs than parenteral drugs. The drug's absorption rate depends on the concentration of the drug, the route of administration, and the solubility of the drug.

Once in the bloodstream, the drug starts circulating throughout the body, which is called systemic circulation. The drug's main purpose is to reach the site of action, but there is not always a free-flowing pathway. The distribution or circulation of drugs depends on blood flow, tissue

Published by Woodhead Publishing Limited

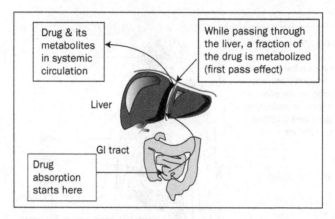

Figure 9.8 The first-pass effect or first-pass metabolism

permeability, the lipophilicity and hydrophilicity of the drugs, and, most importantly, the drug–plasma protein binding (Figure 9.9).

If the drug molecules bind with macromolecular plasma protein, they cannot penetrate the tissues to reach the target, instead they will stay in the blood plasma longer, which slows the time until elimination. This drug–protein binding is reversible, so the process can prolong action. The free drug molecules then pass through the cell membranes, which are made of a lipid bilayer with a hydrocarbon chain inward and a hydrophilic end outward. Thus the drug molecules' ability to penetrate cell membranes depends on the molecules' nature. Highly polar molecules cannot penetrate membranes, but highly non-polar molecules can be distributed widely in tissues and deposited in body fats.

After making the long journey that begins at the mouth, the drug molecules finally reach the site of the target and exert their therapeutic

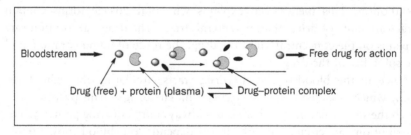

Figure 9.9 Drug–protein (plasma) binding

Published by Woodhead Publishing Limited

effects. After that, the body recognizes the drug molecules as xenobiotics (foreign substances) and wants to get rid of them by transforming them to more water-soluble products, a process known as metabolism. The drug molecules can be metabolized by enzymes anytime and anywhere in the body but are mainly metabolized in the liver. In this biotransformation, the drugs may be converted to less toxic or more toxic metabolites, which can exert different types of effects. The biotransformation is mainly of two types: phase I reactions and phase II reactions.

A phase I metabolic reaction changes the drug by generating a new functional group for a phase II reaction. The reactions include oxidation, reduction, hydroxylation, and hydrolysis. The phase I reactions are catalyzed by the enzymes (e.g. cytochrome P450 enzymes), which are available in subcellular systems, including cytoplasm, mitochondria, and endoplasmic reticulum (Figure 9.10).

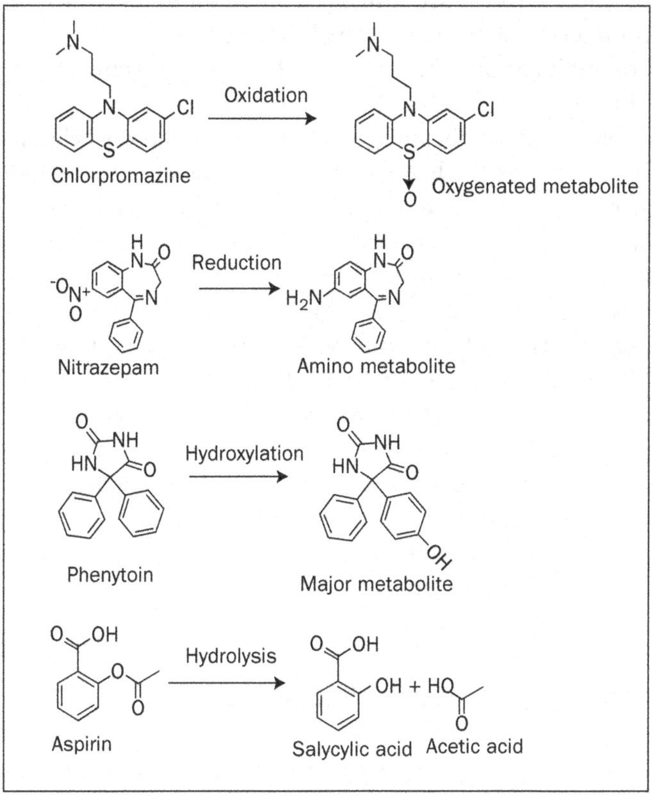

Figure 9.10 Examples of phase I metabolic reactions

Published by Woodhead Publishing Limited

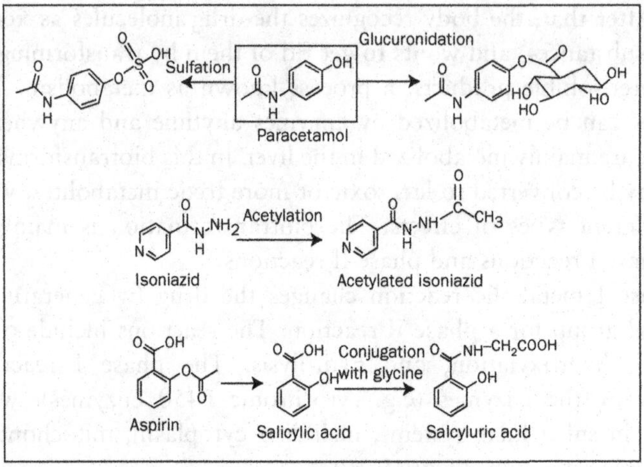

Figure 9.11 Examples of phase II metabolic reactions

Phase II metabolisms are usually conjugation reactions of mostly phase I products. The reactions include glucuronidation, acetylation, sulfation, or conjugation with amino acids, such as glycine or glutathione (Figure 9.11).

The ultimate end of the drug and its metabolites is elimination or removal from the body, which is carried out mostly by the kidneys via urine. Other pathways of excretion include the lungs, bile, sweat, saliva, feces, exhaled air, and breast milk. Hydrophilic or polar drugs have a shorter half-life and are eliminated rapidly compared with lipophilic drugs. In metabolism, lipophilic drugs are slowly converted to hydrophilic drugs and are excreted through the kidneys (Figure 9.12). Lipid-soluble drugs remain in the body for longer amounts of time.

After performing its function, the drug or its broken-down products (metabolites) should be eliminated from the body quickly, otherwise side effects can occur. The elimination of drugs depends on the structure and nature of drug molecules, especially their hydrophilicity or lipophilicity, acidity or basicity, and molecular weight. Drug-protein binding also regulates the elimination of drugs from the body.

9.4 Drug absorption, bioavailability, and activity

Drug absorption is the first step of action for all routes of drug administration except the parenteral route. When a tablet is taken it must undergo disintegration and dissolution within the gastrointestinal media.

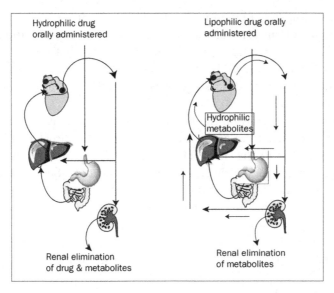

Figure 9.12 The elimination of hydrophilic and lipophilic drugs

Capsules undergo dissolution directly (the gelatin shell dissolves immediately when in contact with gastric fluid) (Figure 9.13). Suspension also needs to undergo dissolution in the GIT.

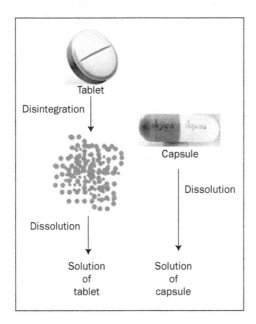

Figure 9.13 The disintegration and dissolution of a tablet and a capsule

Published by Woodhead Publishing Limited

Once the drug is a solution in the small intestine, it is absorbed into the bloodstream and quickly reaches a peak level of drug concentration. Then its level starts decreasing as the drug starts metabolizing and being eliminated from the body. The generalized profile of drug absorption and elimination after a single dose is shown in Figure 9.14 as drug concentration versus time (in hours).

Drug activity depends on the bioavailability of the drug. The available amount of the active form of the drug in general blood circulation is called the bioavailability of the drug. The extent of drug concentration in the bloodstream indicates the therapeutic level or effective dose of the drug. Drugs administered at a concentration below the correct level of dosage are less effective than those administered at the correct dose level, but a higher level concentration can have toxic side effects.

Drugs are usually taken in multiple doses a day, though sometimes single doses are taken. The following abbreviations are used by physicians for doses:

- *bid* – twice a day
- *tid* – three times a day
- *qid* – four times a day.

When a drug is taken in multiple doses, it is essential to maintain a minimum effective blood concentration of the drug. The drug concentration–time curve for multiple doses is shown in Figure 9.15.

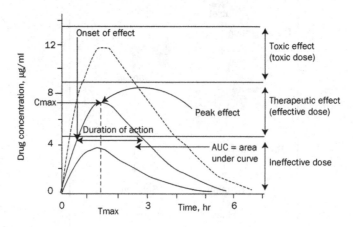

Figure 9.14 Drug concentration in blood serum and drug effects over seven hours after a single dose

Published by Woodhead Publishing Limited

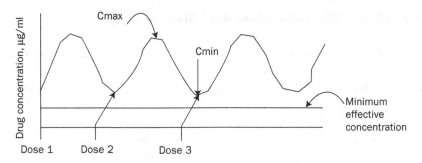

Figure 9.15 A kinetic profile of multiple doses of a drug

9.5 Pharmacokinetic profile of oral and IV dosage forms

We have already seen that oral dosage forms are slower in drug action because they must reach a particular area of the organ to be absorbed into the blood circulation system, known as systemic effects or distribution. Intravenous dosage forms can put drugs directly into blood circulation, bypassing the absorption step, so the IV route is faster in action. Kinetic profiles of oral and IV routes of administration are shown in Figure 9.16.

For patients who need emergency medication or are unable to take medicine orally, the IV route is the best choice of administration. The outcomes produced by drugs circulated in the blood are known as systemic effects. Most drugs have systemic effects, but some have local effects, such as ophthalmic (eye), otic (ear), and topical (skin) drugs.

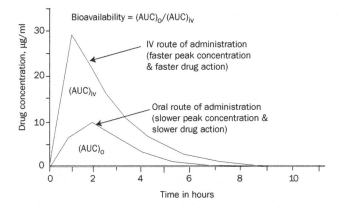

Figure 9.16 A pharmacokinetic profile of oral and IV routes of administration

Published by Woodhead Publishing Limited

9.6 Metabolism, or biotransformation of drugs

Metabolism is a process by which the body acts on drugs to get rid of them. The body recognizes drugs as foreign materials and wants to convert them so it can eliminate them easily. The biotransformation of drugs mostly takes place in the liver, but can occur in other organs, such as the kidneys, GIT, and lungs, and in the blood.

The body's enzymes catalyze these biotransformations. Through this biotransformation drugs can become inactive or more active, or more toxic or less toxic, depending on the nature of the drug. The biotransformed products of drugs are called metabolites. For example, aspirin (acetylsalicylic acid) is metabolized into salicylic acid, the active metabolite of aspirin. For excretion, this metabolite is further transformed into more water-soluble products for elimination purposes. The metabolic reactions are divided into two classes: phases I and II.

9.6.1 Phase I reaction

The first conversion of a drug that takes place in the body is known as a phase I metabolic reaction and its purpose is to make the drug either more active or more inactive. This reaction also makes the drug ready for further polar reactions (phase II). Phase I reactions mostly take place in the liver, caused by the enzyme cytochrome P450 (CYP-450) (Figure 9.17).

If the drug is lipophilic in nature, it is converted to more hydrophilic compounds by CYP-450, the biological oxidative enzyme. The phase I

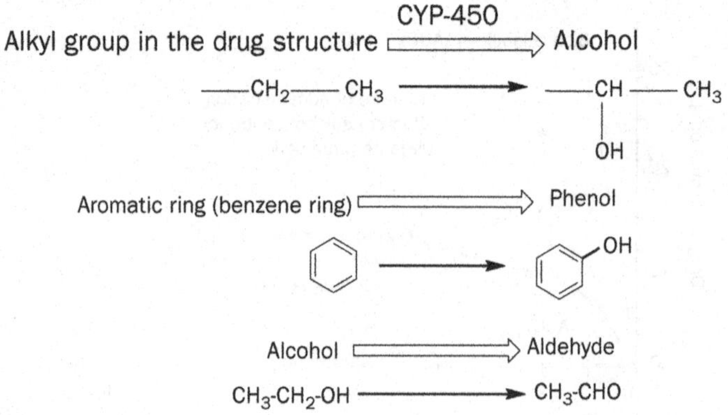

Figure 9.17 Phase I oxidation reactions catalyzed by CYP-450

Published by Woodhead Publishing Limited

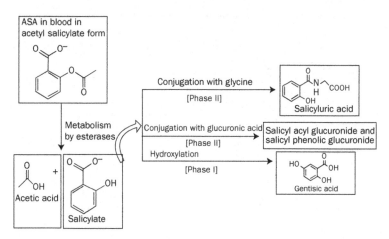

Figure 9.18 The metabolism of aspirin

metabolism also includes hydroxylation, reduction, and hydrolysis. Phase I metabolic reactions are shown in Figure 9.18.

9.6.2 Phase II reaction

This metabolic reaction is the final biotransformation of phase I metabolites making more water-soluble products for excretion purposes. The most common phase II biotransformations are conjugation reactions, such as glucuronation, sulfation, acetylation, or glucothione conjugation. The metabolic reactions of paracetemol in phases I and II are shown in Figure 9.19.

Metabolic reactions can also occur in blood plasma after absorption. The hydrolysis of a drug by esterases is shown in Figure 9.18. Many factors affect metabolism reactions, including race, age, sex, diet, and physiological body conditions.

9.7 Bioavailability, bioequivalence, and generic drugs

The US FDA defines bioavailability, as 'the rate and extent to which the active ingredient or active moiety is absorbed from a drug product and becomes available at the site of action'.[1] The bioavailability of non-intravenous drugs, such as orally or rectally administered drugs, inhaled dosage forms, and patch dosage forms, is the most important factor when assessing a new drug or a generic drug.

Published by Woodhead Publishing Limited

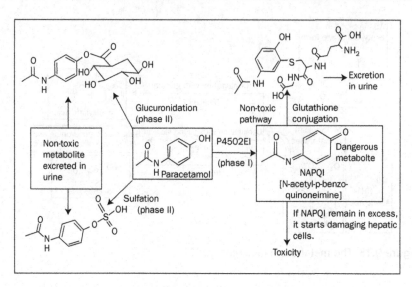

Figure 9.19 Phase II metabolic reactions of paracetamol

We have seen in Figure 9.14 that there is a range of drug concentration in blood serum that determines the therapeutic effectiveness of the drug. Drug concentrations higher or lower than the therapeutic level are unacceptable. From the bioavailability of a drug, we can learn how fast and how much of the drug goes into systematic circulation, but there are a number of factors that can affect the bioavailability of a drug.

9.7.1 Dosage forms

There are different dosage forms in orally administered drugs, such as tablets, capsules, syrups, and suspensions. Syrup is supplied as a solution form, and is therefore faster to be absorbed than the other three forms. Tablet forms are the slowest to be absorbed because they undergo disintegration and dissolution before they are absorbed.

9.7.2 Manufacturing qualities

Different pharmaceutical companies manufacture generic drugs, but the bioavailability of a drug, for example tablets, depends on the particle size of the active pharmaceutical ingredient (API), manufacturing processes, excipients, tablet hardness, and so on.

Published by Woodhead Publishing Limited

9.7.3 Drug users

The patient's age, genetic makeup, and stomach contents (full or empty) also affect the bioavailability of drug.

9.7.4 Bioequivalence

The bioequivalence of a drug is an assessment of its bioavailability when produced by different manufacturers. If two products drugs are bioequivalent, to all intents and purposes they are expected to be the same.[2] The US FDA defines bioequivalence as:

> the absence of a significant difference in the rate and extent to which the active ingredient or active moiety in pharmaceutical equivalents or pharmaceutical alternatives becomes available at the site of drug action when administered at the same molar dose under similar conditions in an appropriately designed study.[3]

After the expiration of a patent, pharmaceutical companies can manufacture and market the generic version of the innovator's drug provided their abbreviated new drug application (ANDA) is approved. To be approved, generic companies must prove that their product is bioequivalent to that of the innovator. For example, Figure 9.20 shows the pharmacokinetic profile of Viagra, a drug manufactured and marketed by Pfizer. The dotted line shows the expected profile for a future generic version of the drug,

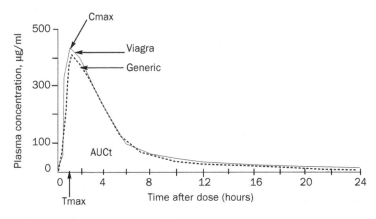

Figure 9.20 The pharmacokinetic profile of Viagra

Source: Redrawn from Viagra website with permission from Pfizer

compared with its existing profile (the unbroken line). In future the generic tablet, sildenafil citrate, should have the same profile as Viagra.

9.8 Safety and the toxic effects of drugs

Safety is important for daily living, regardless of health, and even more important for the sick, especially when they take medicine as treatment. However, the body's infrastructure is complicated, although it can be explained in simple terms. For example, it can be said that once a person takes medicine orally, it goes to the stomach, then to the small intestine, where it is absorbed (absorption) into the blood circulation (distribution) and starts working for the person's well being. Finally the medicine undergoes biotransformation (metabolism) and is eliminated (excretion) from the body.

In reality, it is not that simple. As it moves through the body the medicine has to interact, bind, or pass through many organs, tissues, cells, proteins, receptors, enzymes, or other molecules present in the body. In most cases, one or two particular interactions could produce beneficial effects, but other interactions may cause bad effects, called side effects or adverse drug reactions, and the drugs may be called toxic. A very simplified version of drug action and adverse drug reaction is shown in Figure 9.21.

Figure 9.21 illustrates how a drug affects the normal signalling pathways that can control the production of the disease-causing molecule X by interfering with A or B. In some cases the drug can directly interact with X to attempt to eliminate it. This system is called a mode of action. The drug

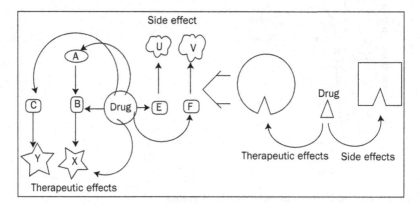

Figure 9.21 Therapeutic and side effects of a drug[4]

Published by Woodhead Publishing Limited

may have effects on other pathways where it can control the production of another disease-causing factor Y from molecule C, which can help control a second beneficial effect. This kind of pathway is classified as alternative medical use. The drug can interact with other pathways too, such as activating E and F and causing some kind of physiological disorder. This kind of system is known as an adverse drug reaction.

These effects are regarded as unwanted. For example, certain antihistamine drugs control the symptoms of allergies but also cause drowsiness. Almost all drugs have common side effects, such as nausea, vomiting, fatigue, dizziness, dry mouth, headache, loss of appetite, weight gain or loss, hair loss, frequent urination, sweating, skin rash, and itching. Sometimes, there are serious adverse drug reactions, which can even be fatal, for example:

- allergies – difficulty in breathing, or a severe skin rash
- stomach, intestinal, or rectal bleeding in the GIT
- fainting, heart attack, high or low blood pressure, anemia, seizures, stroke caused by side effects in the brain or blood
- mental disorders – anxiety, depression, or hallucination
- liver damage, jaundice, hepatitis, or acute kidney failure caused by side effects in the liver or kidney
- back pain, tremor, or spasm caused by side effects in a muscle.

The severity of these side effects depends on the length and dose of medication, patient age, weight, gender, ethnicity, and general health. Hardly any medicine is free of side effects.

It is important to see the benefit–risk ratio of medicines. The benefit is a measure of efficacy, and the risk is a measure of toxicity; if a drug has a large benefit–risk ratio it indicates it is a successful drug. There is no standardized, widely accepted quantitative measurement of this benefit–risk ratio. European pharmaceutical legislation states that the benefit–risk balance is

> an evaluation of the positive therapeutic effects of a medicinal product in relation to any risk relating to the quality, safety or efficacy of the medicinal product as regards patients' health or public health. A marketing authorisation shall be refused if the risk-benefit balance is not considered to be favourable.[5]

Figure 9.22 shows some hypothetical benefit–risk ratios for drugs.

Published by Woodhead Publishing Limited

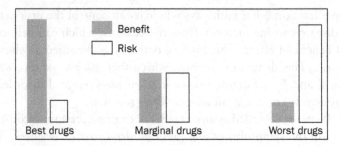

Figure 9.22 Hypothetical benefit–risk ratios for drugs

9.9 The ideal pharmacokinetics and pharmacodynamics of a drug

This chapter started with the concept of pharmacokinetics and pharmacodynamics for a drug, and after discussing the important aspects of a drug and its pharmacology (pharmacokinetic and pharmacodynamic), we will now try to characterize the ideal drugs. The pharmacokinetic and pharmacodynamic profiles of a drug are shown graphically in Figure 9.23.

From the pharmacokinetic profile, it appears that drug plasma concentration increases with time until it reaches the peak concentration and begins falling. Similarly, the pharmacodynamic profile shows that the drug effects start with the increase of drug plasma concentration. It reaches the peak of effectiveness, but then ultimately diminishes unless it is maintained with multiple doses.

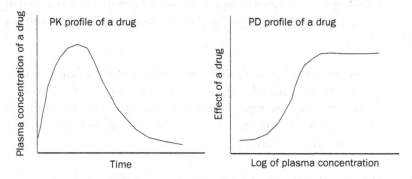

Figure 9.23 General pharmacokinetic and pharmacodynamic profiles of a drug

In summary, an ideal drug should have the following characteristics:

- *Efficacy* – If the drug is not efficacious for the symptoms or disease it is intended to treat, it should not be called a drug.
- *Safety* – Safety is the primary criteria the drug must meet to be considered a drug. A drug can be efficacious in treating a disease but not safe, or it could cause fatal side effects. In these cases, the drug should not be launched at all. Some drugs are withdrawn from the market because of safety concerns.
- *Low toxicity* – The drug is efficacious and safe but still has some toxicity. The lower the toxicity level, the safer and more effective the drug will be.
- *Fewer doses per day* – A 'once daily' dose is the best choice.
- *Larger therapeutic window* – With a smaller therapeutic window (Figure 9.24), the drug could be fatal if it is overdosed. The LD_{50} (lethal dose 50) should be higher.
- *Consistent plasma concentration* – The efficacy of a drug depends on the bioavailability or plasma concentration of the drug.
- *Rapid onset of action* – The drug should work immediately after being administered – the sooner the bloodstream acquires an effective drug concentration, the sooner the drug action will take place.
- *No drug accumulation in the body* – After the drug acts on the target, the drug should be eliminated from the body. Drug accumulation in the body will prolong the drug's side effects, which is not desirable.
- *Minimum drug–drug interactions* – In many cases, patients take multiple drugs, and it is important that there is not much interaction between the drugs any individual patient takes. Drug–drug interactions often lead to serious side effects or toxicity.
- *Stability* – The drug stability or the dosage form's stability is very important. If the drugs start degrading because of environmental conditions or other reasons, the drugs cannot be taken. The more distant the expiration date of a drug, the better for the patient.
- *Linear dose-response and kinetics* – There should be a linear relationship between dose amount (strength of drug) and its response or effectiveness (magnitude of effects). Based on the severity of the disease condition, physicians sometimes determine the dose amount for patients or start with higher dose load then continue with a maintenance load.
- *Inexpensiveness* – One of the most important criteria of an ideal drug is affordability. It should be inexpensive and affordable for common people.

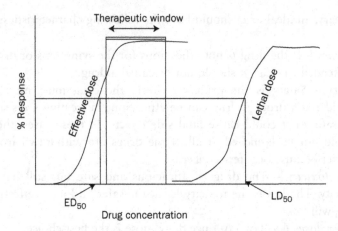

Figure 9.24 The concentration of a therapeutic window and a lethal dose

Practice questions

1. What are the advantages and disadvantages of oral and parenteral dosage forms?
2. Using a flow-sheet, show how drugs act in our body.
3. Discuss metabolic reactions using paracetamol as an example.
4. If you check the oral dosage form and injectable dosage form of the same drug, you will find the amount of the oral dosage form is much higher than that for the injectable form. Rationalize this observation.
5. Why does the overdose of drugs or alcohol affect the liver?
6. Which is good for a drug: a higher LD_{50} value or a higher ED_{50} value?
7. Arrange these dosage forms according to how fast they act, with the fastest one first: tablet, capsule, solution, suspension, and injection.
8. Describe the difference between orally administered and parenteral dosage forms, and list the advantages and disadvantages of each.
9. What is the half-life of a drug?
10. What are ED_{50} and LD_{50} on the therapeutic index?

Answers to some practice questions

8. There are various forms of orally administered medicines, such as fast release, sustained release, enteric-coated tablets, syrup, and suspension, which are available for patients or doctors to prescribe. Advantages of oral forms of dosage:

•   They are inexpensive, convenient, easy to carry, and easy to swallow.

Disadvantages:

•   They have a relatively delayed onset of action because the drugs need to be absorbed in the systemic circulation.
•   They go through a fast pass metabolism at the liver, so higher dose amounts are required.
•   Food can affect drug absorption.

Parenteral dosage forms, especially the IV route, deliver drugs directly into the blood stream and thus provide rapid action. In emergencies, this is the only option. Advantages of parenteral dosage forms:

•   There is no fast pass metabolism.

Disadvantages:

•   IV drugs are relatively expensive.
•   Some patients are scared of needles.
•   A trained professional is required to administer injection.

9. The time required for the body to eliminate one-half or 50% of the administered drug by a normal excretion process. If the drug has six hours of half-life, it will take six hours for 50% of the drug to be eliminated, so the other 50% will remain in the body. The half-life of a drug represents the duration of drug action.

10. An effective dose (ED) is one that produces a specific given effect; when it is ED_{50}, it means there is a 50% response. A lethal dose (LD) is the dose level that would be fatal for the subject; LD_{50} means a dose level at which 50% subjects are expected to die. For an ideal drug, there should be very low ED_{50} and very high LD_{50}. The therapeutic index is the measure of safety and it is a ratio of LD_{50}–ED_{50}.

Published by Woodhead Publishing Limited

Notes

1. US Food and Drug Administration, CFR Code of Federal Regulations Title 21, 'Part 320 – Bioavailability and bioequivalence requirements', April 2010, www.accessdata.fda.gov/scripts/cdrh/cfdocs/cfcfr/CFRSearch.cfm?fr=320.1 (accessed December 5, 2010).
2. Dale P. Conner, *General BA/BE Issues*, [n.d.], www.aapspharmaceutica.com/meetings/files/90/19Conner.pdf (accessed February 11, 2011).
3. US Food and Drug Administration, CFR Code of Federal Regulations Title 21, 'Part 320 – Bioavailability and bioequivalence requirements', April 2010, www.accessdata.fda.gov/scripts/cdrh/cfdocs/cfcfr/CFRSearch.cfm?fr=320.1 (accessed December 5, 2010).
4. I appreciate the help given to me by Kakon Nag in creating this figure.
5. 'Guideline on the definition of a potential serious risk to public health in the context of Article 29(1) and (2) of Directive 2001/83/EC – March 2006', *Official Journal of the European Union*, June 8, 2006, http://ec.europa.eu/health/files/eudralex/vol-1/com_2006_133/com_2006_133_en.pdf (accessed February 12, 2011).

10

The top five most common or long-selling drugs

Amoxicillin   Aspirin   Paracetamol   Ranitidine   Ciprofloxacin

Learning objective

This chapter is the heart of this book. It discusses some drugs that have either been widely used, used for many years, or achieved blockbuster status (Figure 10.1). Students will learn:

- how the drugs amoxicillin, aspirin, paracetamol, ranitidine, and ciprofloxacin were discovered
- how these drugs are manufactured
- what the dosage forms for these drugs are
- how the dosage forms are manufactured
- about pharmacology and pharmacokinetic

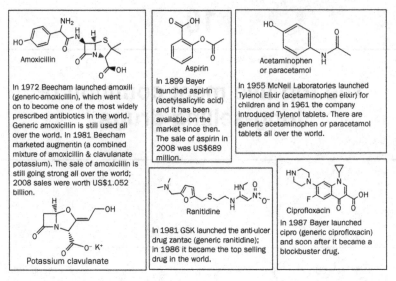

Figure 10.1 The structure of and brief information on five common or long-selling drugs

10.1   Amoxicillin – the largest-selling β-lactam antibiotic

Key concept terms

6-APA: 6-aminopenicillanic acid, an intermediate for many semi-synthetic types of penicillin

Antibiotic: a substance produced by or derived from certain microorganisms that can kill or inhibit the growth of other pathogenic microorganisms

API: active pharmaceutical ingredient

Capsule: a solid dosage form employing a hard gelatin shell filled with an API

Compacted powder: powder with high bulk density suitable for making tablet or capsule dosage forms

Published by Woodhead Publishing Limited

Dane salt: a suitable intermediate, side chain compound used in the production of amoxicillin

Dosage form: physical form of a dose of medicine made for administration

Dry syrup: a dosage form supplied in powdered form but converted to liquid form by adding water before ingestion

Excipient: therapeutically inactive pharmaceutical ingredient used with an API to make dosage forms

GIT: gastrointestinal tract

Heterocyclic ring: a ring containing atom(s) other than carbon

Injectable: parenteral dosage form; gives faster action than other forms

Micronized powder: powder with low bulk density; the particle size is smaller (micron size) and suitable for dry syrup preparation

Pen G: penicillin G or benzylpenicillin; parenteral dosage form

Pen V: penicillin V or penoxymethylpenicillin; oral penicillin

Semi-synthetic: part of the processes of drug production carried out by laboratory synthesis

Serum concentration: blood or plasma concentration

Tablet: a solid-dosage form of medicine made by compression; pill form

Trihydrate: three molecules of water

β-lactam: four-member heterocyclic ring containing lactam functional group (cyclic amide)

10.1.1 Introduction

Amoxicillin is a semi-synthetic penicillin that has been on the market consistently since its introduction in 1972. The chemical name of amoxicillin is 6-[D(-)β-amino-p-hydroxyphenyl-acetamido.] penicillanic acid. The International Union of Pure and Applied Chemistry (IUPAC) lists its

Published by Woodhead Publishing Limited

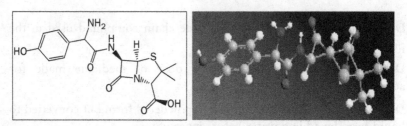

Figure 10.2 2D structure and 3D structure of amoxicillin

systematic name as (2S,5R,6R)-6-[[(2R)-2-amino-2-(4-hydroxyphenyl)acetyl.]amino.]-3,3-dimethyl-7-oxo-4-thia-1-azabicyclo[3.2.0.] heptane-2-carboxylic acid. Figure 10.2 illustrates the 2D structure and 3D structure of amoxicillin.

Some time ago amoxicillin was off-patented, so it goes by numerous brand names around the world. However, its original brand name was Amoxil, which was used by Beecham until Beecham merged with GlaxoSmithKline (GSK). Therapeutically, amoxicillin is used as a broad spectrum of bactericidal activity against many gram-positive and gram-negative microorganisms. In general, amoxicillin is produced as amoxicillin trihydrate. During the crystallization of amoxicillin from its solution form, it picks up three molecules of water as water of crystallization, although anhydrous amoxicillin can also be made and used. It is a fine, white to off-white crystalline powder, which is sparingly soluble in water.

To understand the full story of this semi-synthetic penicillin, amoxicillin we need to go back to the fascinating discovery of penicillin.

10.1.2   The discovery of penicillin

Sir Alexander Fleming (a bacteriologist at St Mary's Hospital in London) and the name of penicillin (the first successful antibiotic) are inseparable. The discovery and development of penicillin are widely considered to be the greatest advances in medical and pharmaceutical sciences. Fleming's curiosity, presence of mind, and subject knowledge helped him discover penicillin in 1928. While working with the cultured petri-dish of *staphylococcus*, he accidently contaminated the dish with blue-green mold.

He observed that the colonies of bacteria nearby were destroyed. Fleming continued his research using the blue mold and different disease-causing bacteria and finally published a paper in the *British Journal of Experimental Pathology* in 1929.

Fleming was not successful in isolating the active compound, but his published research paper led a team of scientists including Australian Howard Florey, German Ernst Chain, and Briton N. G. Heatley to extract penicillin from mold, *penicillium notatum*, while working at Oxford University. In this team, Florey was the clinician, and Chain and Heatley were the chemists. The team conducted clinical trials in different parts of the world on patients with war injuries in 1941–1943. They were a huge success, but the large-scale production of penicillin was found to be very difficult, until, eventually, a joint effort between industries and government institutes in Britain and the USA succeeded in overcoming them. Fleming, Florey, and Chain were jointly awarded the 1945 Nobel Prize for medicine (see Figures 10.3 and 10.4).

The discovery of penicillin was a revolutionary step in treating infectious diseases. Humans had won the first battle in the war against pathogenic bacteria. The penicillin antibiotics used in therapy were penicillin G (Pen-G) or benzyl penicillin (parenterally administered) and its close biosynthetic relative penicillin V (Pen-V), or phenoxymethyl penicillin (orally administered). For a long time, these antibiotics were the treatment choices for infections caused by most gram-positive and gram-negative bacteria.

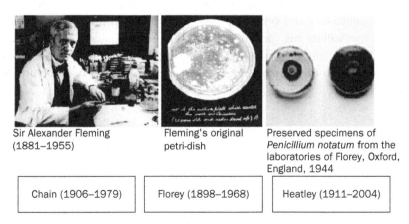

Sir Alexander Fleming (1881–1955)

Fleming's original petri-dish

Preserved specimens of *Penicillium notatum* from the laboratories of Florey, Oxford, England, 1944

Chain (1906–1979)   Florey (1898–1968)   Heatley (1911–2004)

Figure 10.3 Illustrations relating to the discovery of penicillin

Published by Woodhead Publishing Limited

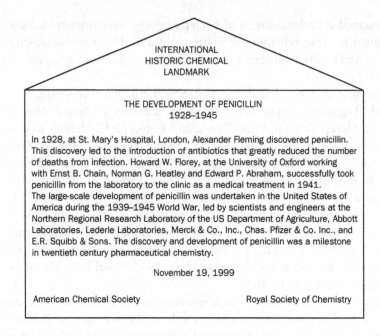

```
INTERNATIONAL
HISTORIC CHEMICAL
LANDMARK

THE DEVELOPMENT OF PENICILLIN
1928–1945

In 1928, at St. Mary's Hospital, London, Alexander Fleming discovered penicillin.
This discovery led to the introduction of antibiotics that greatly reduced the number
of deaths from infection. Howard W. Florey, at the University of Oxford working
with Ernst B. Chain, Norman G. Heatley and Edward P. Abraham, successfully took
penicillin from the laboratory to the clinic as a medical treatment in 1941.
The large-scale development of penicillin was undertaken in the United States of
America during the 1939–1945 World War, led by scientists and engineers at the
Northern Regional Research Laboratory of the US Department of Agriculture, Abbott
Laboratories, Lederle Laboratories, Merck & Co., Inc., Chas. Pfizer & Co. Inc., and
E.R. Squibb & Sons. The discovery and development of penicillin was a milestone
in twentieth century pharmaceutical chemistry.

November 19, 1999

American Chemical Society                        Royal Society of Chemistry
```

Figure 10.4 Plaque commemorating the development of penicillin

Source: Royal Society of Chemistry and American Chemical Society[1]

The development and successful therapeutic use of Pen-G and Pen-V has opened the door for pharmaceutical researchers to find better penicillanic derivatives or β-lactam derivatives. This kind of pharmaceutical research around the world, especially in the UK and the USA, has produced semi-synthetic penicillins and cephalosporins (also β-lactam antibiotics). Semi-synthetic penicillins are produced by changing the side chain on the intermediate, 6-aminopenicillanic acid (6-APA). In penicillins, the β-lactam ring is fused with the thiazolidine ring. Figure 10.5 shows the structure of amide to 6-APA.

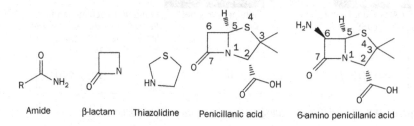

Figure 10.5 The structure of amide to 6-aminopenicillanic acid

6-APA is a stable intermediate that consists of a β-lactam ring, which can be produced through fermentation. Figure 10.6 shows the structural relationship and conversion of b-lactam drugs.

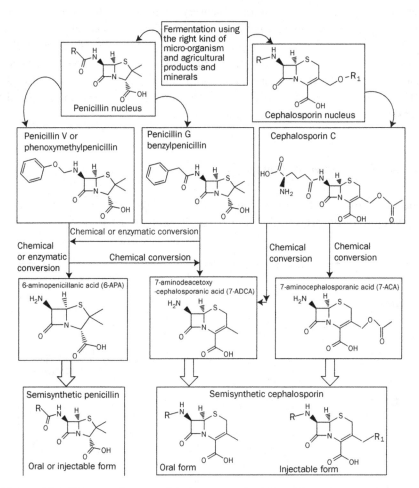

Figure 10.6 β-lactam drugs and their structural relationship and conversion

Source: Adapted with permission from DSM[2]

10.1.3 The production of β-lactam raw materials, intermediates, and end products

The active part of the molecule responsible for the bactericidal action of penicillins and cephalosporins is the β-lactam ring structure. β-lactam is a four-membered cyclic amide. After the discovery of penicillin, the second major breakthrough in β-lactam antibiotics was the introduction of cephalosporins. As 6-APA led to the development of dozens of semi-synthetic penicillins, similarly 7-aminocephalosporanic acid (7-ACA) or 7-aminodeacetoxycephalosporanic acid (7-ADCA) led to different cephalosporin antibiotics (see Figures 10.1 and 10.2). Figure 10.7 shows a family tree of β-lactam antibiotics, including natural and semi-synthetic penicillins and cephalosporins.

10.1.4 The discovery of amoxicillin

The development of semi-synthetic penicillin took place in the Beecham Research Laboratories Ltd operated in Brockham Park in Surrey, UK,

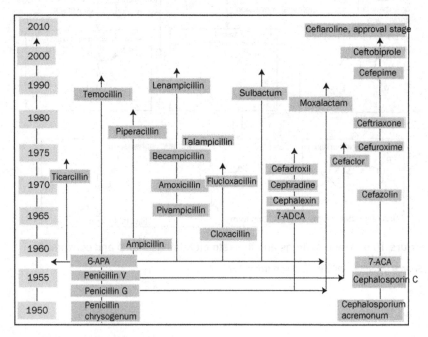

Figure 10.7 Family tree of natural and semi-synthetic β-lactam antibiotics

Source: Adapted and expanded with permission from DSM[3]

Published by Woodhead Publishing Limited

which then merged with Smith & Kline in 1989, and later became SmithKline Beecham. In 2000, SmithKline Beecham and Glaxo Wellcome merged to form GlaxoSmithKline (GSK). In 1959 Beecham scientists discovered the penicillin nucleus 6-APA, and this discovery played a pivotal role in developing semi-synthetic penicillin. The same year, Beecham marketed pheneticillin, followed by another semi-synthetic penicillin, meticillin. Finally, in 1961 Beecham hit the market with the blockbuster drug ampicillin (brand name Penbritin), which continued successfully for several decades. Although ampicillin did not last longer because it developed bacterial resistance, amoxicillin, which is structurally similar to ampicillin, has been in production since its introduction in 1972. Figure 10.8 shows the development of semi-synthetic penicillins at Beecham Laboratories.

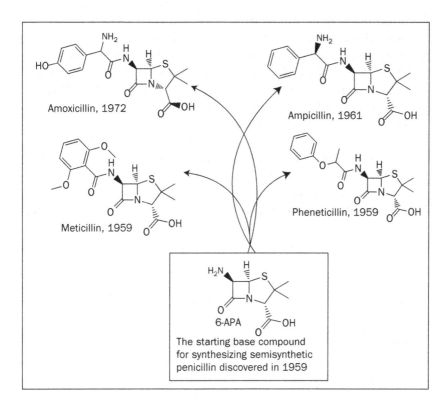

Figure 10.8 The development of semi-synthetic penicillins at Beecham Laboratories

Published by Woodhead Publishing Limited

10.1.5 Manufacturing of amoxicillin trihydrate

All semi-synthetic penicillins manufactured starting from 6-aminopenicillanic acid (6-APA) are produced through a fermentation process. The semi-synthetic part of production of amoxicillin trihydrate is discussed here. Starting from 6-APA, a side chain (specific for amoxicillin) is joined to the amino group of 6-APA. This conjunction may seem simple, but it is not.

10.1.6 Manufacturing amoxicillin using the Dane salt method

10.1.6.1 Industrial synthesis of amoxicillin

Figure 10.9 illustrates the construction of amoxicillin. It has two parts – 6-APA on the right and p-hydroxyphenylglycine. 6-APA and a precursor of p-hydroxyphenylglycine are available from chemical suppliers.

Your synthetic job is to combine these two in the highest possible yield and purity. For a reaction in a solution, you need to choose the correct, cost-effective, and recyclable solvent or solvents. In addition, catalytic amounts of other reagents and the maintenance of proper pH balance are required for a smooth reaction (Figure 10.10).

In this process, the side chain of amoxicillin comes from para-hydroxy phenylglycine, which is used as Dane salt where the amino group is protected as enamine. Dane salt is not used directly to react with 6-APA. It is activated by reacting with pivaloyl chloride, which results in a mixed anhydride that undergoes a reaction with 6-APA. The process flow sheet Figure 10.11 and the flow diagram Figure 10.12 illustrate the following steps:

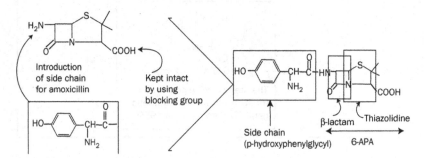

Figure 10.9 The structural construction of amoxicillin

Published by Woodhead Publishing Limited

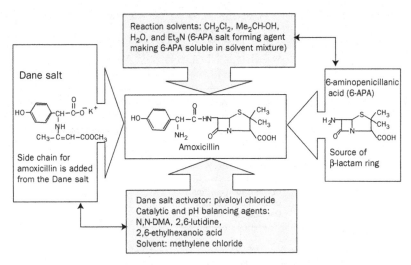

Figure 10.10 A strategic outline of the synthesis of amoxicillin

- 6-APA dissolution
- acylation of Dane salt
- condensation at very low temperature
- hydrolysis
- extraction
- crystallization.

There are two critical factors during production:

- The semi-synthetic penicillin containing the β-lactam ring is very sensitive to acids and alkalis as well as to high temperatures. Thus during production, parameters such as temperature and resident time have to be strictly maintained.
- Washing and drying of the final product are very important because residual solvents and other reagents may affect product quality and stability.

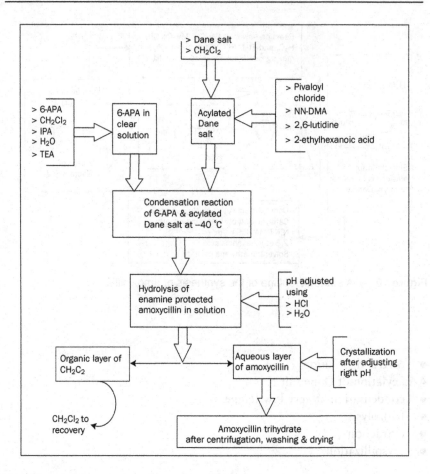

Figure 10.11 The manufacture of amoxycillin

10.1.7   Reaction chemistry of synthesis of amoxicillin

Amoxicillin is synthesized in four steps: through dissolution, acylation, condensation, and hydrolysis followed by crystallization.

10.1.7.1   Step 1 The dissolution of 6-APA

Figure 10.13 illustrates the dissolution of 6-APA.

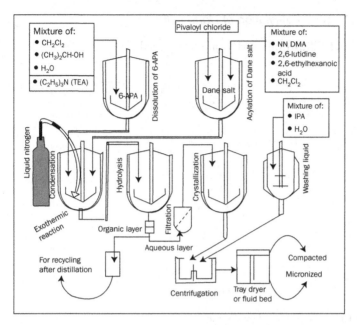

Figure 10.12 The production of bulk amoxicillin through the reactors – reactions, crystallization, centrifugation, and drying followed by compaction or micronization

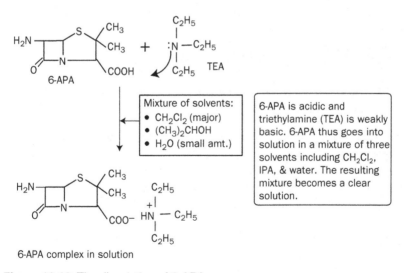

6-APA complex in solution

Figure 10.13 The dissolution of 6-APA

10.1.7.2 Step 2 Acylation of Dane salt

Figure 10.14 illustrates acylation of Dane salt.

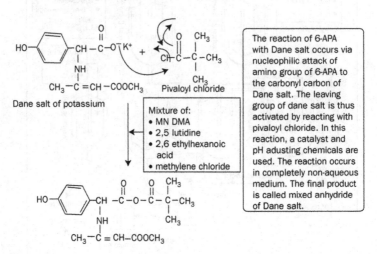

Dane salt of potassium

Mixture of:
• MN DMA
• 2,5 lutidine
• 2,6 ethylhexanoic acid
• methylene chloride

The reaction of 6-APA with Dane salt occurs via nucleophilic attack of amino group of 6-APA to the carbonyl carbon of Dane salt. The leaving group of dane salt is thus activated by reacting with pivaloyl chloride. In this reaction, a catalyst and pH adusting chemicals are used. The reaction occurs in completely non-aqueous medium. The final product is called mixed anhydride of Dane salt.

Figure 10.14 Acylation of Dane salt

10.1.7.3 Step 3 Condensation reaction between 6-APA complex and acylated Dane salt

Figure 10.15 illustrates the condensation reaction between 6-APA complex and acylated Dane salt.

10.1.7.4 Step 4 Hydrolysis of enamine protected amoxycillin followed by crystallization

Figure 10.16 illustrates hydrolysis of enamine protected amoxycillin followed by crystallization.

A critical factor in the reaction chemistry of the synthesis of amoxycillin is that it is always possibility that the amoxicillin will degrade (because of the presence of highly sensitive β-lactam ring) producing a lower yield.

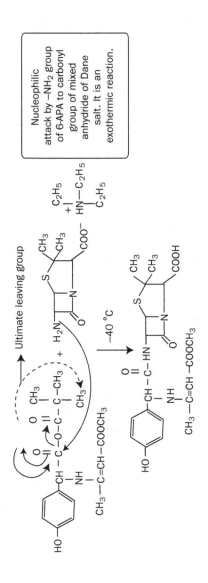

Figure 10.15 Condensation reaction between 6-APA complex and acylated Dane salt

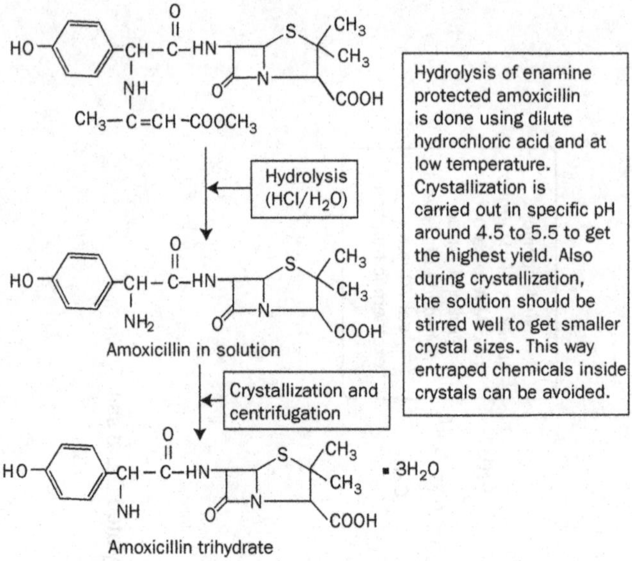

Hydrolysis of enamine protected amoxicillin is done using dilute hydrochloric acid and at low temperature. Crystallization is carried out in specific pH around 4.5 to 5.5 to get the highest yield. Also during crystallization, the solution should be stirred well to get smaller crystal sizes. This way entraped chemicals inside crystals can be avoided.

Figure 10.16 Hydrolysis of enamine protected amoxycillin followed by crystallization

10.1.8 Formulation of dosage forms using the active pharmaceutical ingredient amoxicillin

Once the pharmaceutical active ingredient is available, the pharmaceutical factory formulates the dosage forms proven to be effective therapeutically. Figure 10.17 illustrates the most common dosage forms available for amoxicillin.

In the oral dosage forms of amoxicillin, only solid forms are available. Liquid dosage forms are not possible because amoxicillin is unstable in this

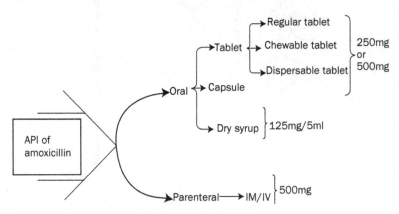

Figure 10.17 Common dosage forms of amoxicillin

Published by Woodhead Publishing Limited

form. However, amoxicillin powder is available in a bottle and can be used to constitute a liquid syrup or put into suspension by adding drinking water. In most cases, pharmacists instantly prepare the liquid form and deliver it to the consumer. This liquid preparation of amoxicillin must be consumed within ten days and be stored in the refrigerator. The β-lactam ring of amoxicillin slowly undergoes degradation (hydrolysis) and the prescribed potency lessens. Fortunately, the degradation products of amoxicillin are not toxic, so 1–2% degradation is acceptable for consumption. The β-lactam ring is unstable in acidic and basic media. It is also sensitive to heat. In acidic and basic media, amoxicillin is broken down into many products, including amoxicillenic acid, amoxillic acid, amoxilloic acid, amoxamaldic acid, amoxicillamine in acid medium, and amoxicilloic acid in water or basic medium (Figure 10.18).

The most common dosage forms of amoxicillin are tablets and capsules, and the capsule form is the simplest and easiest to produce in the manufacturing scale. Not many excipients are required to make this form. In addition to hard gelatin capsules, excipients may include magnesium silicate and talc to improve the flow of the powder in filling up the capsules. Tablet production requires many more excipients, such as filler, binder, disintegrant, or gliding agent. Once the tablets are produced, there are many quality checks, such as for hardness, friability, disintegration time, and dissolution profile, which ensure the uniformity and potency of the tablets.

The parenteral or injectable dosage form requires the API to be water-soluble. Amoxicillin trihydrate is not very water-soluble, so this form of

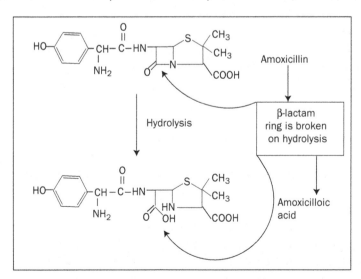

Figure 10.18 Hydrolysis of amoxicillin produces amoxicilloic acid

Published by Woodhead Publishing Limited

amoxicillin cannot be used in injectable form. The API for injectables has to be manufactured in an aseptic environment, and the powder has to be transferred to the container in an aseptic condition. Amoxicillin trihydrate is converted to sodium salt of amoxicillin, which is water-soluble and can be injected.

10.1.9 Pharmacology, the kinetics of amoxicillin

Amoxicillin is bactericidal, and works by inactivating an enzyme necessary for the cross linking of bacterial cell walls. The inhibition of the bacterial enzyme, transpeptidase, takes place by forming a covalent bond through a β-lactam ring of amoxicillin with an amino acid residue at the active site of the enzyme. The four-membered β-lactam ring of amoxicillin, any penicillin, or any semi-synthetic penicillin is highly strained and thus very reactive. Because of the inhibition of enzyme, bacterial cell walls cannot be formed so the bacteria cannot reproduce and start dying.

Before marketing dosage forms of any drug, the pharmacology and pharmacokinetics of the dosage forms are studied in detail. Amoxicillin has been on the market for about 40 years and there have been many studies on it. Amoxicillin is rapidly absorbed after oral administration, and reaches average peak serum levels within 1–2 hours. In the late 1970s Eshelman and Spyker and Spyker et al. investigated the pharmacokinetic profiles of amoxicillin (oral, intramuscular, and intravenous).[4] Spyker et al. compared the pharmacokinetics of amoxicillin among different dosage forms and showed that the pharmacokinetic parameters are nearly identical for intramuscular and orally administered 500 mg single doses of amoxicillin. They found, as expected, that an intravenous injection of amoxicillin starts with an instantaneous highest peak serum level and gradually decreases with time.

10.1.10 The packaging of amoxicillin dosage forms

The quality assurance of medicine until its expiration date is considered an absolute necessity for the survival of a pharmaceutical company, so the packaging of formulated dosage forms is a significant part of the total quality assurance system. Tablets and capsules are packed in blister or strip packs or put into a container. Injectables are put into a vial. Dry syrups are packaged in a container with enough volume to add water to make a specific amount of syrup or put into suspension (Figure 10.19).

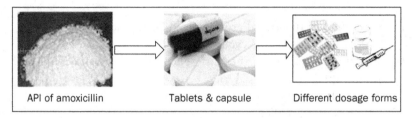

| API of amoxicillin | Tablets & capsule | Different dosage forms |

Figure 10.19 Packaging of different dosage forms of amoxicillin

Practice questions

1. What does parenterally administered mean?
2. Why is Pen G injected and not orally administered?
3. What are natural antibiotics and semi-synthetic antibiotics?
4. Why is amoxicillin called β-lactam antibiotic?
5. Ampicillin and amoxicillin are both β-lactam antibiotics. What is the difference between them?
6. If a carboxylic acid functional group is not protected, what can happen?
7. What is the role of urea in the synthesis of amoxicillin?
8. What type of reaction happens when an amino group of 6-APA attacks the carbon of an acyl group:
   (a) S_N1 (b) S_N2 (c) E1 (d) E2
9. How many functional groups are there in the amoxicillin molecule:
   (a) 3 (b) 4 (c) 5 (d) 6
10. For a serious infection, what dosage form of amoxicillin would be best and why?
11. In the structure of amoxicillin, which functional group is not there:
   (a) phenol (b) amide (c) ketone (d) carboxylic acid (e) amine
12. How many chiral centers are there in amoxicillin:
   (a) 2 (b) 3 (c) 4 (d) 5
13. How many heterocyclic rings are there in amoxicillin? Which one is in a β-lactam ring? What is the name of the other fused heterocyclic ring?
14. Structurally, what is common to penicillin and cephalosporins:
   (a) both are bicyclic (b) both have amino group (c) both have β-lactam ring

Published by Woodhead Publishing Limited

15. What kind of functional group does β-lactam have:
    (a) ketone (b) amine (c) cyclic amide (d) amide
16. Structurally, what is the difference between ampicillin and amoxicillin:
    (a) no difference (b) difference in side chain
17. Which is more acidic:
    (a) ampicillin (b) amoxicillin (c) meticillin (d) phenticillin
18. When the side chain for amoxicillin is joined with 6-APA, what functional group is formed:
    (a) substituted amine (b) amide (c) ketone (d) phenol
19. There are four non-cyclic functional groups in amoxicillin. How many are acidic and basic functional groups:
    (a) 1 and 3 (b) 2 and 2 (c) 3 and 1 (d) 4 and 0 (e) 0 and 4
20. What are two cyclic functional groups in amoxicillin? Which one acts against bacteria?
21. Methylene chloride is a recyclable solvent. How can you get it back to reuse it:
    (a) Separate it from aqueous layer and use it directly.
    (b) Separate it from aqueous layer and use it after purification by extraction process.
    (c) Separate it from aqueous layer and use it after purification by distillation.
22. What the ultimate objective in choosing the best process for manufacturing of amoxicillin:
    (a) to get the highest yield of amoxicillin
    (b) to get the highest purity of amoxicillin
    (c) to get the highest yield as well as purity of amoxicillin
    (d) to get the highest yield and purity as well as cost-effectiveness for amoxicillin
23. In the production of amoxicillin, why does the temperature of condensation step start from –40 °C:
    (a) The condensation reaction is endothermic, so starting at a low temperature is good.
    (b) The condensation reaction is exothermic, so starting at a low temperature is good.
24. High temperature speeds up the reaction, but in the production of amoxicillin low temperature is used. Why:
    (a) the thiazolidine ring breaks down (b) the β-lactam ring breaks down

Published by Woodhead Publishing Limited

25. In steps 2 and 3 of the reaction chemistry of amoxicillin, what type of reaction takes place:
    (a) nucleophilic substitution
    (b) electrophilic substitution
    (c) nucleophilic addition
    (d) electrophilic addition
26. What is the purpose of centrifugation in the last step of the production process of an active pharmaceutical ingredient (API):
    (a) to isolate solid products by filtration
    (b) to evaporate the solvent and isolate product
27. Many pharmaceutical manufacturers use liquid nitrogen in the manufacturing process of amoxicillin. Why:
    (a) to maintain inert atmosphere in the reactor
    (b) to lower the reaction temperature
28. What is the role of pivaloyal chloride in the synthesis of amoxicillin:
    (a) in the reaction it forms hydrochloric acid (HCl), which maintains pH balance for the reaction
    (b) to activate the Dane salt for nucleophilic substitution reaction
29. Why is triethylamine used in the synthesis of amoxicillin?
30. Why is there no pre-made liquid dosage form in amoxicillin formulation:
    (a) the liquid dosage form is messy
    (b) the liquid dosage form is bitter in taste
    (c) amoxicillin is unstable in liquid dosage form
    (d) the liquid dosage form has delayed action
31. Which one of the following dosage forms of amoxicillin acts fastest:
    (a) a tablet
    (b) a capsule
    (c) dry syrup (instantly made liquid form)
    (d) an injectable form
32. Arrange these dosage forms in order of the quickest action times (quickest first):
    (a) a>b>c>d (b) d>c>b>a (c) c>b>a>d (d) b>c>a>d
33. After the administration of amoxicillin, how long does it stay in the blood stream:
    (a) 2 hrs (b) 4 hrs (c) 6 hrs (d) 8 hrs

Published by Woodhead Publishing Limited

34. After the administration of amoxicillin solid dosage forms, what is the peak blood level:
    (a) 2–3 µg/ml (b) 4–5 µγ/ml (c) 7–8 µg/ml (d) 7–8 mg/ml

Answers to some practice questions

29. Triethylamine helps the reaction in three ways: amoxicillin is weakly acidic and triethylamine is weakly basic, thus it helps in dissolution of 6-APA. It forms a salt with carboxylic acid and thus protects the group during further reactions. It also neutralizes HCl that forms during the reactions and maintains pH balance.

10.2   Aspirin – the longest-selling drug on the market

Key concept terms

Acetylsalicylic acid: acetylated salicylic acid; common generic name of aspirin; the IUPAC name is 2-acetoxybenzoic acid

Analgesic: a pain reliever

Anti-inflammatory: a drug that reduces inflammation

Antiplatelet action: action to block platelets from aggregating into harmful clots

Antipyretic: fever reducer

API: active pharmaceutical ingredient

Aspirin: aspirin is the brand name of acetylsalicylic acid (ASA); this name is now treated as generic too

Branded generic drug: a generic drug given a pharmaceutical manufacturer sponsored name

Buffered aspirin: aspirin coated with an acid neutralizing substance

Chewable aspirin: aspirin that is chewed

Enteric coated: special polymeric coating given to aspirin tablets so they pass through the highly acidic stomach and start dissolving in small intestine

Published by Woodhead Publishing Limited

Salicin: antipyretic active ingredient isolated from willow tree; made of salicylic acid

Salicylic acid: precursor of aspirin

Suppository: drug system intended for insertion into rectum

Aspirin was introduced to the commercial market in 1899, and since then its worldwide popularity has grown steadily. According to one estimate, about 30 million Kg of aspirin are consumed annually worldwide. Aspirin is the brand name, given by its originator Bayer of Germany, for what is generically known as acetylsalicylic acid (Figure 10.20). Chemically, its IUPAC name is 2-acetoxybenzoic acid, and structurally it is one of the simplest molecules used as medicine for more than a century. Aspirin is used as an analgesic, antipyretic, and anti-inflammatory agent.

10.2.1   The discovery of aspirin

The story of aspirin is also the story and development of Bayer – a German pharmaceutical company. Felix Hoffman, a chemist working at Bayer during 1890s, is known as the father of aspirin because of his synthetic work on aspirin from salicylic acid. However, the original idea of the active form of aspirin comes from Hippocrates (400 B.C.), the father of modern medicine, who used the bark and leaves of the willow tree to help heal headaches, pains, and fevers. Since then, the bark of willow tree has traditionally been used to treat pains, fevers, and rheumatic fever. Around

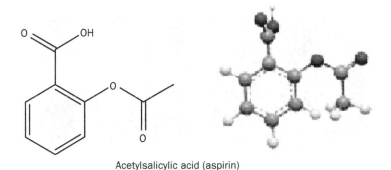

Acetylsalicylic acid (aspirin)

Figure 10.20 The structure of acetylsalicylic acid (aspirin)

Published by Woodhead Publishing Limited

1763, Reverend Edward Stone of Oxford, England, informed the Royal Society of London about the efficacy of willow bark in treating rheumatic fever.

After some 60 years, in 1823, Italian scientists isolated the active ingredient within willow tree bark and named it salicin. Salicin had also been isolated from the meadow sweet flower by Swiss and German researchers. In 1853, French scientists made salicylic acid from salicin and found that it worked as a pain reliever but irritated the gut. Finally, in 1897, Bayer scientist Hoffman synthesized aspirin from salicylic acid by treating it with acetic anhydride. In 1899, Bayer launched the aspirin after successful animal testing and clinical trials. Since 1930, aspirin has become generic, and the pharmaceutical companies around the world started producing aspirin as a branded generic drug. Figure 10.21 illustrates some pictures relating to the discovery of aspirin.

Many drugs become obsolete after being on the market for a couple of decades because of the availability of newer and better drugs, but aspirin has been produced since 1899 and is the only drug that has been on the

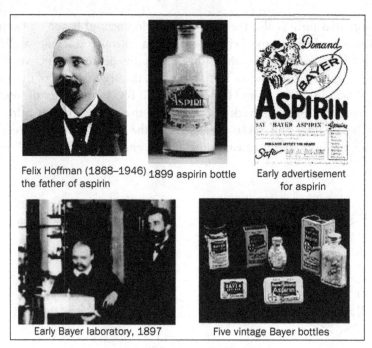

Felix Hoffman (1868–1946) the father of aspirin 1899 aspirin bottle Early advertisement for aspirin

Early Bayer laboratory, 1897 Five vintage Bayer bottles

Figure 10.21 Pictures relating to the discovery of aspirin

Source: Bayer's website[5]

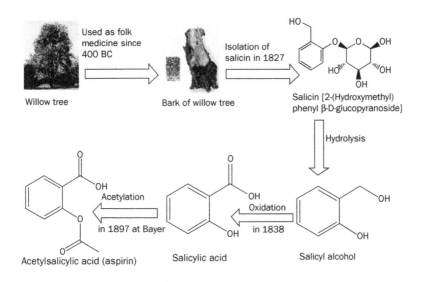

Used as folk medicine since 400 BC

Willow tree

Isolation of salicin in 1827

Bark of willow tree

Salicin [2-(Hydroxymethyl) phenyl β-D-glucopyranoside]

Hydrolysis

Acetylation in 1897 at Bayer

Acetylsalicylic acid (aspirin)

Oxidation in 1838

Salicylic acid

Salicyl alcohol

Figure 10.22 The historical development of aspirin

market for more than a century. In 1974 scientists found that aspirin could be used for other purposes than pain relief, such as preventing heart attacks. Aspirin was first marketed in powder form in 1899; a tablet form was only introduced in 1915. Currently aspirin is marketed as enteric-coated tablets, which have been found to be the safest form for oral dosage.

Once a folk remedy, aspirin has become the most successful drug in the world, and according to one estimate, almost 100 billion tablets are produced each year.[6] The use of aspirin continues to evolve. A low-strength dose of aspirin (75–80 mg per tablet) is widely used to prevent heart attacks and strokes. More research is under way to find other potential uses of aspirin, such as in treating diabetes, colon cancer, and dementia (including Alzheimer's disease). Figure 10.22 illustrates the historical development of aspirin.

10.2.2 The production of aspirin

Chemically, aspirin is a very simple aromatic molecule with a benzene ring, a carboxylic acid group, and an acetate group (Figure 10.23).

Starting from phenol, aspirin can be easily synthesized by introducing a carboxylic group followed by acetylation, and not the other way around (Figure 10.24).

Published by Woodhead Publishing Limited

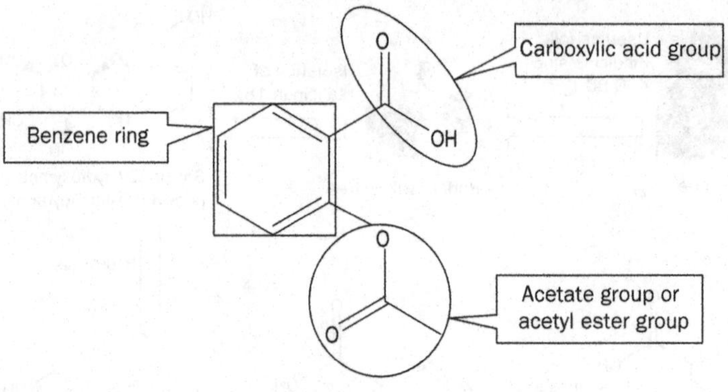

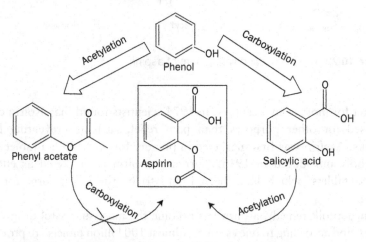

Figure 10.23 Functional groups in aspirin molecule

Figure 10.24 How aspirin is synthesized starting from phenol

In 1898 Hoffmann, a researcher at Bayer, developed the process to make aspirin from salicylic acid by causing it to react with acetic anhydride, which eliminated the corrosive side effects of salicylic acid on the mouth and stomach. The industrial synthesis of salicylic acid had already been streamlined by Kolbe and Schmitt (1874–1884) from sodium salt of phenol using carbon dioxide gas at 150–160 °C under pressure of 5 bar (7 atm). Figure 10.25 shows the industrial production of aspirin from salicylic acid by acetylation.

Aspirin can also be shown to be produced from benzene. Phenol is produced from benzene using different routes, such as benzene to chlorobenzene and chlorobenzene to phenol, or benzene to isopropylbenzene (commonly called cumene) to phenol. The reaction steps are shown in Figure 10.26.

Published by Woodhead Publishing Limited

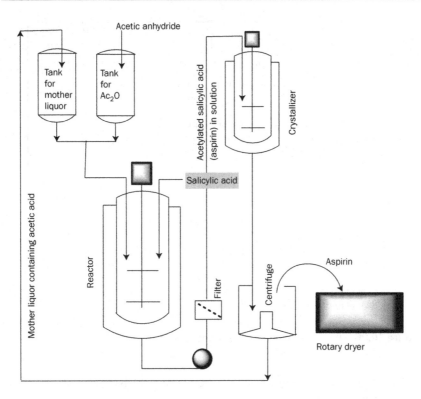

Figure 10.25 Industrial production of aspirin from salicylic acid by acetylation

The conversion of phenol to salicylic acid is a high pressure and temperature reaction with carbon dioxide gas. Most pharmaceutical bulk drug industries get the supply of salicylic acid from the chemical industry and complete the last step of aspirin production themselves. The last step, the acetylation of salicylic acid, is tricky because for the production of bulk drugs, yield and purity are essential to achieve cost-effectiveness.

College laboratory experiments include the reaction of salicylic acid with acetic anhydride using acidic catalysts, such as sulfuric acid or phosphoric acid. Some manufacturers use non-aqueous solvents, or salicylic acid and excess acetic anhydride, as a medium and heat the mixture to around 98 °C in a pressure reactor for 2–3 hours, then crystallize it at around 0 °C to get a reported yield of 90%. An even higher yield of 98% is possible if calcium oxide or zinc oxide is used as a catalyst. As shown in Figure 10.25, the mother liquor can be recycled over and over because the by-product, acetic acid, can also acetylate salicylic acid. It is critical to avoid water or

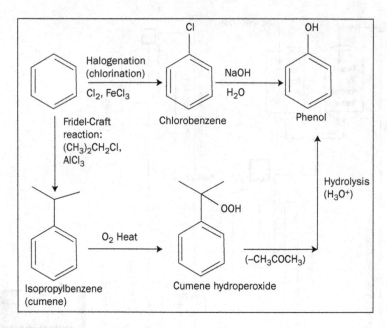

Figure 10.26 The conversion of benzene to phenol

moisture, which can hydrolyze acetylsalicylic acid back to salicylic acid (Figure 10.27).

The overall reactions starting from phenol are shown in Figure 10.28, in which curve arrows illustrate the mechanism. The first step is to make salt of phenol by reacting phenol with sodium hydroxide, and the benzene ring becomes activated for electrophillic aromatic substitution with carbon dioxide. On acidification, sodium salicylate forms salicylic acid. Then the phenolic oxygen of salicylic acid acting as a nucleophile attacks the carbonyl carbon of acetic anhydride, a nucleophilic center.

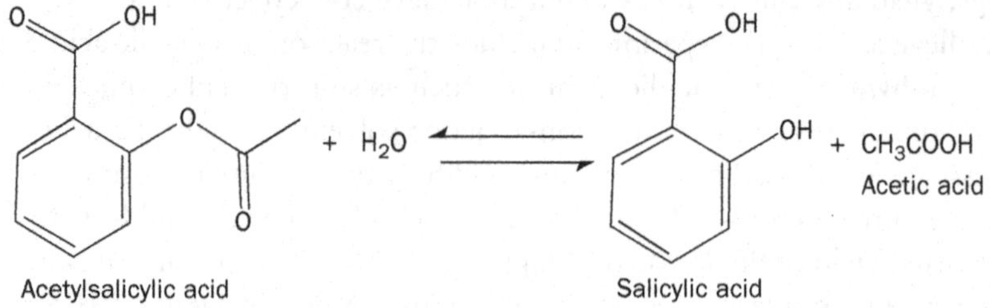

Acetylsalicylic acid   + H$_2$O   Salicylic acid   + CH$_3$COOH
                                                                                          Acetic acid

Figure 10.27 How hydrolysis of aspirin produces salicylic acid and acetic acid in a reversible reaction

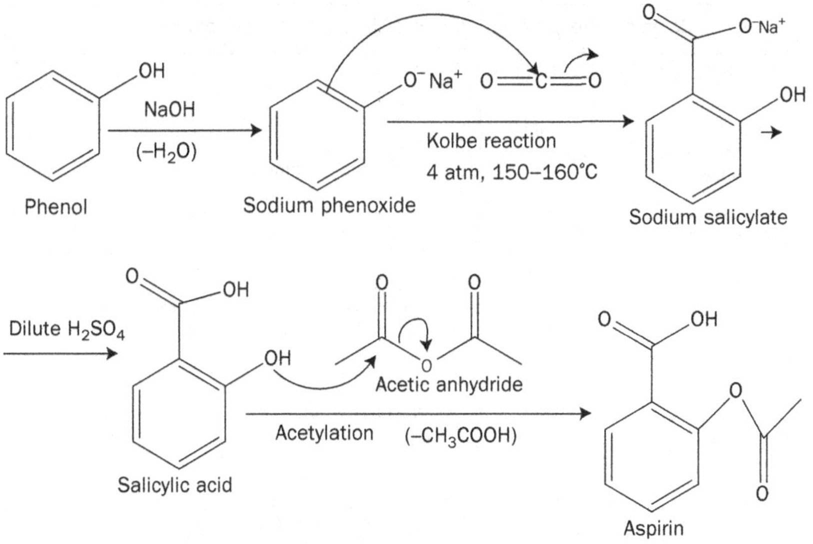

Figure 10.28 The reaction mechanism of production of aspirin

10.2.3 Dosage forms of aspirin

Aspirin is not available in many dosage forms. Because of the nature of acetylsalicyclic acid, which is hydrolyzed easily, no liquid dosage forms are available on the market, but an instant solution can be prepared from a buffered tablet or quick release crystals in powder. Different dosage forms and their strengths are shown in Figure 10.29.

Tablets of aspirin are enteric coated (Figure 10.30). Other than tablets and powder forms, aspirins can be taken as suppositories, insertion into the rectum. This is useful if the patient is unable to take the medicine orally, or if quick action is needed, as the suppository is fast-acting.

10.2.4 The making of aspirin dosage forms

The API of aspirin is acetylsalicylic acid, which is sensitive to moisture and heat. It undergoes hydrolysis in the presence of moisture to produce salicylic acid and acetic acid (Figure 10.31).

Thus in making dosage forms of aspirin, humidity control in the process room is essential and wet processing is not recommended. The dry

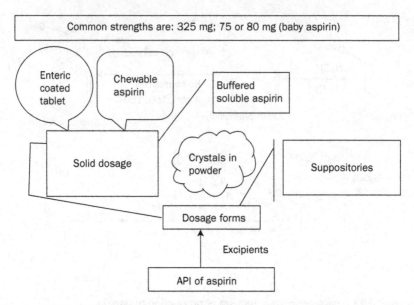

Figure 10.29 Different dosage forms and strength of acetylsalicylic acid

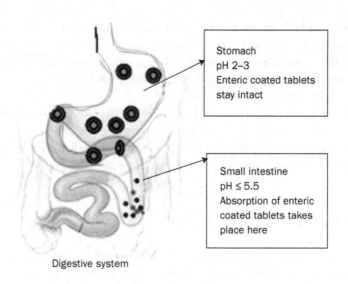

Figure 10.30 Enteric coated tablets and our digestive system

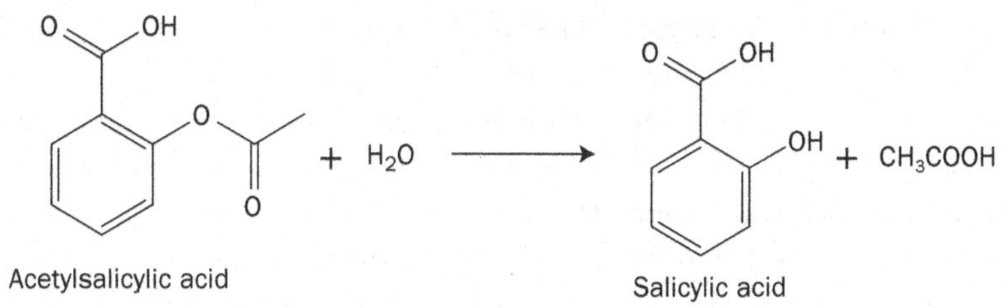

O
‖
   C—OH
      O
      ‖
      O—C—CH₃
                    + H₂O ⟶

O
‖
   C—OH
      OH
                    + CH₃COOH

Acetylsalicylic acid   Salicylic acid

Figure 10.31 Hydrolysis of acetylsalicylic acid in presence of water

compression method is universally used to make different dosage forms of aspirin (Figure 10.32).

Acetylsalicylic acid (ASA) tablets are usually coated with enteric materials. The enteric-coated tablet can pass through the stomach without releasing the active material until it reaches the small intestine, where the tablet starts dissolving. Research studies indicate that enteric-coated tablets of ASA provide a lower incidence of gastrointestinal discomforts or complications than uncoated ASA tablets. Similarly buffered ASA tablets also help prevent stomach discomfort by only dissolving in the higher pH level of the small intestine.

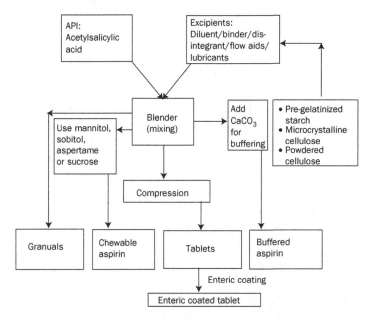

Figure 10.32 How common dosage forms of aspirin are made

Published by Woodhead Publishing Limited

10.2.5 Pharmacology and the kinetics of aspirin

The normal aspirin tablet (without enteric coating), once orally taken, goes into dissolution in the stomach, releasing ASA. In the acidic medium of the stomach, the active ingredient ASA remains ASA (not a salt form) and is absorbed (as it is in the form of ASA) in the stomach and small intestine. Once the ASA is in the blood, it forms acetylsalicylate at the blood pH of 7.4; then its concentration slowly decreases as it starts to convert to salicylate and acetic acid (Figure 10.33). The metabolism of ASA to salicylate is achieved by the enzyme esterases, and the concentration of salicylate slowly increases until within less than an hour it reaches the peak concentration. The salicylate stays in the body for almost 24 hours afterwards.

Before excretion in urine, most salicylates are further converted to different polar water soluble products. About 75% of salicylates are conjugated with the amino acid glycine, forming salicyluric acid, and are then excreted via the kidney. About 10% of salicylates are conjugated with glucuronic acid as salicyl acyl glucuronide and salicyl phenolic glucuronide. A very small portion (1%) is hydroxylated to gentisic acid. The rest is eliminated as free salicylic acid.

Aspirin has been on the market for almost 110 years. Hundreds of scientists have discussed this drug, and research on it continues. Low dose aspirin (baby aspirin, 75 mg or 81 mg) has been developed for antiplatelet action, which is caused by the acetyl group of ASA.

10.2.6 Uses or functions of acetylsalicylic acid

Acetylsalicylic acid has four established functions: acting as an anti-inflammatory, an analgesic, an antipyretic, and an antiplatelet. Recently Prof. K. Schror confirmed the structure and activity relationship for aspirin.[7] The presence of an acetyl group in aspirin not only makes it safe for oral ingestion, but has increased the anti-inflammatory, analgesic, and antipyretic action of salicylic acid. At the same time, the acetyl group has created a new pharmacological action: antiplatelet activity (Figure 10.34).

10.2.7 The mechanism of action of aspirin

The mechanism of aspirin was first described by John Robert Vane, in 1971.[8] Aspirin acts by suppressing the production of prostaglandins and

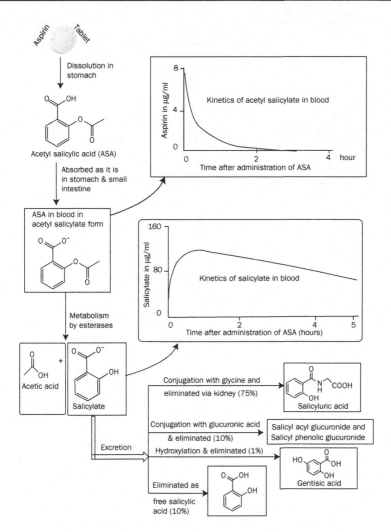

Figure 10.33 The pharmacology and kinetics of acetyl salicylic acid

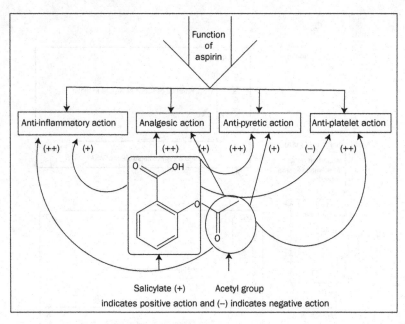

Figure 10.34 The pharmacologic action of aspirin

thromboxane. Prostaglandins are chemical messenger hormones, biochemically produced from membrane phospholipids via arachidonic acid. They have many physiological effects, such as activating inflammatory responses and inducing pain and fever. Thromboxane is also a type of prostaglandin that stimulates aggregation of platelets in response to blood vessel damage or for some other reason. For the biosynthesis of these prostaglandins, the enzyme cyclooxygenase (COX-1 and COX-2) is essential. Aspirin can irreversibly block these COX enzymes, and as a result stop prostaglandin production. Thus anti-inflammatory, antipyretic, analgesic, and antiplatelet actions are achieved. Figure 10.35 illustrates the mechanism of action of aspirin.

Recently, a British pharmacologist named Derek Gilroy discovered an additional pathway for the action of aspirin. Aspirin induces the production of nitric oxide in the blood, which helps to reduce inflammation.

10.2.8   What's new with aspirin after 110 years

It is exciting to think that even after 110 years, research is still being carried out to discover aspirin's additional applications. Studies sponsored by Bayer

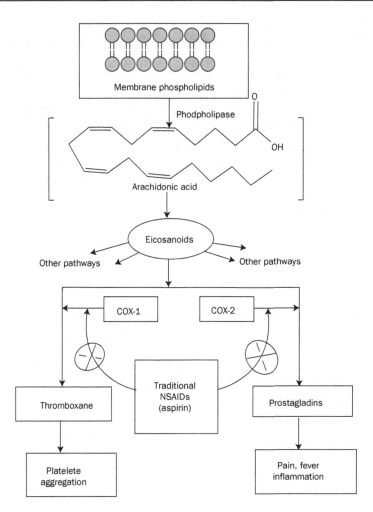

Figure 10.35 The mechanism of the action of aspirin

HealthCare are currently under way on cardiovascular diseases, strokes, pregnancy complications, certain cancers, and dementia. The US FDA has already approved aspirin as treatment for different diseases, including heart attacks, recurrent heart attacks or angina, and stroke prevention.

Practice questions

1. The active metabolite or active form of aspirin is salicylic acid. Why is salicylic acid acetylated to make acetylsalicylic acid (aspirin)?

2. Willow tree barks have salicylic acid but not aspirin. How is aspirin developed?
3. If you store aspirin tablets in an open humid area, the tablets may smell like vinegar. Explain why.
4. The pharmacology and kinetics of aspirin have been well studied. Discuss briefly what happens to aspirin in the body and show the pharmacokinetic profile of aspirin.
5. How do you synthesize aspirin, starting from benzene?
6. Use a flow diagram to show how aspirin is manufactured on a large scale.
7. How does aspirin act as an antiplatelet drug?
8. Discuss low dose aspirin.
9. Can you figure out why the other pathway (acetylation first and carboxylation second) does not work when aspirin is synthesized?
10. Why does phenol form sodium salt of phenol with sodium hydroxide?
11. In the second step in the production aspirin, sodium phenoxide is converted to sodium salicylate reacting with carbondioxide. What type of reaction is it:
    (a) electrophilic aromatic addition
    (b) nucleophilic aromatic addition
    (c) electrophilic aromatic substitution
    (d) nucleophilic aromatic substitution
12. What is the enteric coating on a tablet of aspirin? What purpose does it serve?
13. How is enteric coating applied?

Answers to some practice questions

2. Aspirin is acetylsalicylic acid. Acetylation of salicylic acid produces aspirin.
9. After acetylation, acetoxybenzene is produced; the acetoxy group is electron withdrawing and thus meta directing.
10. Phenol is a weak acid and NaOH is a strong base, thus it forms salt and water.
12. In Greek, enteric means intestine. When a tablet is enteric coated (has a plasticized material coating it), it does not dissolve in the stomach's strong acidic medium and passes unaltered to the small

intestine, where it starts dissolving in the relatively higher pH. Absorption of aspirin takes place in the small intestine. The purpose is to prevent the upset stomach and discomfort possible if aspirin tablets start dissolving in the stomach.

13. After making regular tablets, enteric coating is applied by spraying the solution of coated materials. The materials used for enteric coatings include synthetic plasticized polymers or polysaccharides. Cellulose acetate phthalate is the most commonly used enteric-coated material, the polymeric structure of which is shown in Figure 10.36.

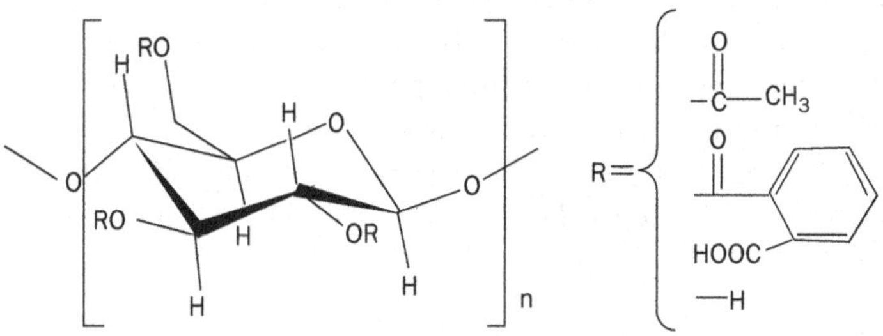

Mixed ester of cellulose: acetate/phthalate/H for R in the structure

Figure 10.36 The polymeric structure of cellulose acetate phthalate

10.3 Paracetemol – the best-selling antipyretic analgesic in the world

Key concept terms

4-Acetamidophenol: the IUPAC name for paracetamol

Acetaminophen: generic name mostly used in USA

Acetylcysteine: antidote for paracetamol overdose or poisoning

Antipyretic: fever reducer

COX: cyclooxygenase

DEG: diethylene glycol (antifreeze); a toxic solvent

EG: ethylene glycol

NAPQI: N-acetyl-p-benzoquinoneimine; a toxic metabolite of paracetamol that can damage hepatic cells

Panadol: brand name of paracetamol used in the UK

Paracetamol: generic name mostly used all over the world except the USA

Tylenol: brand name of acetaminophen used in the USA

There are two generic names for antipyretic analgesics: acetaminophen in the USA (after 4-acetamidophenol) and paracetamol in the UK (after para-acetylaminophenol). Paracetamol is widely used all over the world; its IUPAC name is N-(4-hydroxyphenyl) acetamide. Other commonly used chemical names are N-acetyl-p-aminophenol and 4-hydroxyacetanilide. Figure 10.37 shows the structure of paracetamol.

Since its introduction in the USA in 1955 as Tylenol and Britain in 1956 as Panadol, this medicine has been found in households all over the world.

10.3.1   The discovery of acetaminophen (paracetamol)

There were a number of antipyretic preparations commonly used before acetaminophen, including a decoction of willow bark or cinchona bark. Willow bark is the source of salicin, or salicylates, and cinchona bark is the source of quinine, popularly known as an antimalarial drug. During the 1880s cinchona barks were in short supply, so scientists looked for alternatives. They discovered two alternative drugs, acetanilide and phenacetin. Figure 10.38 shows the early uses of antipyretic drugs.

The introduction of acetanilide in 1886 and phenacetin the following year opened up the road to paracetamol's discovery. The structural similarity of these three drugs is shown in Figure 10.39.

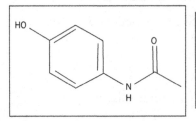
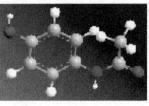

Figure 10.37 The structure of acetaminophen or paracetamol

Published by Woodhead Publishing Limited

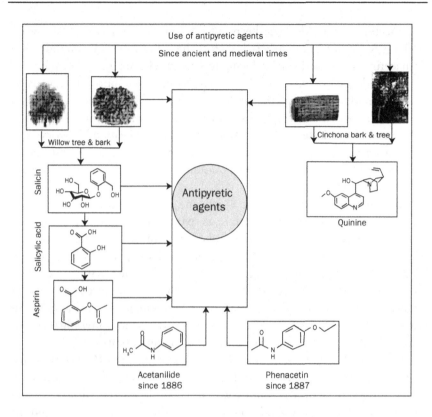

Figure 10.38 Use of antipyretic agents before the introduction of acetaminophen on the market

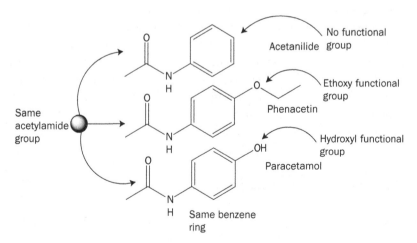

Figure 10.39 The structural similarity between acetanilide, phenacetin, and paracetamol

Paracetamol should have been introduced earlier than 1953, when Sterling & Winthrop marketed it for the first time. Acetanilide and phenacetin were effective in reducing fever and relieving pain, but they had a high incidence of toxic side effects. The former was more toxic, causing cyanosis resulting from methemoglobinemia. It was reported that French chemist Charles Gerhardt synthesized paracetamol in 1852 but did not test it for medical use. Later, in 1878, American chemist Harmon N. Morse also synthesized paracetamol by reducing p-nitrophenol, using tin and glacial acetic acid. Once again, the scientific community did not work to discover the medical uses of the product.

More than a decade later, in 1889, one of the major metabolites of acetanilide was identified in urine as paracetamol. Similar results of metabolic paracetamol were also found in the urine of the patient who had taken phenacetin. Joseph Von Mering published a paper in 1893 based on his clinical research using paracetamol, and he concluded that paracetamol, unlike phenacetin, caused methemoglobinemia. This discovery was a setback in the manufacture of paracetamol, and remained so for another 50 years until Brodie and Axelrod began a systematic investigation of paracetamol and published a paper in 1948 (Figure 10.40).[9]

Brodie and Axelrod's two publications on acetanilide in 1948 in the same journal convinced the medical and scientific community that paracetamol, a major metabolite of acetanilide, was responsible for the antipyretic and analgesic action of acetanilide. However, aniline, a minor metabolite of acetanilide, is responsible for causing methemoglobin formation. The work with phenacetidine also confirmed that phenacetidine is a prodrug and acts via paracetamol. Brodie and Axelrod started advocating the use of paracetamol, and ultimately Sterling Winthrop introduced paracetamol to the market in 1953. Soon after, in 1955, McNiel Laboratories marketed Tylenol, the US brand of paracetamol. The following year, Frederick Stearns & Co, a subsidiary of Sterling Drug Inc, marketed the brand name Panadol in Britain. For the last half century, Tylenol, Panadol, and the generic paracetamol have become household names around the world and can be found in most household medicine cabinets.

10.3.2 The production of bulk paracetamol

Paracetamol is a structurally a simple molecule with two functional groups attached to benzene (Figure 10.41).

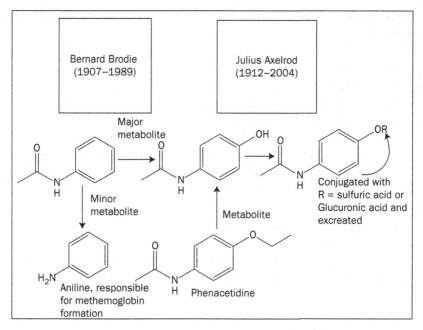

Figure 10.40 Summary of the research by Brodie and Axelrod on paracetamol

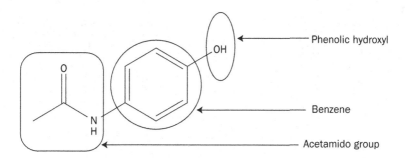

Figure 10.41 The structure of paracetamol

Bulk paracetamol can be produced through different manufacturing routes:

- from p-nitrochlorobenzene
- from phenol
- through the electrolytic reduction of nitrobenzene
- from p-hydroxyacetophenone.

All these methods are currently used to produce paracetamol, but the first route (from p-nitrochlorobenzene route) is the most cost-effective and widely used. All routes have a common method of synthesis, except for the fourth route, which produces p-aminophenol, from which paracetamol is finally manufactured. From p-aminophenol, it is only a one step method, called acetylation.

Figures 10.42–10.44 show the three steps of producing paracetamol from p-nitrochlorobenzene.

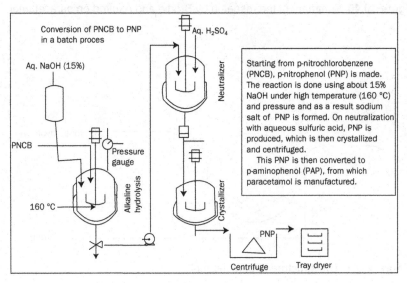

Figure 10.42 The conversion of p-nitrochlorobenzene to p-nitrophenol

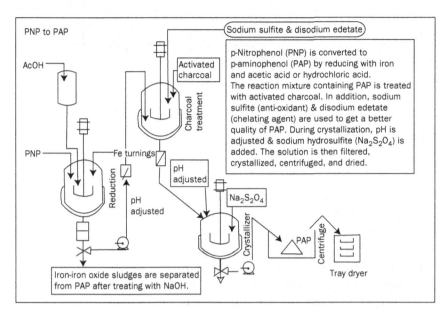

Figure 10.43 The conversion of p-nitrophenol to p-aminophenol

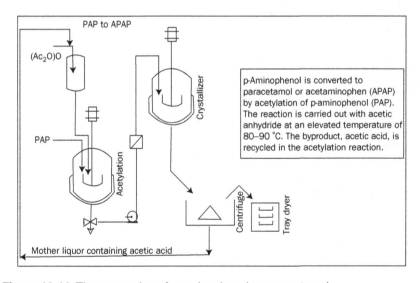

Figure 10.44 The conversion of p-aminophenol to paracetamol

Figure 10.45 shows the reaction chemistry of the production of paracetamol from p-nitrochlorobenzene.

Published by Woodhead Publishing Limited

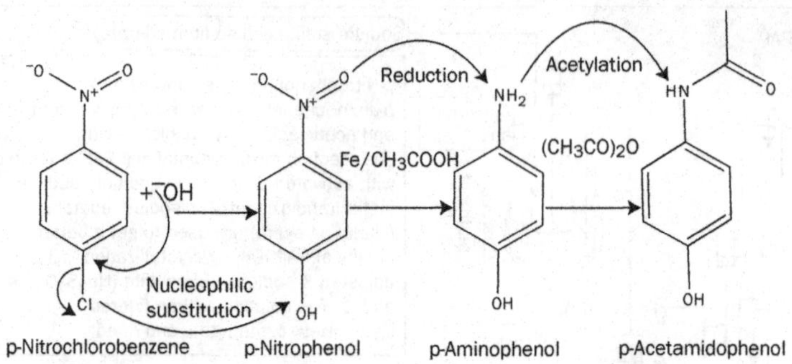

Figure 10.45 Reaction chemistry of the production of paracetamol from p-nitrochlorobenzene

The phenol route (Figure 10.46) is comparatively easy, but produces lower yields than the other routes and is hazardous. The intermediate, nitrosocompound, can explode unless a cool temperature is maintained.

Electrolytic reduction of nitrobenzene to p-aminophenol (Figure 10.47) is pollution-free and produces comparatively higher yields of p-aminophenol. Aniline and acetic acid are by-products, but the process depends on a deoxygenated acid solution, cathode potential, materials, and temperature.

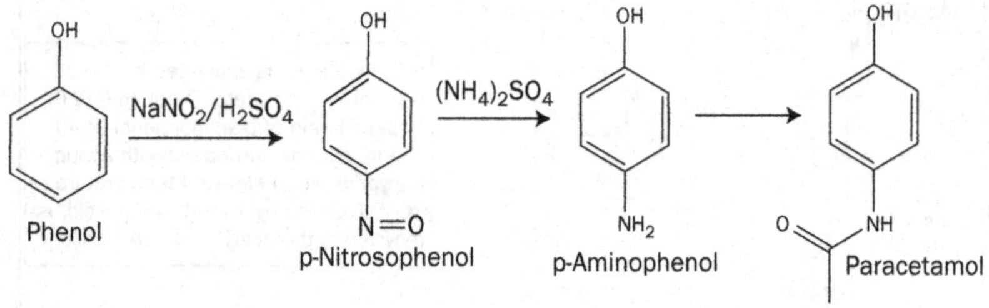

Figure 10.46 The conversion of phenol to paracetamol

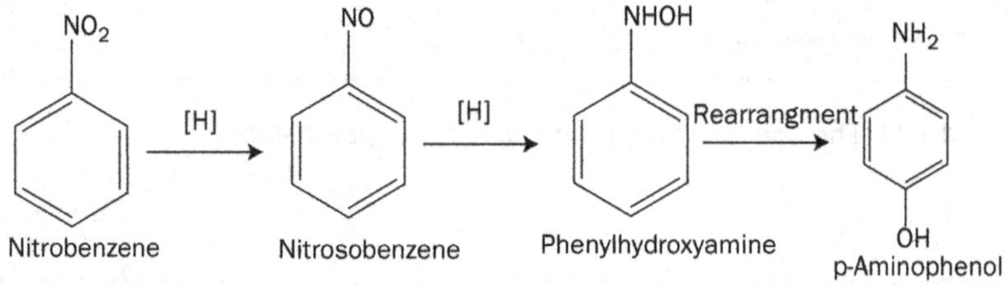

Figure 10.47 Electrolytic reduction of nitrobenzene to p-aminophenol

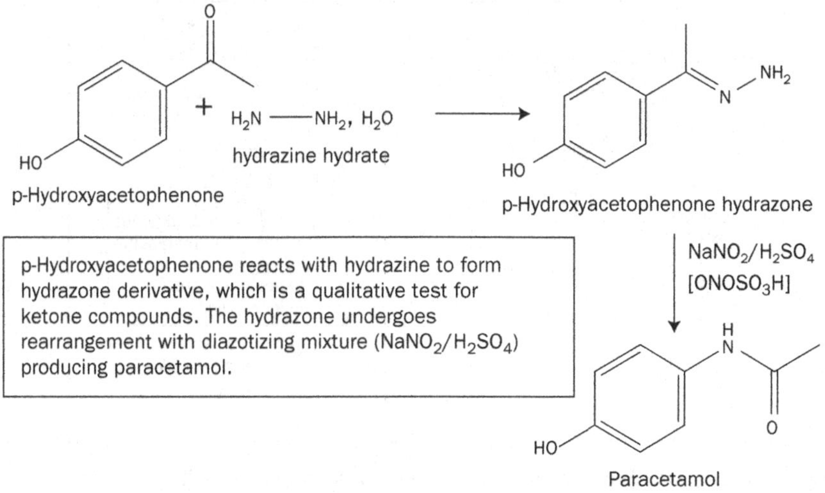

Figure 10.48 Synthesis of paracetamol from p-hydroxyacetophenone

Figure 10.48 illustrates the synthesis of paracetamol from p-hydroxyacetophenone.

10.3.3 Paracetamol toxicity

In general, paracetamol is a relatively safe antipyretic analgesic over-the-counter drug, which has been on the market for more than half a century. However, paracematol has one minor metabolite that is extremely toxic to the liver, and an overdose can be fatal. Normally, 90% of a therapeutic dose is metabolized into a sulfate form, and glucuronide conjugates in the liver and is excreted in urine. The other 10% of the drug is converted to toxic N-acetyl-p-benzoquinoneimine (NAPQI) by the enzyme cytochrome P4502EI. NAPQI can damage hepatic cells, leading to serious liver problems. Fortunately, there is a liver protector called glutathione, which can bind NAPQI, form non-toxic conjugates, and be excreted from the body, but if a person has less glutathione or overdoses on paracetamol, NAPQI will be free to attack the liver. Figure 10.49 illustrates the metabolic pathways of paracetamol and its toxicity.

Acetylcysteine is known to be an antidote for paracetamol poisoning. An injectable form of acetylcysteine (brand name Acetadote) is available in Australia to treat paracetamol overdose.

Published by Woodhead Publishing Limited

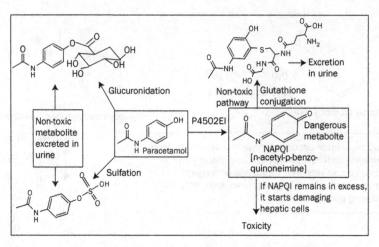

Figure 10.49 Metabolic pathways of paracetamol and its toxicity

10.3.4 The paracetamol tragedy

The deaths from paracetamol that have occurred in many countries are sometimes referred to as the paracetamol tragedy, but the drug itself was not responsible for them. For any dosage form's formulation, excipients need to be added. Paracetamol is not soluble in water, so to make a liquid dosage form of paracetamol, the pharmaceutical industry uses propylene glycol as one excipient to solubilize paracetamol. Some manufacturers with no quality control use a similar type of solubilizing solvent, such as diethylene glycol (DEG) or ethylene glycol (EG), commonly known as antifreeze, which are inexpensive and very toxic. The paracetamol liquid syrup made using toxic DEG or EG is fatal if ingested. The use of these excipients is what caused the deaths. There have been many DEG and EG related deaths since those caused by sulfanilamide elixir in the USA in 1937, some of which are listed in Table 10.1.

Table 10.1 Some diethylene glycol related incidents, 1990–1998

Year	Country	Incident
1990	Nigeria	Acetaminophen syrup containing DEG; 40 deaths
1990–2	Bangladesh	Paracetamol syrup containing DEG; 339 deaths
1998	Bangladesh	Paracetamol syrup for children containing DEG; 24 deaths

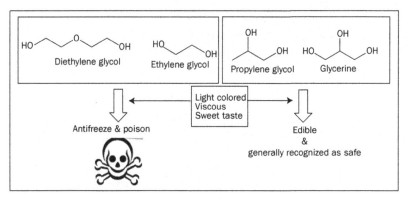

Figure 10.50 The structure and properties of diethylene glycol, ethylene glycol, propylene glycol, and glycerine (glycerol)

DEG and EG are known as nephrotoxins and hepatotoxins and are considered poisonous. Industrially, they are used as antifreeze. In contrast, propylene glycol and glycerine are edible and generally accepted as safe. Propylene glycol and glycerine are used in pharmaceutical formulation, especially in preparing liquid dosage forms, such as syrup. Figure 10.50 illustrates the structure and properties of diethylene glycol, ethylene glycol, propylene glycol, and glycerine (glycerol).

10.3.5　Mechanism of action

Paracetamol is analgesic and antipyretic, but it does not have any significant anti-inflammatory effects. We have seen that aspirin uses all three actions and works by inhibiting the cyclooxygenase (COX) enzymes, COX-1 and COX-2, so that prostaglandins cannot be produced. It seems that paracetamol does not work the same way as aspirin.

Another important fact about paracetamol is that it does not have the gastrointestinal side effects that non-steroidal anti-inflammatory drugs (NSAIDs) usually have. However, recent research has identified a new cyclooxygenase enzyme, COX-3, found in the brain and spinal cord.[10] This COX-3 enzyme can also produce prostaglandins, which ultimately cause pain and fever in the body. Paracetamol can selectively inhibit COX-3 in the brain and spinal cord and thus reduce pain and fever. Figure 10.51 illustrates paracetamol's mechanism of action.

Published by Woodhead Publishing Limited

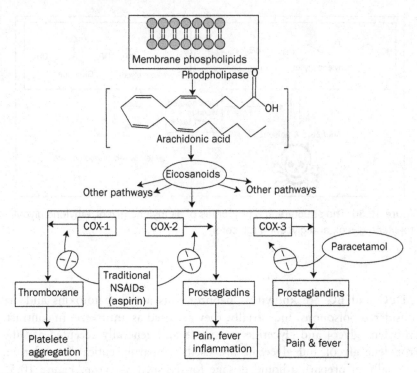

Figure 10.51 The mechanism of action of paracetamol

10.3.6   The dosage forms and kinetic profile of paracetamol

Paracetamol is available in solid dosage forms, such as tablets and capsules, liquid dosage forms, such as solution and suspension, and a semi-solid dosage form (as a suppository). Injectable or infusion paracetamol is not available, although research literature suggests it is possible to make injectable dosage form of paracetamol.[11] When orally taken, paracetamol is rapidly absorbed from the gastrointestinal tract. The maximum blood concentration occurs within 10–90 minutes. A pharmacokinetic profile of paracetamol (Tylenol) is presented in Figure 10.52.

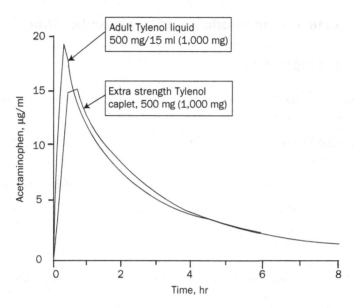

Figure 10.52 Mean pharmacokinetic profile for 24 fasting subjects who received 1,000 mg of acetaminophen dosed as liquid or caplets

Source: Tylenol website[12]

Practice questions

1. Find out the structural similarity of acetanilide, phenacetine, and paracetamol.
2. Synthesize paracetamol starting from benzene.
3. Paracetamol is manufactured using different routes. Name all of them and discuss one particular method of manufacturing paracetamol.
4. Why is the liquid preparation of paracetamol absorbed more quickly than the solid dosage form?
5. Do you think paracetamol toxicity and the paracetamol tragedy have the same causes? Explain both. Is there any antidote for paracetamol toxicity?

Published by Woodhead Publishing Limited

10.4 Ranitidine – the world's leading prescribed drug

Key concept terms

Anti-ulcer drug: histamine H2 receptor antagonist such as ranitidine; used to treat ulcers

Effervexcent tablet: tablet made up of organic acid and bicarbonate that bubbles up when taken in a glass of water

Heartburn: a burning sensation in the chest because of hyperacidity

Histamine: a chemical stimulator released from the main source; mast cells of the gastrointestinal tract

IR: infrared

Mannich reaction: an organic named reaction used in the synthesis of ranitidine; see Figure 10.56

NMR: nuclear magnetic resonance

OTC: over the counter; an OTC drug is one that can be bought over the counter without a prescription

Polymorphism: different physical forms or crystalline forms of the same drug substance; ranitidine has two polymorphs

Tautomer: constitutional isomer; see Figure 10.58

Ranitidine is the generic name of the brand name drug Zantac, an anti-ulcer drug, developed and marketed by GSK in 1981. Hydrochloric acid is produced in the stomach to help digest food, but excess acid causes heartburn. If there is a consistently high acidity in the stomach, ulcers can develop. Ranitidine treats this heartburn-related acidity problem by controlling gastrointestinal acidity.

Pharmacologically, ranitidine is called histamine H2 receptor antagonist. Ranitidine (Zantac) is widely recognized as the 'golden egg' of the pharmaceutical industry, which single-handedly made Glaxo the world's largest pharmaceutical company in 1992. Chemically ranitidine is N[2-[[[5-[(dimethylamino)methyl.]-2-furanyl.]methyl.]thio.]ethyl.]-N'-methyl-2-nitro-1,1-ethenediamine, HCl. It is available over the counter. The structure with its identified functional groups is shown in Figure 10.53.

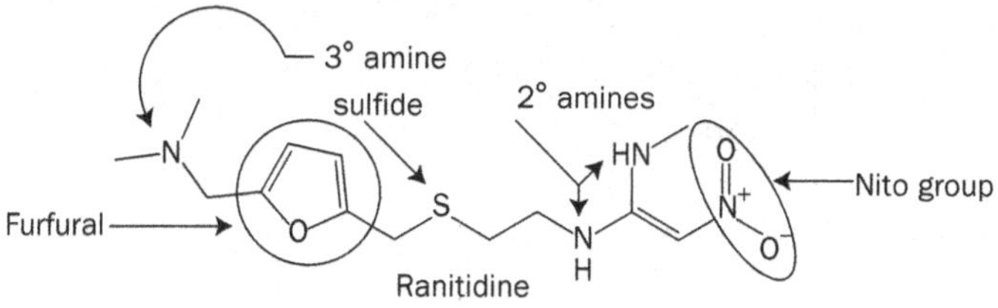

Figure 10.53 The structure of ranitidine

10.4.1 The discovery of ranitidine

A peptic ulcer used to be a common gastrointestinal tract problem. In the 1960s, pharmaceutical companies started to develop medicines to treat them. In this competitive race, the then Smith, Kline & French laboratory (SK&F), led by James Black – a Nobel prize winner, Scottish physician, and pharmacologist, was carrying out the most important research. Black and his co-workers showed for the first time that the histamine H2 receptor influences the secretion of gastric acid, and they began investigations to find a drug that could block the H2 receptor to slow down acid secretion. Figure 10.54 shows how scientists developed cimetidine and ranitidine, and summarizes the characteristics of the drugs.

Black's team synthesized about 200 compounds, structures related to histamine, and surprisingly, only one compound with a guanidine side chain showed some blocking activity in *in-vitro* assays; this small success led the team to find a better analog, which ultimately became the drug called cimetidine. Smith, Kline & French launched cimetidine with the brand name Tagamet in 1976. Thus it took almost 12 years to commercialize the drug after its creation in 1964. Tagamet was the first drug to become a blockbuster drug within six years of being on the market.

The success of cimetidine encouraged other pharmaceutical companies to develop similar ('me-too' drugs) types of drugs with better efficacy. Researchers at the Glaxo Group, led by Sir Jack David, made several H2 receptor antagonists, and one was found to inhibit gastric acid secretion. Not only did the compound inhibit gastric acid secretion, it performed better than cimetidine. The compound called ranitidine, with the trade name Zantac, was introduced to the drug market in Europe in 1981 and 1984 in the USA. During the final stage of manufacturing development, Glaxo had to solve a salt formation from a ranitidine base compound. The initial method involved the use of hydrogen chloride gas from a compressed

Published by Woodhead Publishing Limited

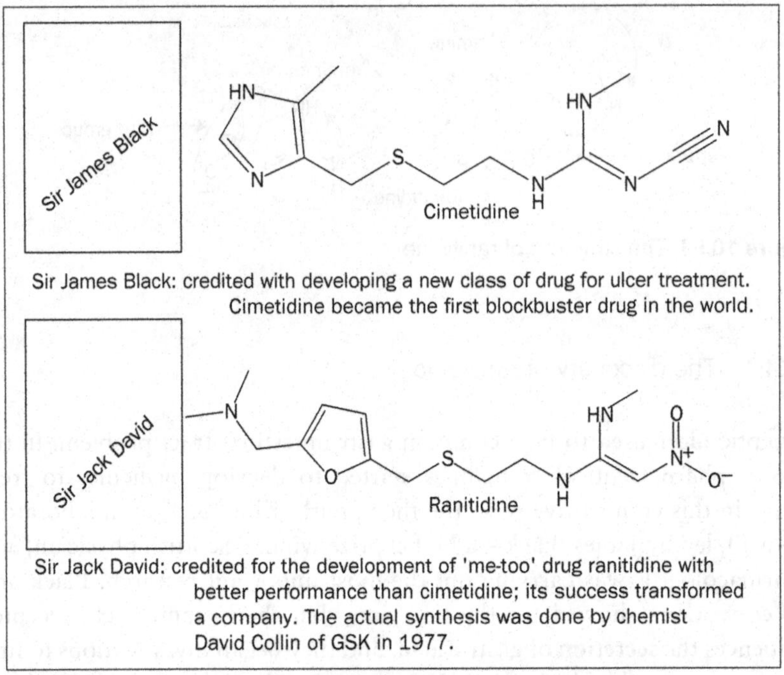

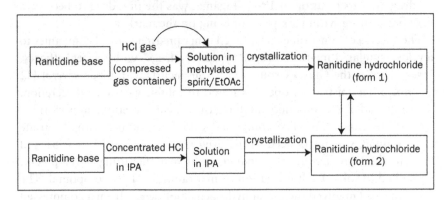

Figure 10.54 Scientists credited with developing cimetidine and ranitidine, and summaries of the characteristics of the drugs

gas container to make ranitidine hydrochloride, known as form 1. This process is hazardous. A better yield and less hygroscopic product was obtained using concentrated hydrochloric acid in isopropyl alcohol, called form 2. Finally, Glaxo used form 2 in its commercial products. The production of polymorphic products is shown in Figure 10.55.

Figure 10.55 The production of polymorphic products of ranitidine

10.4.2   The synthesis of ranitidine

There are many different methods to synthesize ranitidine, most of which have been patented. One of the best methods is described in this section. The starting material for this synthetic process is furfural. All the steps involved are shown in Figure 10.56.

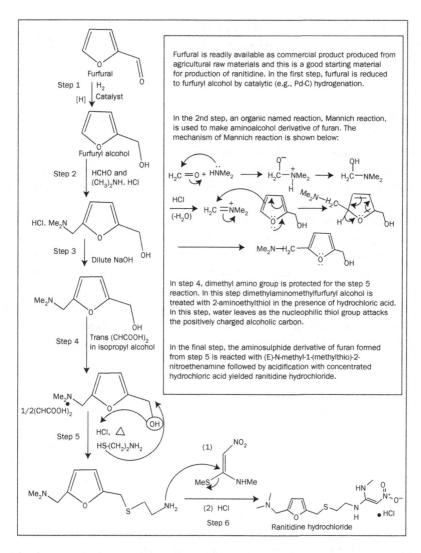

Figure 10.56 The total synthesis of ranitidine starting from furfural

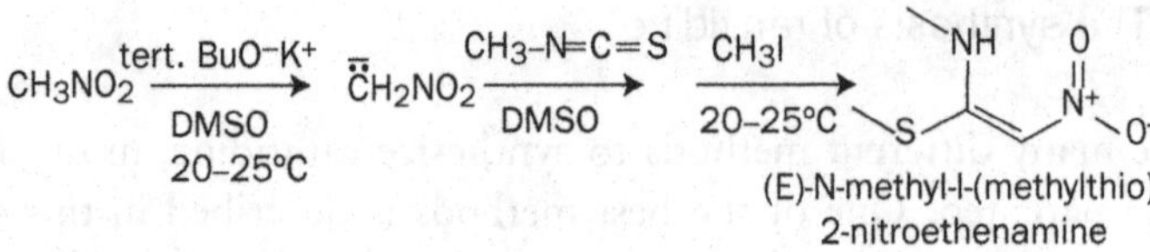

CH₃NO₂ →(tert. BuO⁻K⁺ / DMSO / 20–25°C) CH₂NO₂⁻ →(CH₃–N=C=S / DMSO) →(CH₃I / 20–25°C) (E)-N-methyl-l-(methylthio)-2-nitroethenamine

Figure 10.57 The synthesis of intermediate (E)-N-methyl-1-(methylthio)-2-nitroethenamine

In the last step, one intermediate, (E)-N-methyl-1-(methylthio)-2-nitroethenamine, is used, which can be prepared from nitromethane as shown in Figure 10.57.

10.4.3 Polymorphism in ranitidine

The phenomenon in which some crystalline chemical compounds can exist in two or more different crystalline phases or physical forms is called polymorphism, and each crystalline form is known as a polymorph. The formation of a polymorph can be controlled by the nature of solvents, crystallization techniques, and rates of cooling during crystallization. Polymorphism is an important aspect of a drug substance because each polymorph of the same drug can be patented. Guidelines of the International Conference on Harmonization of Technical Requirements for Registration of Pharmaceuticals for Human Use (ICH) classify the features of solid drug substances as solvated forms and amorphous forms. There are no polymorphs in amorphous powders. Sometimes polymorphs can have slightly different melting points, chemical properties, solubility characteristics, dissolution rates, and bioavailability.

Ranitidine hydrochloride exists as two polymorphs, popularly called form 1 and form 2. GSK has the US patent for both forms – form 1 in 1978 and form 2 in 1985 – and GSK markets exclusively form 2. A number of generic pharmaceutical companies, including NovoPharm and GenPharm, wanted to market a generic version of form 1 immediately after the expiry of the form 1 patent in 1995. GSK sued these two companies on the grounds that their generic products contained a mixture of form 1 and form 2 and not a pure form 1. GSK won the case and continued its marketing exclusivity until 2002 when the patent of form 2 expired.

Ranitidine form 1 is crystallized from ethylacetate and has a melting point of 134–140 °C; form 2 is crystallized from a mixture of isopropyl alcohol and hydrochloric acid and has a melting point of 140–144 °C.

There is no difference in solubility and bioavailability between the two forms, or in therapeutic efficacy, but there are some advantages in the production of form 2 ranitidine, especially during filtration and drying of bulk powders. Structurally, ranitidine has two tautomeric forms (Figure 10.58); form 1 is an enamine tautomer and form 2 is mostly a nitronic acid tautomer.

The two forms of ranitidine can be identified by infrared (IR), nuclear magnetic resonance (NMR), Raman spectroscopy, and X-ray powder diffractometry. It was found that X-ray diffraction, Raman spectroscopy, and Diffuse Reflectance Infrared Fourier Transform Spectroscopy (DRIFTS) are all suitable to distinguish between form 1, and form 2 of ranitidine HCl.

10.4.4 Mechanism of action and metabolism

There are parietal cells in the stomach, which make and secrete hydrochloric acid. There are three receptors in parietal cells, which can be stimulated for acid secretion by:

- acetylcholine
- gastrin
- histamine (H2 type receptor).

One of the stimulators, a common chemical, such as a histamine, is released from the main source – the mast cells of the gastrointestinal tract (GIT). The histamine then binds with the H2 receptor of parietal cells and starts

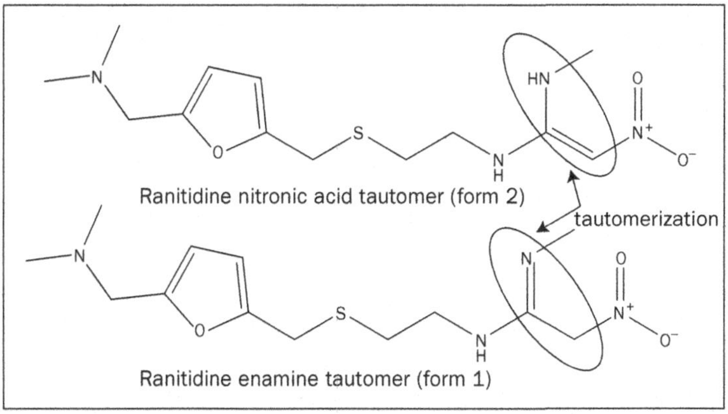

Ranitidine nitronic acid tautomer (form 2)

tautomerization

Ranitidine enamine tautomer (form 1)

Figure 10.58 Tautomeric forms of ranitidine

Published by Woodhead Publishing Limited

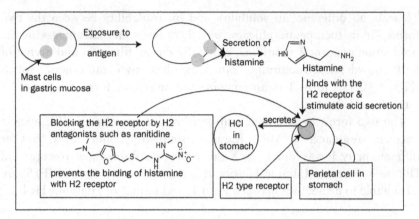

Figure 10.59 The mechanism of action of ranitidine

secreting hydrochloric acid. The detailed mechanism is somewhat complex; a simplified flow sheet of acid secretion is presented in Figure 10.59. Interestingly, the thought, taste, and smell of food as well as eating food can instigate this stimulation and enhance the secretion of histamine, which helps to initiate secretion of acid via the H2 receptor.

Ranitidine, as an H2 blocker or antagonist, can block the H2 receptor so that histamine cannot bind with the receptor and as result acid secretion is reduced in the stomach. Hyperacidity can thus be controlled.

Ranitidine is quickly absorbed after oral administration and reaches peak concentration within a couple of hours. Most of the ranitidine is eliminated and ends up as stool, but 10–35% of the ranitidine is metabolized in the liver and produces a derivative of N-oxide, S-oxide, and N-desmethyl ranitidine (Figure 10.60).

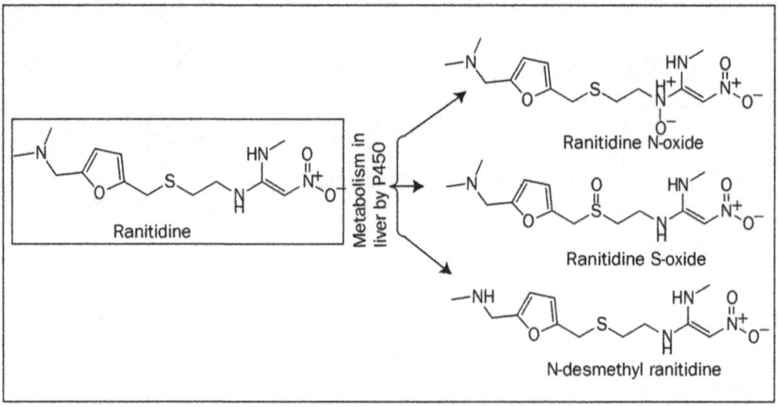

Figure 10.60 The metabolism of ranitidine

10.4.5 Dosage forms of ranitidine

There are different dosage forms of ranitidine (Zantac), which are shown in Figure 10.61.

The tablet form has different strengths, ranging from 25 mg to 300 mg. There are also 25 mg effervescent tablets that need to be dissolved in water before consumption. One important aspect of ranitidine is its approval as an over-the-counter (OTC) product since it was previously a prescription-only medicine (POM). After reviewing the overall safety of marketed ranitidine, the US Food and Drug Administration (FDA) has given it an OTC approval in 75 mg tablets.

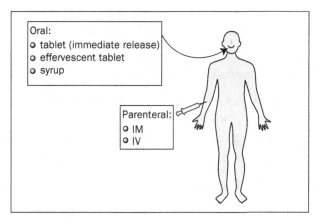

Figure 10.61 Dosage forms of ranitidine

Practice questions

1. Do you think ranitidine is one of the 'me-too' drugs? Explain.
2. Polymorphism is an important phenomenon used in the marketing of Zantac (ranitidine). Discuss the situation in relation to the polymorphic forms of ranitidine.
3. Why is Zantac (ranitidine) now an OTC drug? On what basis does the US FDA approve which drugs should be available on prescription only and which available over the counter?

Published by Woodhead Publishing Limited

4. What happens to ranitidine molecules in the body? Discuss its metabolism.
5. Why is ranitidine called antihistamine?

10.5   Ciprofloxacin – the best-selling antibacterial in the world

Key concept terms

Fluoroquinolone: fluorinated quinolone compound, for example ciprofloxacin

Grohe cycloaracyclation: one cyclic reaction in the synthesis of ciprofloxacin developed by Grohe while working in Bayer

Immediate release tablet: regular tablet that undergoes disintegration and dissolution immediately after being taken

Klauke compound: 2,4-dichoro-5-fluorobenzoyl chloride, the starting intermediate for synthesizing ciprofloxacin

Malonic ester synthesis: a simple textbook type of reaction used in the synthesis of ciprofloxacin; see Figure 10.65

Nalidixic acid: the first quinolone antibacterial drug developed by Lesher

Norfloxacin: the first fluoroquinolone antibacterial drug developed in Japan

NSAID: non-steroidal anti-inflammatory drug

Structure and activity: when each functional group of a molecule has some activities in the overall drug action, for example ciprofloxacin

XR tablet: extended release tablet; a tablet that works for a longer period of time than usual as the drug is released slowly at a predetermined rate

Ciprofloxacin is the generic name of a widely used antibacterial, known by the brand names Cipro, Ciprobay, and Ciproxin, and discovered by Bayer of Germany. It is a fluoroquinolone drug available as monohydrochloride monohydrate. Chemically, it is named 1-cyclopropyl-6-fluoro-1, 4-dihydro-4-oxo-7-(1-piperazinyl)-3-quinolinecarboxylic acid. Figure 10.62 illustrates the structure of ciprofloxacin indicating all different groups.

Ciprofloxacin is a completely synthetic product, thus it is termed as antibacterial rather than antibiotic, which means that part of or the full product comes from a living organism. However, antibacterials and antibiotics are similar in function.

10.5.1   The discovery of ciprofloxacin

The discovery of ciprofloxacin was the result of continuous efforts to find a better fluroquinolone since the discovery and development of nalidixic acid – a quinolone drug developed in 1962 by George Lesher and his co-workers. Lesher was an organic chemist who used to work at the Sterling Winthrop Institute, an American subsidiary of Bayer. While working to synthesize chloroquine in 1946, Lesher's team isolated a by-product called nalidixic acid. Later, they confirmed the antibacterial activity of nalidixic acid. After almost 16 years, Lesher organized clinical trials for kidney infection. Finally, nalidixic acid with the brand name Neggram became the first quinolone drug available in 1964 for urinary tract infections.

Since the introduction of nalidixic acid in 1964, there had been over 10,000 analogues of quinolones and fluroquinolones synthesized before Bayer introduced the super fluoroquinolone ciprofloxacin to the market in 1987. The scientist who began working on the fluoroquinolone project

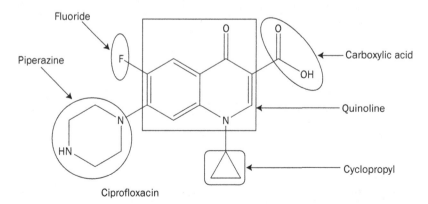

Figure 10.62 The structure of ciprofloxacin

was not successful initially and was transferred to another project. However, Klaus Grohe did not quit his earlier project and continued working without his superior's knowledge. Meanwhile, in 1978 a Japanese firm, Kyorin Pharmaceuticals, discovered the first fluoroquinolone, norfloxacin. In 1980 Dr Grohe attended a conference in Japan where a scientist from Kyorin Pharmaceuticals gave a talk on norfloxacin. The structure of norfloxacin is very similar to ciprofloxacin, except that an ethyl group, instead of cyclopropyl group, is attached to a nitrogen ring of norfloxacin (Figure 10.63). From earlier work experiences with fluoroquinolones, Dr Grohe knew that a cycloproyl group attached to the fluoroquinolones enhanced antibacterial activity. Klaus Grohe was excited and decided to introduce a cyclopropyl group in the N-ring of the structure of norfloxacin. He enlisted the help of another chemist, Hans-Joachim Zeiler, and together they were successful in synthesizing norfloxacin with a cyclopropyl ring attached to nitrogen of bicyclic ring. Thus, Bayer created ciprofloxacin.

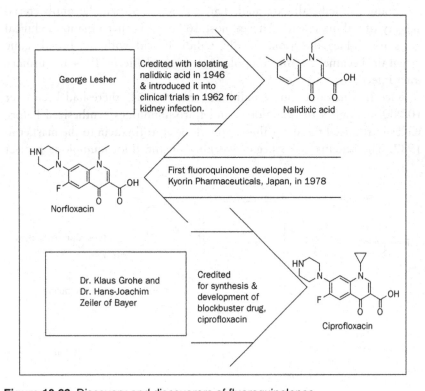

Figure 10.63 Discovery and discoverers of fluoroquinolones

10.5.3 The synthesis of ciprofloxacin

The synthesis of ciprofloxacin is fairly simple and straightforward. It starts from 2,4-dichloro-5-fluorobenzoyl chloride (known as the Klauke compound) except for a cyclization reaction (Figure 10.64), which was discovered at the Bayer laboratories by Grohe (known as Grohe cycloaracyclation reaction).

The starting intermediate, 2,4-dichloro-5-fluorobenzoyl chloride, can be synthesized from another intermediate, 2,4-dichloro-5-aminotoluene. The very first reaction of 2,4-dichloro-5-aminotoluene is a textbook reaction of diazotization, which is then coupled with a dimethylamine. The triazine compound reacts with an anhydrous hydrogen fluoride at elevated temperatures to produce 2,4-dichloro-5-fluorotolune. The next reaction is a light-induced free radical reaction followed by acidification, which is then treated with thionyl chloride to produce 2,4-dichloro-5-fluorobenzoyl chloride (Figure 10.65).

In the next phase of synthetic reactions, beginning with 2,4-dichloro-5-fluorobenzoyl chloride (Klauke compound) (Figure 10.65), there are basically two important objectives: synthesis of 6-fluoroquinolinic acid (6-FQA) via cycloaracyclation of the Klauke compound, and addition of piperazine to 6-FQA to synthesize ciprofloxacin. Figure 10.66 illustrates all the synthetic reactions used in the production of ciprofloxacin.

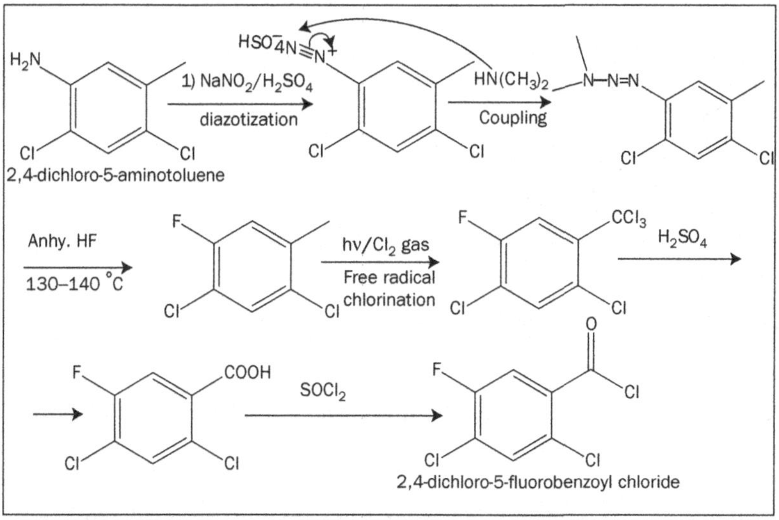

Figure 10.64 The synthesis of ciprofloxacin

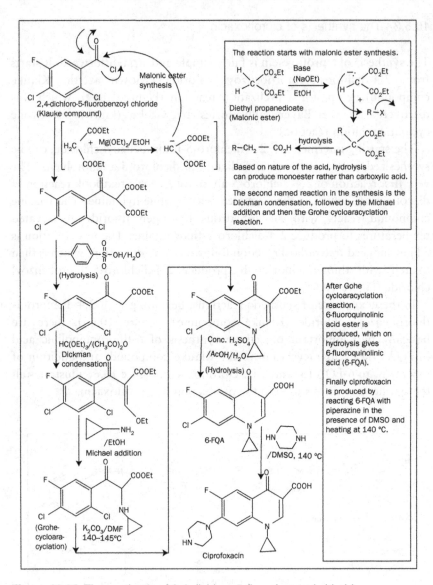

Figure 10.65 The synthesis of 2,4-dichloro-5-fluorobenzoyl chloride

10.5.4 The mechanism of action and structure and activity relationship of ciprofloxacillin

Ciprofloxacillin is a broad spectrum fluoroquinolone antibacterial. It is bactericidal (it kills bacteria). Bacteria use their own enzymes for different

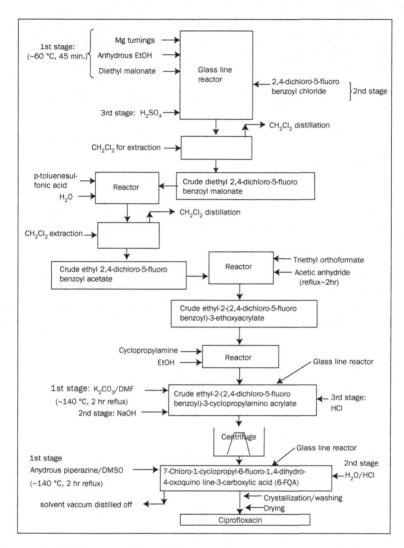

Figure 10.66 The production of ciprofloxacin

functions, such as the formation of cell walls, synthesis of protein or replication, repair, and the transcription of DNA. In DNA-related activities, bacteria use DNA gyrase enzymes. Ciprofloxacin in its action inhibits or blocks DNA gyrase enzymes and topoisomerase, and as a result the bacteria's cell death occurs.

There are a number of functional groups in the ciprofloxacin molecule, each of which is important in the molecule's overall performance. Actual

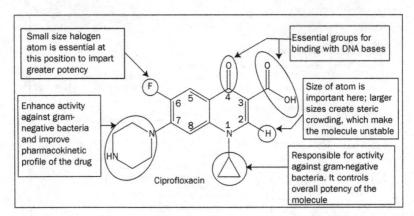

Figure 10.67 The structure and activity relationship of ciprofloxacin

binding takes place through the polar carboxylic and ketone groups with the DNA gyrase. The structures and the activity relationship of ciprofloxacin are shown in Figure 10.67.

10.5.5 Dosage forms of ciprofloxacin

Ciprofloxacin has been on the market since 1987 and generic versions of ciprofloxacin are available. Figure 10.68 illustrates the dosage forms available for ciprofloxacin.

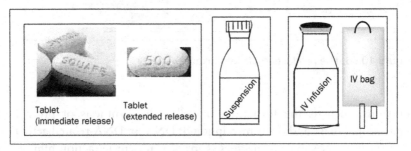

Figure 10.68 Different dosage forms of ciprofloxacin

Tablets have:

- *an active ingredient* – ciprofloxacin
- *excipients* – cornstarch, microcrystalline cellulose, silicon dioxide, crospovidone, magnesium stearate, hypromellose, titanium dioxide, and polyethylene glycol.

Tablets with extended release have:

- *an active ingredient* – ciprofloxacin
- *inactive ingredients* – crospovidone, hypromellose, magnesium stearate, polyethylene glycol, silica colloidal anhydrous, succinic acid, and titanium dioxide.

Oral suspension has:

- *an active ingredient* – ciprofloxacin micronized
- *excipients* – povidone, methacrylic acid copolymer, hypromellose, magnesium stearate, and Polysorbate 20; diluent is medium-chain triglycerides, sucrose, lecithin, water, and strawberry flavor.

Intravenous forms have:

- *an active ingredient* – ciprofloxacin
- *excipients* – lactic acid as a solubilizing agent, and hydrochloric acid for pH adjustment.

Practice questions

1. Find out what functional groups are present in the ciprofloxacin molecule. What functions do each of the functional groups have in the overall drug action of ciprofloxacin?
2. The synthesis of ciprofloxacin involves many textbook type reactions as well as a few interesting newly developed reactions. Describe the total synthesis of ciprofloxacin.
3. Why is ciprofloxacin called an antibacterial drug rather than an antibiotic?
4. Explain how ciprofloxacin kills bacteria.

Notes

1. Royal Society of Chemistry, 'Discovery and Development of Penicillin', www .rsc.org/Chemsoc/Activities/ChemicalLandmarks/International/Penicillin.asp, and American Chemical Society, 'Discovery of Penicillin', http://portal.acs.org/ portal/acs/corg/content_nfpb=true&_pageLabel=PP_ARTICLEMAIN&node_ id=926&content_id=CTP_004451&use_sec=true&sec_url_var=region1&__ uuid=98624b40-bcf9-49bb-8b70-4cfe04bc6a77.
2. R. van Furth, *β-lactam Antibiotics: Past, Present And Future*, Delft: Gist Brocades (DSM), [n.d.].
3. Ibid.
4. Fred N. Eshelman and Daniel A. Spyker, 'Pharmacokinetics of amoxicillin and ampicillin: crossover study of the effect of food', *Antimicrobial Agents and Chemotherapy*, Vol. 14, No. 4, 1978, pp. 539–43; Daniel A. Spyker et al., 'Pharmacokinetics of amoxicillin: dose dependence after intravenous, oral, and intramuscular administration', *Antimicrobial Agents and Chemotherapy*, 1977, pp. 132–41.
5. See Bayer, 'Expect wonders', 2010, www.wonderdrug.com/historical_photos .html (accessed October 5, 2010).
6. Aspirin Foundation, 'What is aspirin?', [n.d.], www.aspirin-foundation.com/ what/100.html (accessed September 25, 2010).
7. Karsten Schror, 'The pharmacology of aspirin', Bayer Healthcare, Aspirin Update at International Press Workshop, Bitterfeld, June 2008, http://news .viva.vita.bayerhealthcare.com/fileadmin/user_upload/Charts_Schroer_ June_19.pdf (accessed February 15, 2011).
8. John R. Vane, 'Inhibition of prostaglandin synthesis as a mechanism of action for aspirin-like drugs', *Nature New Biology*, Vol. 25, No. 231, 1971, pp. 232–35.
9. Bernard B. Brodie and Julius Axelrod, 'The fate of acetanilide in man', *Journal of Pharmacology and Experimental Therapeutics*, Vol. 94, No. 1, 1948, pp. 29–38; and Bernard B. Brodie and Julius Axelrod, 'The estimation of acetanilide and its metabolic products, aniline, N-acetyl p-aminophenol and p-aminophenol (free and total conjugated) in biological fluids and tissues', *Journal of Pharmacology and Experimental Therapeutics*, Vol. 94, No. 1, 1948, pp. 22–28.
10. N. V. Chandrasekharan et al., 'COX-3, a cyclooxygenase-1 variant inhibited by acetaminophen and other analgesic/antipyretic drugs: cloning, structure, and expression', *Proceeding of National Academy Science*, 99, 2002, pp. 13926–31.
11. FreshPatents.com, 'Patent application title: injectable liquid paracetamol formulation', Patent # 20090215903, August 27, 2009.
12. Redrawn from www.tylenolprofessional.com/pharmacology.html#Pharmaco kineticData (accessed October 5, 2010), with permission from Johnson & Johnson (McNeil Consumer Healthcare).

11

Life-style drugs, statins, and COX-2 drugs

Sildenafil citrate

Atorvastatin

Celebrex

Vioxx

Learning objective

In this chapter students will find out about life-style drugs, statins, and COX-2 drugs:

- how these drugs were discovered
- who directed the research towards successes
- how the drugs are synthesized
- how they work
- what dosage forms are available.

Key concept terms

Blockbuster drug: sale of a drug reaching US$1 billion per annum

COX-2 drug: cyclooxygenase-2 inhibitor drug used for treating pain and inflammation

HMGCoAR: hydroxymethylglutaryl coenzyme A reductase, which is involved in the production of cholesterol; Lipitor inhibits the action of this enzyme

Life-style drug: drugs used for non-medical or minor conditions, e.g. Viagra and other erectile dysfunction drugs such as livitra and cialis

'Me-too' drug: a drug that is structurally similar to a known marketed established drug; livitra and cialis are 'me-too' drugs of Viagra

NSAID: non-steroidal anti-inflammatory drug

Paal-Knorr pyrrole synthesis: when 1,4-dicarbonyl compounds react with ammonia or primary amines to produce pyrrole; this reaction is used in the synthesis of Lipitor

PDF5: phosphodiesterase-5 enzyme; Viagra acts by inhibiting this enzyme

Statin drug: a new class of cholesterol reducing drugs; Lipitor, a statin drug became a super blockbuster drug

Stereoisomer: three dimensional aspects of an organic molecule; one stereoisomer, 3R, 5R, is active out of four stereoisomers of Lipitor

11.1   An introduction to sildenafil citrate (Viagra)

Sildenafil citrate is a generic name for Pfizer's brand name drug Viagra. Its chemical name is 1-[[3-(6,7-dihydro-1-methyl-7-oxo-3-propyl-1*H*pyrazolo [4,3-*d*.] pyrimidin-5-yl)-4-ethoxyphenyl.] sulfonyl.]-4-methylpiperazine citrate. Figure 11.1 shows its structural formula.

Sildenafil citrate is the citrate salt of sildenafil and as a result it is water-soluble (3.5 mg/ml). Pfizer's Viagra tablet is blue in color but sildenafil citrate's actual color is white to off-white. This drug created a new therapeutic field and was the first drug to make US$1 billion in sales in the first full year after marketing.[1] It is a drug for men only, for adult males with erectile dysfunction. For a drug with a limited consumer base, it is a huge success, continuing with billion dollar sales every year.

There are two other 'me-too' drugs (structurally similar to known marketed established drugs) on the market: vardenafil (Livitra) and tadalafil (Cialis) (Figure 11.2).

Published by Woodhead Publishing Limited

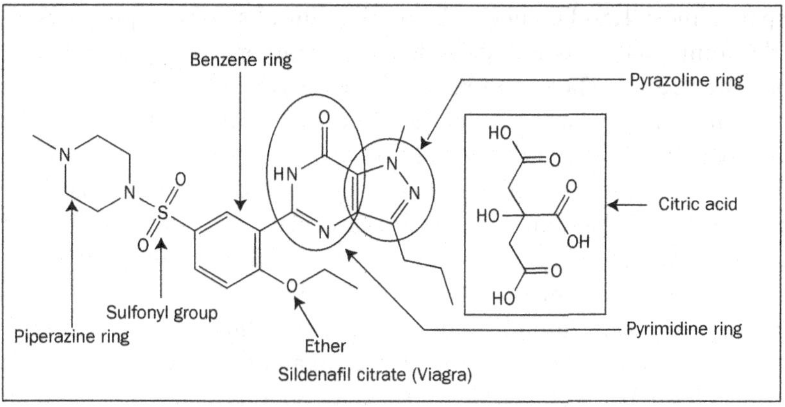

Figure 11.1 The structure and functionality of sildenafil citrate

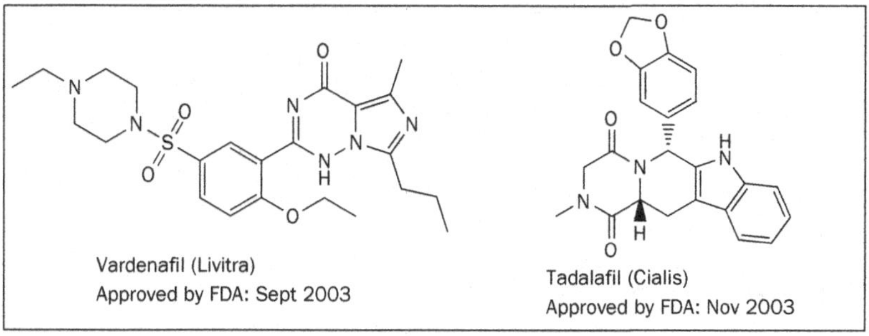

Figure 11.2 The life-style drugs vardenafil and tadalafil

11.2 Discovery of sildenafil citrate

The discovery of sildenafil citrate (Viagra) is a unique and fascinating story. From the Viagra story, new generations of pharmaceutical scientists can learn how prepared minds and scientific knowledge can turn a failure into a success. The history of the discovery of Viagra is also a good example of teamwork and connecting the dots of interdisciplinary sciences.

In 1985, scientists at Pfizer's research facility in Sandwich, England, decided to start a project of finding a new chemical entity to treat cardiovascular diseases, especially hypertension, but later on focused on angina, a symptom of ischaemic heart disease. Simon Campbell, head of the research division, initiated the project proposal. A team of 15 chemists and biologists started working, increasing to 40 by 1989. The team managed to

Published by Woodhead Publishing Limited

prepare almost 1,500 compounds for pre-clinical screening purposes. One of the compounds was today's sildenafil citrate, or Viagra, given the code name UK-92,480. The team finally selected only one compound (sildenafil citrate) for clinical trials. Sildenafil citrate was synthesized by Peter Dunn and Albert Wood in 1989 (Figure 11.3).

It was a nine-step synthesis, and they produced enough material to perform the clinical test. In choosing this particular UK-92,480 compound, the team used previously discovered information of the pyrazolopyrimidinone class of compounds made by Peter Ellis, David Brown, and Nicholas Terrett, which were found useful in treating angina. Pre-clinical studies with the compound showed a very powerful and selective inhibitor for the phosphodiesterase type-5 (PDE5) enzyme. So this new compound of a

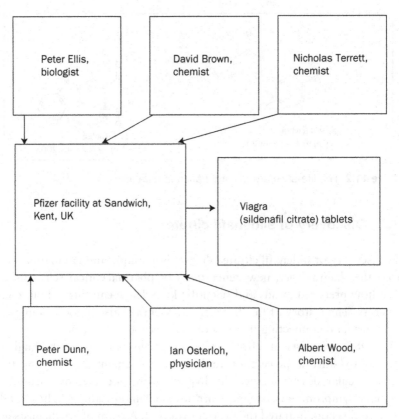

Figure 11.3 Key persons involved in the development of sildenafil citrate (Viagra)

Published by Woodhead Publishing Limited

similar class may treat angina better by inhibiting the PDE5 enzyme, which breaks down the cyclic guanosine monophosphate.

The phase I clinical trial began in early 1991, using single dose regimens in healthy volunteers to find out the compounds' safety and vasodilating effects. After completion of phase I trial, the team concluded that the compound was fairly safe to use and had a moderate effect on the blood vessel for a short time in the healthy volunteers. It was considered promising and the team decided to use multiple dose regimens.

The team tried the second phase I clinical trial using multiple doses (three times a day) on healthy volunteers. Although some unexpected side effects of penile erection were reported from the results of that trial, no one took the side effect seriously at that time. The Pfizer team tried for phase II with a small number of patients using multiple doses. Ian Osterloh, who was studying the effect of UK-92,480 with nitrates, the standard treatment for angina, directed one of two clinical trials.

The results indicated that UK-92,480 did enhance the effect of the nitrates, but blood pressures went down too low. The prospect for angina treatment using UK-92,480 was no longer encouraging enough to continue further clinical trials. Pfizer was about to close down the angina project because by that time millions of dollars had already been spent. However, the team had observed unusual behavior in patients. Patients did not want to return the unused tablets of UK-92,480, in fact, some wanted to have more of the medicine. The side effect of penile erection was such that patients wanted to continue taking the medicine, especially those who had problems with impotency. The team members considered future courses of action.

Team members Peter Ellis, Nicholas Terrett, and Ian Osterloh thought that the compound UK-92,480 might work for erectile dysfunction, and fortunately there were other studies around that time revealing more information about the biochemical pathways of penile erection. The team also understood how their drug could help in stimulating penile erection and finally decided to go forward with a clinical trial, using patients with erectile dysfunction.

A new chapter in the clinical trials had begun as no one had conducted this type of trial before. The researchers set up a control group for the first pilot study. According to Osterloh's own language, 'In the initial study, the men watched erotic videos while a device monitored girth and hardness of their penises. The initial results were encouraging and showed the drug was much more effective than a placebo.'[2]

Pfizer did not want to miss the opportunity to become a pioneer by quickly marketing the drug in the fairly open field of impotency. The company accelerated its research, and gradually increased staff numbers to

Published by Woodhead Publishing Limited

get the drug to the market quickly: 15 people were working on the drug in 1985, and 500 in 1997, when Pfizer applied for registration with the US Food and Drug Administration (FDA). Figure 11.4 gives a summary of the discovery of soldenafil citrate.

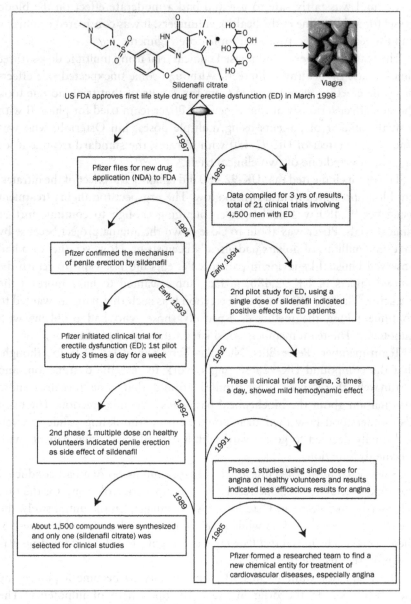

Figure 11.4 Summary of the development of soldenafil citrate

11.3   Synthesis of sildenafil citrate

The synthesis of sildenafil (Viagra) can be started with a simple molecule of 2-pentanone (I). In the presence of base (NaOEt/EtOH), a Claisen ester condensation with diethyloxalate (II) produces 1,3-diketo ethylester (III) (Figure 11.5). The International Union of Pure and Applied Chemistry's (IUPAC's) name of this compound is ethyl 2,4-diketoheptanoate.

The diketoester reacts with simple hydrazine, producing a cyclic five-membered heterocyclic ring called a pyrazole ring, which is the key intermediate in this synthesis. The mechanism of the pyrazole ring formation involves the nucleophilic attack of nitrogen of hydrazine to carbonyl carbon followed by dehydration. The actual name of the compound (IV) is 3-propylpyrazole-5-carboxylic acid ester. The methylation of the compound IV using dimethylsulfate at a temperature of 20–60 °C produces N-methyl pyrazole ester (V), which in alkaline hydrolysis yields a stable compound commonly known as pyrazolic acid (VI) (Figure 11.6).

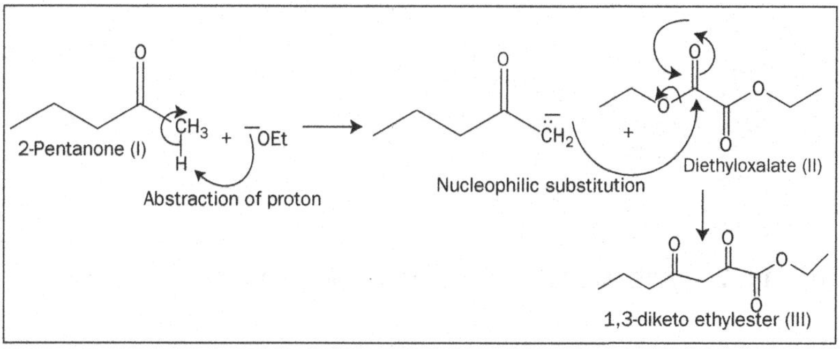

Figure 11.5 Claisen condensation in the initial synthesis of soldenafil citrate

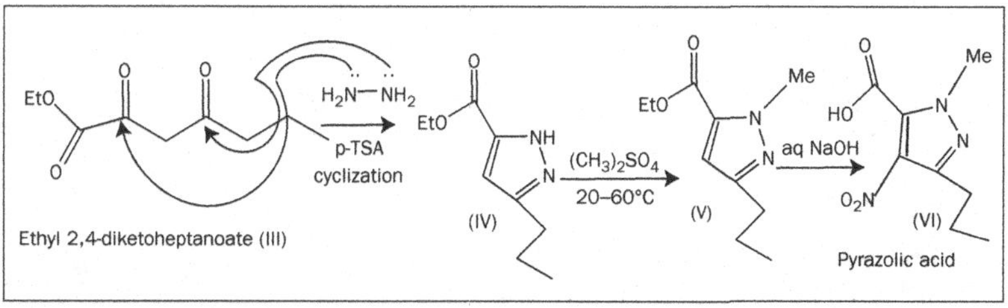

Figure 11.6 Synthesis of pyrazolic acid, the key compound of sildenafil citrate

Published by Woodhead Publishing Limited

The pyrazolic acid (VI) is then nitrated using a mixture of concentrated nitric acid and concentrated sulfuric acid. Nitro pyrazolic acid (VII) is then converted to the corresponding amide (VIII) by treating it with thionyl chloride and then with ammonia, which is reduced in the next step to aminopyrazolamide (IX) (Figure 11.7).

The IUPAC name of this compound is 4-amino-1-methyl-3-propylpyrazole-5-carboxamide. These reactions seem to be very simple, but on a manufacturing scale, the product yield in each step is low. There are thus many alternative routes. One of the best is shown in Figure 11.8.

Another intermediate is produced starting with 2-ethoxybenzoic acid. This reacts with chorosulfonic acid and then N-methylpiperazine to produce the intermediate (B). This second intermediate (B) is condensed with the first intermediate (A). The cyclization of the condensed product in the presence of a strong base, potassium tert-butaoxide yields sildenafil. On acidification with citric acid, a salt form of sildenafil (sildenafil citrate) is produced. The total systhesis is presented in Figure 11.9.

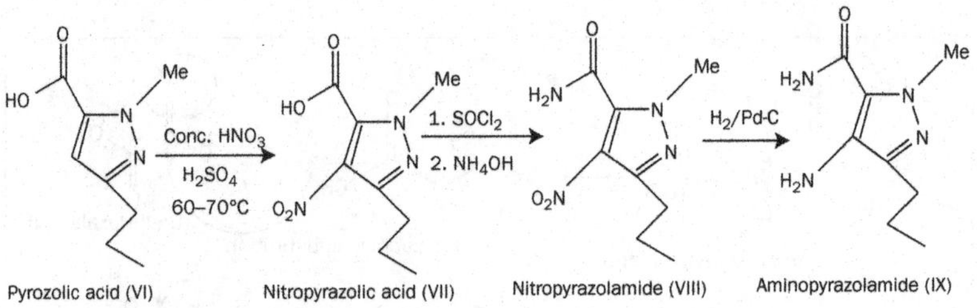

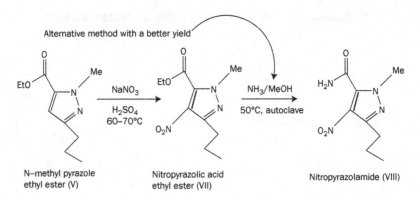

Figure 11. 7 Synthesis of aminopyrazolamide from pyrazolic acid

Figure 11.8 Alternative method to make nitropyrazolamide (VIII)

Published by Woodhead Publishing Limited

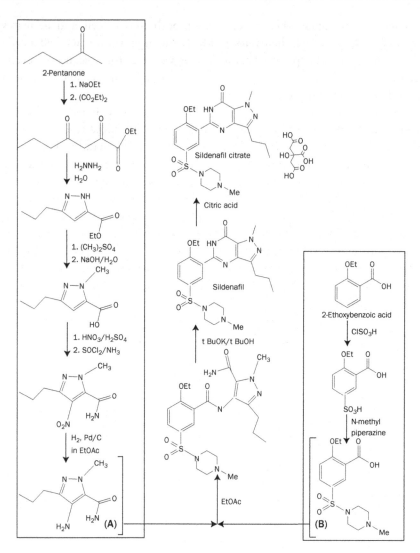

Figure 11.9 Total synthesis of sildenafil citrate

11.4 How does sildenafil work in the body?

One simple gaseous compound, nitric oxide (NO), the biomolecule, cyclic guanosine monophosphate, and the PDE5 enzyme are instrumental in the mechanism of sildenafil. Whenever a man is sexually stimulated, the brain sends signals through the nerves ending in the corpus cavernosum tissue around the penis. Immediately, a biochemical reaction takes place where L-argenine is deaminated to citruline and NO by NO synthase. The chemical nitric oxide then enters the smooth muscle cell and activates guanyl cyclase, which helps to produce the important chemical cyclic guanosine monophosphate. This acts as a vasodialator. Because of cyclic guanosine monophosphate, the blood vessels in the penis become wider and blood gushes in and there is an erection.

An important consideration is how long an erection will last, and nature comes to the rescue. There is an enzyme called phosphodiesterase-5, which regulates the concentration of cyclic guanosine monophosphate by hydrolyzing it to guanosine 5'monophosphate (5'-guanosine monophosphate) and the erection disappears. Normally this is what happens to the able adult male. However, in the case of men with erectile dysfunction, the presence or concentration of cyclic guanosine monophosphate is very important and can only occur by inhibiting PDE5 so that it cannot hydrolyze cyclic guanosine monophosphate. When the optimal concentration of cyclic guanosine monophosphate accumulates, it does its job to widen the blood vessels so that blood can cause the erection. The mechanism is presented in Figure 11.10.

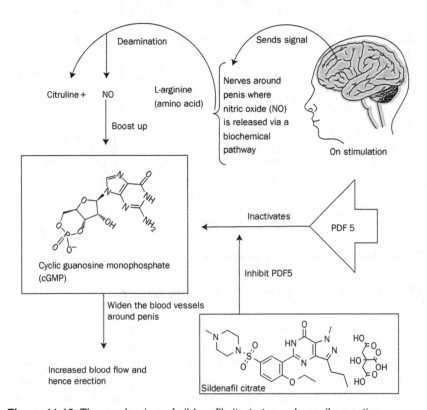

Figure 11.10 The mechanism of sildenafil citrate towards penile erection

Published by Woodhead Publishing Limited

11.5   Dosage form of sildenafil citrate

Sildenafil is only available in a tablet solid dosage form, with three different strengths – 25 mg, 50 mg, and 100 mg (Figure 11.11). The tablets are film coated a blue color and are diamond shaped.

By 2012, Pfizer's patent for sildenafil will expire and there will be generic versions available on the market. One pharmaceutical company has already developed an oral spray form of sildenafil citrate to market immediately after the Pfizer's patent expiration. The US FDA has already approved sildenafil citrate to treat other conditions, such as pulmonary hypertention, and Pfizer started marketing a 20 mg tablet with the brand name Revatio. Recently an injectable form of Revatio (10 mg) was made available on the market.

Once swallowed, Viagra tablets undergo rapid absorption with a peak plasma concentration within 30–120 minutes (median 60 minutes). Figure 11.12 shows the pharmacokinetic profile after the administration of a single oral dose of 100 mg to a healthy male volunteer.

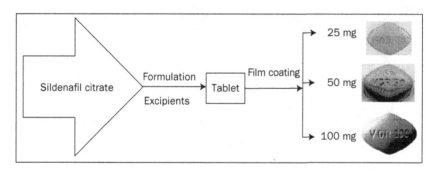

Figure 11.11 The tablet dosage form of Viagra

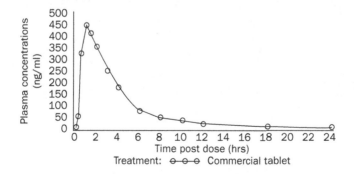

Figure 11.12 Mean sildenafil plasma concentrations in healthy male volunteers

Source: Reproduced with permission from Pfixer's Viagra website[3]

11.6　Atorvastatin – a brief introduction

Atorvastatin (brand name Lipitor) is a cholesterol-reducing drug. This lipid-lowering medicine has become the most successful and biggest blockbuster drug in the world. In 2009, Lipitor brought in over US$13 billion dollars in sales for Pfizer. Lipitor's sales since its introduction in 1997 are shown in Figure 11.13.

Though the development of anticholesterol drugs started with the compounds isolated from fungus, Lipitor is a synthetic drug. The chemical structure with its functional groups is shown in Figure 11.14.

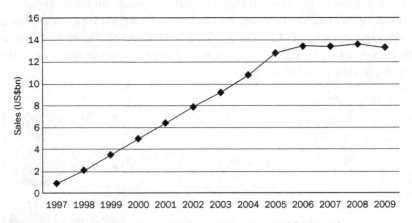

Figure 11.13 Worldwide sales of Lipitor, 1997–2009 (US$ billion)[4]

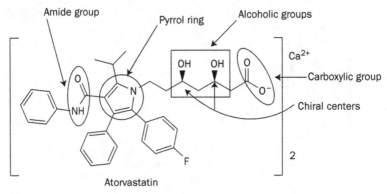

Figure 11.14 Structure of atorvastatin calcium salt (Lipitor)[5]

Published by Woodhead Publishing Limited

11.7 Discovery of atorvastatin

Many heart-related problems start with an increased level of blood cholesterol, so a drug to reduce blood cholesterol level would be a big revenue earner. Pharmaceutical scientists know that hydroxymethylglutaryl-coenzyme A reductase (HMG CoAR or HMGCR) catalyzes the biosynthesis of cholesterol. An effective inhibitor of HMGCR is able to reduce cholesterol formation. The person credited with the development of the first HMGCR inhibitors is Akira Endo, a Japanese biochemist who screened 600 fungal metabolites to find one during 1971–1973 while working at the Sankyo Co. One of the metabolites from *Penicillium citrinum* was mevastatin, the first compound of the statin class to inhibit HMGCR.

Endo's work inspired Merck. Merck's natural product division headed by Roy Vagelos started working on a statin project in 1976, and after two years researchers identified lovastatin from *Asperigillus terreus* in 1978. Nine years later, Merck introduced lovastatin as mevacor in 1987. After only one year, Merck launched another statin drug, simvastatin, with the brand name Zocor. A simple analogue of lovastatin, simvastatin earned blockbuster status within a few years. Meanwhile, Sankyo and BMS together developed and marketed pravastatin (brand name Pravacol) in 1991 and Novartis launched fluvastatin (brand name Lescol) in 1994. The statin market was no longer empty – four brands shared the market, with Zocor in the leading position. Figure 11.15 summarises the contributions of some scientists responsible for developing statin drugs.

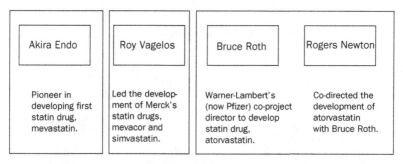

Figure 11.15 Scientists responsible for the development of statin drugs

Published by Woodhead Publishing Limited

The story of another statin drug begins with Bruce D. Roth. After finishing one year of a post-doctoral fellowship at Rochester University, Roth, an organic chemist, joined Parke Davis, a division of Warner-Lambert around 1982. He worked on pyrrole synthesis and was interested in anticholesterol drugs; he was soon made co-chair of the statin project. Roth and his colleagues became successful in synthesizing one drug in 1985 that inhibited HMGCR. However, the compound was a racemic mixture, and they found that the (–) stereoisomer was inactive and only the (+) stereoisomer was 100% active. To make the drug more potent, they needed to get only the (+) stereoisomer, which was not simple at that time. Roth's team spent a couple of months looking for a methodology to make the stereo-selective product. Finally they solved the problem by causing a reaction under a very low temperature (80°C). Scaling up was also a tedious job; it took 3 weeks to get from the raw materials to the final product of (+) atorvastatin calcium.

Donald Black, vice president of clinical research, guided the clinical trials. The initial trial started with 10 mg and 80 mg tablets on 24 employees or volunteers. The results were astonishing when compared with those of competitors such as Zocor and mevacor. A titanic drug was born. Almost a small library's worth of documents was created for its new drug application (NDA) to the US FDA (Figure 11.16).

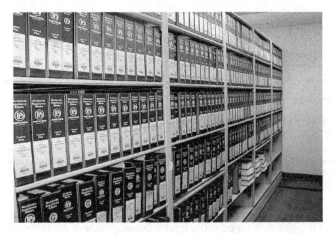

Figure 11.16 Files submitted for a new drug application for Lipitor

Source: Reproduced with permission from Pfizer

11.8   Synthesis of atorvastatin calcium

The commercial synthetic route developed by Pfizer:

- is highly convergent
- uses Paar-Knorr pyrrole synthetic process
- has one cryogenic reaction (around minus 90 °C)
- requires a special jacketed reactor to perform cryogenic reaction.

11.8.1 The Paal-Knorr pyrrole synthesis

Carl Paal and Ludwig Knorr published the Paal-Knorr pyrrole synthesis, a process used in the synthesis of atorvastatin, in 1885. Pyrrole is a condensation or cyclization of 1,4-dicarbonyl compounds with excess of ammonia or primary amines. The total synthesis is illustrated in Figure 11.17.

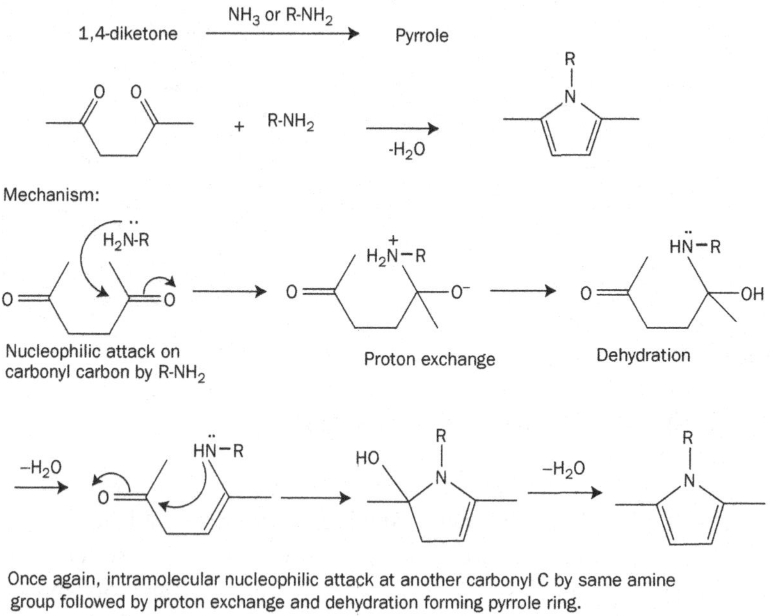

Once again, intramolecular nucleophilic attack at another carbonyl C by same amine group followed by proton exchange and dehydration forming pyrrole ring.

Figure 11.17 The total synthesis of atorvastatin calcium

Published by Woodhead Publishing Limited

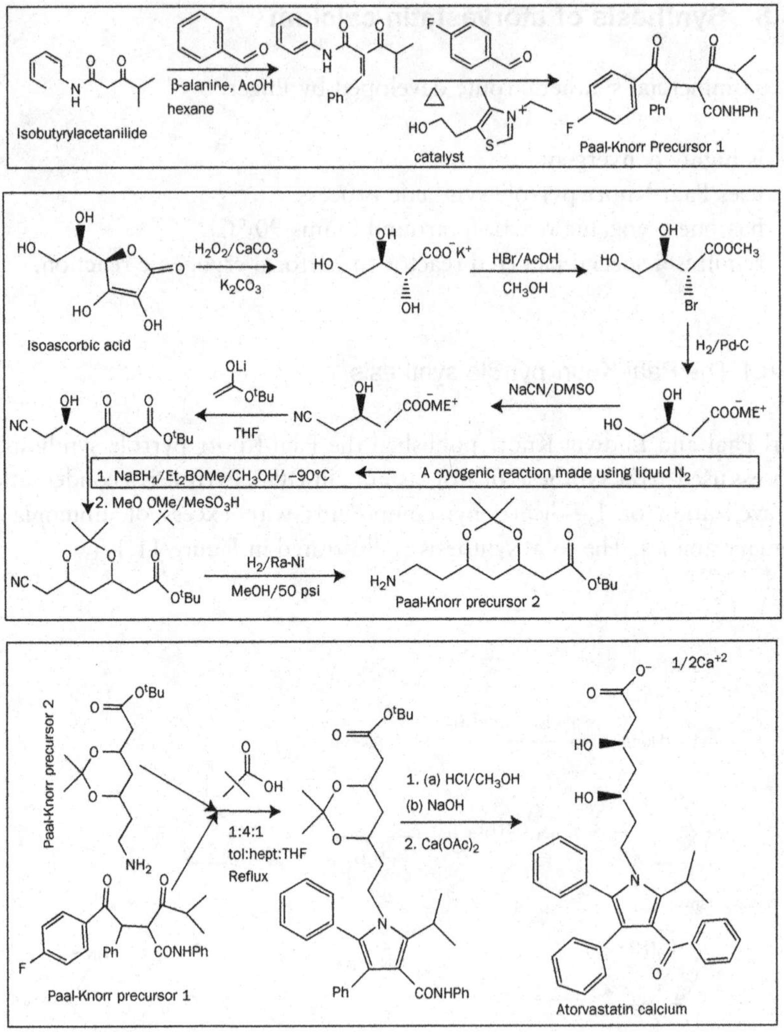

Figure 11.17 (Cont'd)

11.9 Stereochemistry and atorvastatin

The stereochemistry and the decision of its inventor Bruce Roth made atorvastatin a US$10 billion per year blockbuster drug. When an organic molecule or drug contains a chiral center, it can have two stereoisomeric forms. Atorvastatin has two chiral centers, so it has four stereoisomers, out of which only one stereoisomer is active in inhibiting HMGCG. Roth decided to use only the active form to have a minimum amount of drug for its action and to avoid side effects from other stereoisomers.

11.9.1 Stereochemistry

Stereochemistry is the study of three-dimensional aspects of an organic compound. The compound in three-dimensional form shows an interesting property when we see the compound in the mirror. For example, left hand becomes right hand in the mirror and they are not superimposable on each other (Figure 11.18).

Certain organic compounds also show this non-superimposability to its mirror image and they become two stereoisomers, which are not identical, called enantiomers. The compound that has this non-superimposable mirror image is called a chiral compound. A chiral molecule must not have the plane of symmetry. There is one distinguishable property of these stereoisomers, called optical activity. The chiral molecules can rotate plane polarized light either clockwise or counter clockwise.

Chemists use different nomenclatures to identify these stereoisomers. If one mirror image is identified as R, the other image will be S. This R and S nomenclature is based on their absolute configuration. Based on their optical rotations, if one is identified as dextro-rotatory or (+) or d, the other one will be levo-rotatory or (−) or l. The enantiomer that rotates plane polarized light clockwise or towards the right is called dextro-rotatory. The number of stereoisomers depends on the number of chiral carbon or center: the number of stereoisomers = 2^n where n is the number of chiral centers.

The four stereoisomers of atorvastatin are shown in Figure 11.19. Only one is active.

The stereoisomer 3R, 5R out of four is biologically active, but the others are not active at all. Human bodies are highly asymmetric or chiral, and it is no wonder that the body's proteins, enzymes, or other receptors are particularly enantiomer selective. The pharmacological activity of drugs depends on how the drugs interact with proteins, enzymes, receptors, nucleic acids, or biomembranes. Figure 11.20 illustrates the interaction

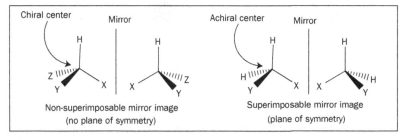

Figure 11.18 Non-superimposable and superimposable mirror images of chiral molecules

Published by Woodhead Publishing Limited

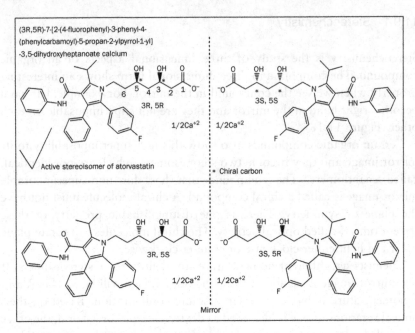

Figure 11.19 Stereoisomers of atorvastatin

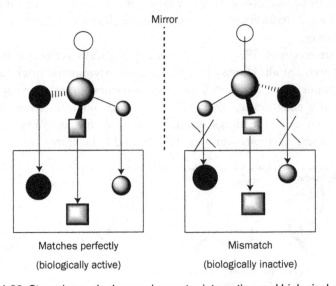

Matches perfectly
(biologically active)

Mismatch
(biologically inactive)

Figure 11.20 Stereoisomeric drug and receptor interaction and biological activity

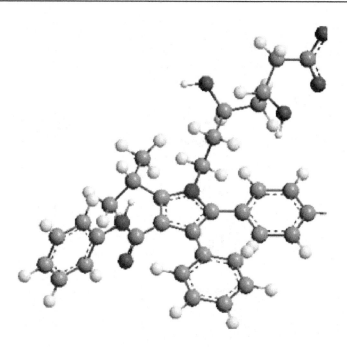

Figure 11.21 3D structure of atorvastatin (anion form)

between stereoisomeric drugs and biological receptors. The left structure has a good fit compared with the right one. See also the 3D structure of atorvastatin shown in Figure 11.21.

11.10   Mechanism of action of atorvastatin

Figure 11.22 presents a family of statin drugs. The journey of developing statin drugs began with the discovery and marketing of mevastatin. Developments of other statins were mainly based on mevastatin and lovastatin. All the structures of statin drugs have similar active sites and work in similar mechanisms.

Cholesterol is a very important biomolecule for our body, but an excess of low-density lipoprotein is bad and can lead to atherosclerosis. To reduce the low-density lipoprotein content in our body and increase the high-density lipoprotein is so far the only solution. The biosynthesis of cholesterol

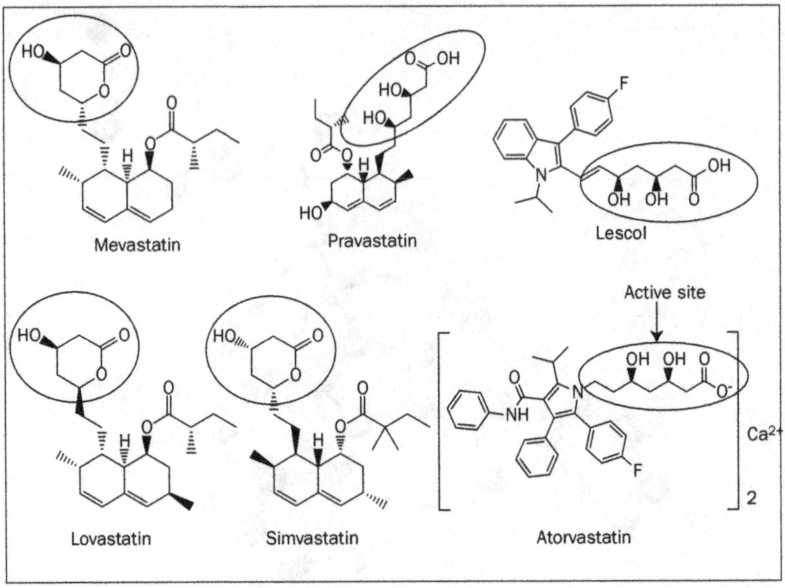

Figure 11.22 A family of statin drugs

illustrates the mechanism of how statins act (Figure 11.23). It involves more than a dozen biosynthetic steps as it has many beneficial effects on our body.

Cholesterol is very vital for the development of memory and function of our brain, and a precursor of important biomolecules such as vitamin D, some hormones, and bile acids.

All steps in the biosynthesis of cholesterol are important, but the production of mevalonate is considered a key step in regulating the biosynthesis. Mevalonate is produced when the HMG-CoA (3-hydroxyl-3-methylglutaryl-CoA) is reduced by the enzyme HMGCR. It is a redox reaction. NADPH is oxidized to NADP+ and HS-CoA while HMG-CoA is reduced to mevalonate. HMG-CoA reductase catalyzes the reaction, and it is the rate controlling enzyme, or this step is rate limiting for the conversion of HMG-CoA to mevalonate. The function of atorvastatin and other marketed statin drugs is to inhibit this HMG-CoA reductase enzyme. Figure 11.24 presents the inhibitory step.

There are many reasons why atorvastatin (Lipitor) is still leading the market. Researchers say it has a much longer inhibitory effect on the HMG Co-A reductase enzymes and may work with fewer side effects.

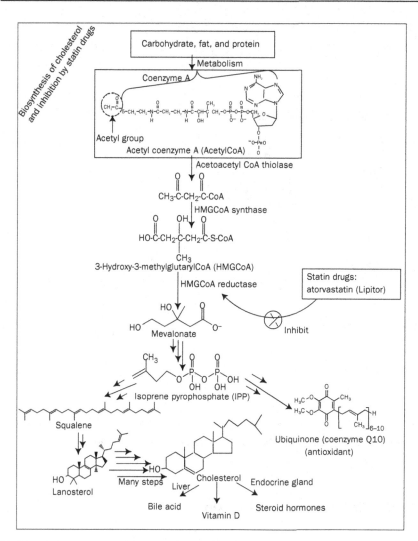

Figure 11.23 A short-cut biosynthesis of cholesterol in the body

11.11   Dosage forms of atorvastatin

Atorvastatin is only available in an oral solid (film coated tablet) dosage form
with different strengths (10 mg, 20 mg, 40 mg, and 80 mg of atorvastatin
calcium). The pharmacologically inactive excipients are calcium carbonate
(USP); candelilla wax (FCC); croscarmellose sodium (National Formulary; NF);
hydroxypropyl cellulose (NF); lactose monohydrate (NF); magnesium stearate
(NF); microcrystalline cellulose (NF); Opadry White YS-1-7040 (hypromellose,
polyethylene glycol, talc, titanium dioxide); and polysorbate 80 (NF).

Published by Woodhead Publishing Limited

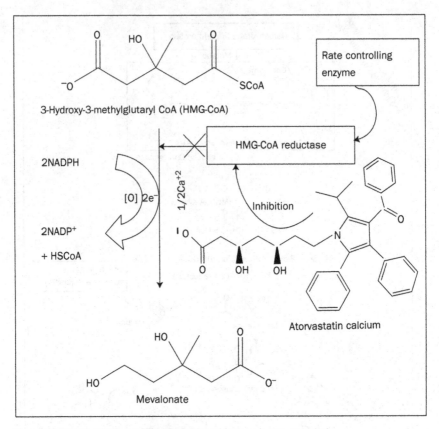

Figure 11.24 Inhibition of HMG-CoA reductase by atorvastatin

11.12 Celecoxib and rofecoxib

Celecoxib (Celebrex) and rofecoxib (Vioxx) are known as non-steroidal anti-inflammatory drugs (NSAIDs) and are also called cyclooxygenase-2 (COX-2) inhibitors based on their functional mechanisms. They are used to relieve pain caused by osteoarthritis, a disease that affects the joint cartilage underlying bone. Many people are affected by osteoarthritis, so there is naturally a huge market for these kinds of drugs. For many years COX-1 NSAID drugs such as aspirin, naproxen, ibuprofen, and a few others have been available on the market. The COX-2 drugs celecoxib and rofecoxib revolutionized the drug market when they were introduced in

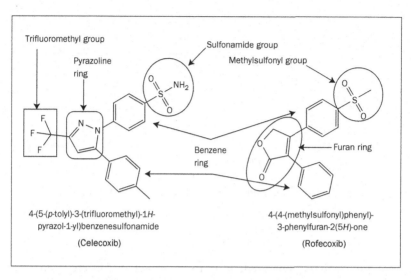

Figure 11.25 Structures of celecoxib and rofecoxib

1999. They were found to be very effective in pain management, especially in arthritis. The structures for celecoxib and rofecoxib are presented in Figure 11.25.

The drugs have some similarities and dissimilarities. Both have two benzene rings and sulfur groups, but there is a sulfonamide group in celecoxib and a methylsulfonyl group in rofecoxib. Among the dissimilarities, celecoxib has a pyrazoline ring and fluoride atoms, but rofecoxib has a furan ring and no fluoride atoms. Structurally, rofecoxib is relatively simpler than celecoxib.

Assessments on hydrophilicity and hydrophobicity, the ability of hydrogen bonding, and areas of electronegativity can be made while looking at the structures. Figure 11.26 illustrates the hydrophilic and hydrophobic sites in celecoxib and rofecoxib. Based on the structures, researchers can predict how they will interact with the COX-2 sites.

11.13   The mechanism of COX-2 inhibition by celecoxib and rofecoxib

The body's cell membranes are made of mostly phospholipid bilayers from which arachidonic acid is formed, catalyzed by phospholipidase during the transformation of cells (old cells die and new cells form). Once the

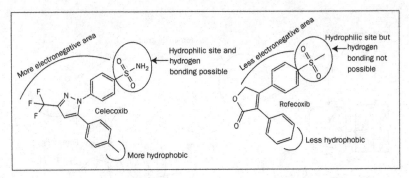

Figure 11.26 The hydrophilic and hydrophobic sites in celecoxib and rofecoxib

arachidonic acid is generated, it is transformed by different enzymatic pathways to a family of compounds called eicosanoids. One of the most prominent pathways is the cycloxygenase (COX) pathway, which produces the prostaglandins, prostacyclins, and thromboxanes. The COX has two forms, COX-1 (the predominant form) and COX-2. Table 11.1 lists the characteristics of these two enzymes.

Prostaglandins and throboxanes are responsible for pain, inflammation, fever, and excessive blood clotting. Traditional NSAIDs such as aspirin, naproxen, and ibuprofen inhibit COX-1 and COX-2, so they can cause peptic ulcers. However, COX-2 NSAIDs such as celecoxib and rofecoxib selectively inhibit COX-2, which is responsible for painful inflammation. Figure 11.27 shows the mechanism of NSAIDs.

Table 11.1 Characteristics of COX-1 and COX-2

COX-1	COX-2
Available in a wide variety of cells	Inducible enzyme
Popularly called 'housekeeping enzyme'	Available in inflammation and immune cells
Gastric cytoprotection	Produces prostaglandins that cause pain and inflammation
Hemostasis	
Produces prostaglandins that protect patient from ulcer formation in gastrointestinal tract	Becomes very active during inflammation

Published by Woodhead Publishing Limited

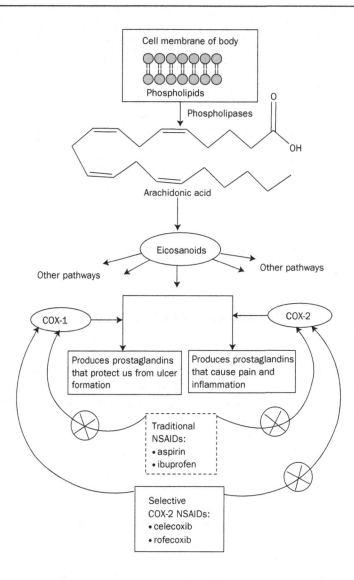

Figure 11.27 The mechanism of action of NSAIDs

Thus selective COX-2 inhibitors have fewer gastrointestinal side effects, but there are other side effects, especially cardiovascular toxicity, such as strokes and heart attacks (Figure 11.28). As a result, rofecoxib was withdrawn from the market. Concern was expressed about celecoxib and the label was changed.

Published by Woodhead Publishing Limited

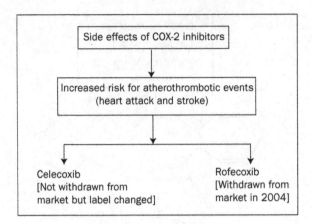

Figure 11.28 Side effects of celecoxib and rofecoxib

11.14 Metabolism and cardiotoxicity of celecoxib and rofecoxib

We know that when the COX-2 inhibitors celecoxib and rofecoxib were marketed in 1999 the public welcomed them and both became blockbuster drugs. However, one of the side effects of rofecoxib is an increased risk of atherothrombtic events with extended use, which led to its withdrawal from the market in 2004.

Mechanistically, celecoxib with its polar sulfonamide group binds with the hydrophilic side pocket of COX-2 enzyme and so did the methylsufonyl group of rofecoxib. No binding occurs with the COX-1 enzyme. Thus, both celecoxib and rofecoxib are selective COX-2 inhibitors. Severe side effects sometimes occur from the biotransformed products or metabolites of the drugs.

Celecoxib is metabolized by the enzyme P450 2C9 to mainly three inactive products (alcohol, carboxylic acid, and glucouronide derivatives of celecoxib), as shown in Figure 11.29.

Rofecoxib is metabolized primarily by cytosolic enzymes to mainly cis-dihydro and trans-dihydro derivatives of rofecoxib in addition to glucuronide of the hydroxy derivative (Figure 11.30).

Intensive investigations were made even after the withdrawal of the rofecoxib to find out what was wrong with the structure of rofecoxib.

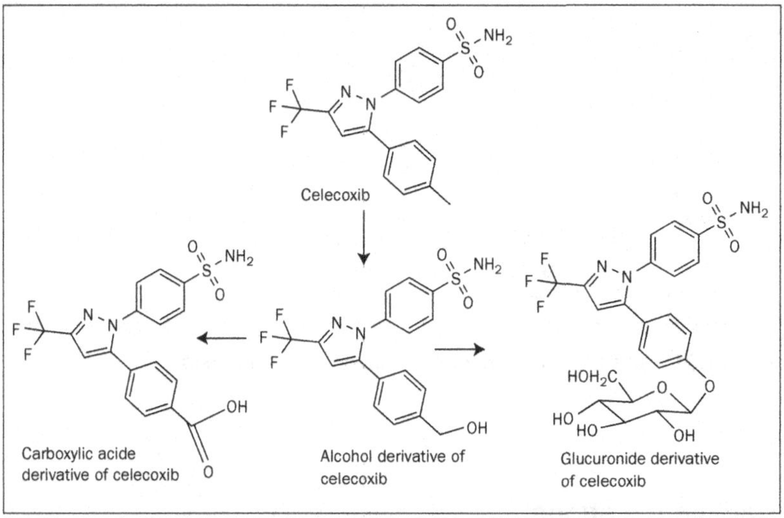

Figure 11.29 Inactive metabolites of celecoxib

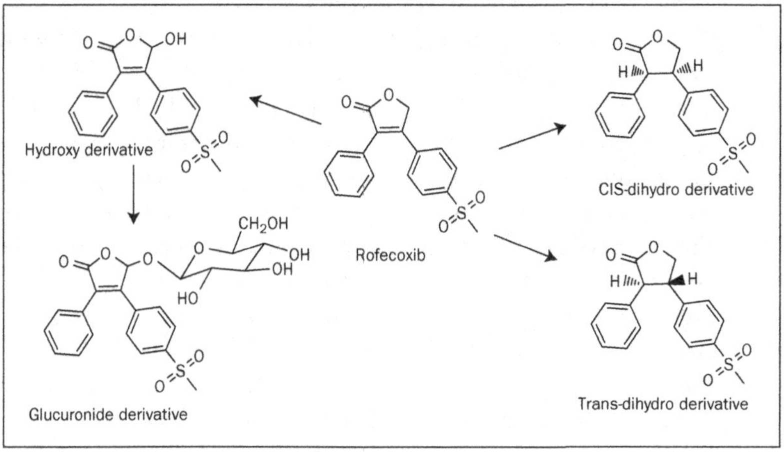

Figure 11.30 Inactive metabolites of rofecoxib

Research indicated that there could be two possible causes: biotransformation of rofecoxib to reactive and toxic maleic anhydride, and the promotion by rofecoxib to the non-enzymatic formation of isoprostane from biological lipids (Figure 11.31).

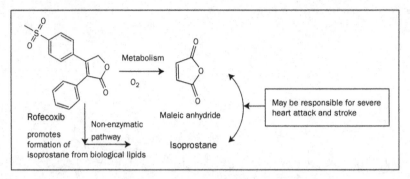

Figure 11.31 Possible reasons for cardiotoxicity of rofecoxib

Practice questions

1. Match the following drug names (a) with their generic names (b):
   (a) Viagra, Lipitor, Vioxx, Celebrex
   (b) atorvastatin, sildenafil, rofecoxib, celecoxib
2. Sildenafil (Viagra) is produced as sildenafil citrate. Explain why. How is sildenafil citrate synthesized?
3. How does Lipitor work in reducing cholesterol? Discuss how Lipitor becomes a drug of choice among all the statin drugs.
4. The introduction of COX-2 drugs brought great relief to millions of people with arthritis, but one COX-2 drug had to be withdrawn from the market. What do research findings suggest should be taken to mitigate the severe side effects of Vioxx?
5. Find out the structural similarities of celecoxib and rofecoxib.
6. Figure out different functional groups present in the Viagra molecule.
7. What functional group or part of the molecule of atorvastatin is responsible for interacting with HMG CoAR?
8. The Viagra tablet contains the following excipients: microcrystalline cellulose, anhydrous dibasic calcium phosphate, croscarmellose sodium, magnesium stearate, hypromellose, titanium dioxide, lactose, triacetin, and FD & C Blue #2 aluminum lake. Classify them into their specific excipient category.
9. Classify these excipients according to their functions: microcrystalline cellulose, anhydrous dibasic calcium phosphate, croscarmellose sodium, magnesium stearate, hypromellose, titanium dioxide, lactose, triacetin, and FD & C Blue #2 aluminum lake.

Published by Woodhead Publishing Limited

Answers to some practice questions

8. They are:

- microcrystalline cellulose – acts as a binder and disintegrating agent; mostly used in direct compression of tablets
- anhydrous dibasic calcium phosphate – diluents or fillers
- croscarmellose sodium – disintegrant
- magnesium stearate – lubricant
- hypromellose – plasticizer in coating tablets
- titanium dioxide – glidant
- lactose – diluents or filler
- triacetin – to maintain flexibility (to avoid cracking) during compression also used during film coating of tablets
- FD & C Blue #2 aluminum lake – color/dye used in tablet coating.

Notes

1. Alex Berenson, 'Sales of impotence drugs fall, defying expectations', *New York Times*, December 4, 2005.
2. Ian Osterloh, 'How I discovered Viagra', *Cosmos*, Issue 15, June 2007, www.cosmosmagazine.com/node/1463/results (accessed July 5, 2010).
3. See www.viagra.com/ (accessed February 6, 2011).
4. Source: IMS Health, Midas, December 2009.
5. 'Lipitor: at the heart of Warner-Lambert', [n.d.], www-personal.umich.edu/~afuah/cases/case25.html#_ednref59 (accessed February 16, 2011).

Published by Woodhead Publishing Limited

12

Counterfeit drugs and drug abuse

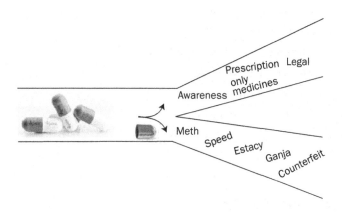

Learning objective

This chapter deals with two important social issues derived from pharmaceutical products: counterfeit drugs and drug abuse. It explains what counterfeit drugs are, how they are used, the prevalence of counterfeiting of medicines around the world, and the anti-counterfeiting measures taken by different agencies. It also examines the origins, categories, and chemistry of abused drugs. Students need to be aware of the difficult situations these drugs can create.

Key concept terms

Abused drug: a drug used in a non-therapeutic way

Active ingredient: active pharmaceutical ingredient

Antihistamine: drug that counteracts the effects of the body's histamine

AIDS: Acquired Immune Deficiency Syndrome

Counterfeit: fake, fraudulent

Crack cocaine: free-base solid cocaine

Depressant: drug that decreases brain activity

Hallucinogen: drug that changes the perception of reality

HIV: Human Immunodeficiency Virus

Internet pharmacy: an online shop for medicine

LSD: lysergic acid diethylamide, hallucinogen

Meth: methamphetamine

RFID: radio-frequency identification

Stimulant: drug that increases brain activity

12.1 Counterfeit drugs

Figure 12.1 shows some counterfeit-drug-related news headlines. They are very straightforward and do not need much explanation. Every week there is somewhere in the world where counterfeit, fake or fraudulent drugs are sold and used. Counterfeit medicine is an important problem and concern for the pharmaceutical industry and regulatory agencies. The World Health Organization defines counterfeit medicine as:

> one which is deliberately and fraudulently mislabeled with respect to identity and/or source. Counterfeiting can apply to both branded and generic products and counterfeit products may include products with the correct ingredients or with the wrong ingredients, without active ingredients, with insufficient active ingredients or with fake packaging.[1]

Figure 12.2 illustrates how a capsule of 500 mg amoxicillin can become counterfeit.

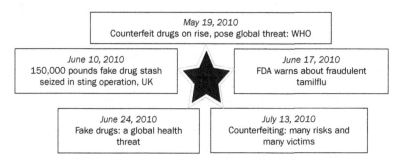

Figure 12.1 Recent news headlines on counterfeit drugs in different news media[2]

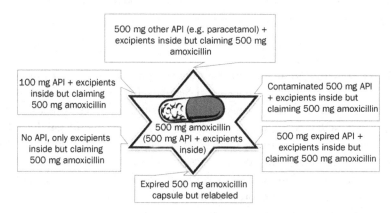

Figure 12.2 How a capsule of 500 mg amoxicillin can become counterfeit amoxicillin

This type of counterfeiting occurs with any products. The difference between counterfeit drugs or medicines and other counterfeit products is that if consumers take counterfeit drugs they can become sick, sometimes fatally (Figure 12.3). Other counterfeit products such as counterfeit purses cannot do any harm to our body.

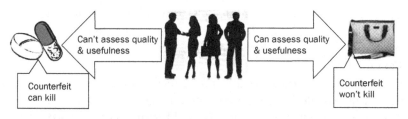

Figure 12.3 The difference between counterfeit medicines and counterfeit handbags

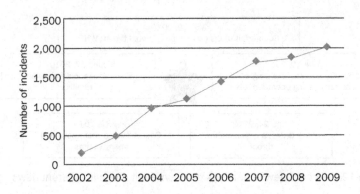

Figure 12.4 Worldwide incidents of counterfeit medicines, 2002–2009

Source: Pharmaceutical Security Institute[3]

There are counterfeit medicines all over the world, and according to the data compiled by the Pharmaceutical Security Institute, the prevalence of counterfeit medicines is increasing at an alarming rate (Figure 12.4).

Of these incidents, which include counterfeits, theft, and illegal diversion, about 48% are on a commercial scale (more than 1,000 dosage units). Incidents of counterfeiting occur in countries or regions that lack strong enforcement of regulatory authority and where legal policing is corrupt.

All kinds of medicines, branded and generic – from medicines for the treatment of life-threatening conditions to inexpensive generic versions of painkillers and antihistamines – have been counterfeited (Table 12.1).

Figure 12.5 shows the market value of counterfeiting incidents around the world.

12.2 Anticounterfeiting strategies

Counterfeit medicines are currently a major patient-safety issue, and a subject of concern for multinational pharmaceutical companies around the world. The Center for Medicines in the Public Interest and other organizations estimated that counterfeit drug sales would reach US$75 billion in 2010.[4]

It is important to know what can be done to mitigate this situation. The first measure should be to increase public awareness. By studying websites on counterfeit medicines, consumers could gain a critical understanding about them.

Table 12.1 Examples of counterfeit medicines

Counterfeit medicine	Country, year	Report
Anti-diabetic traditional medicine (used to lower blood sugar)	China, 2009	Contained six times the normal dose of glibenclamide (two people died, nine people hospitalized)
Metakelfin (antimalarial)	United Republic of Tanzania, 2009	Discovered in 40 pharmacies; lacked sufficient active ingredient
Viagra and Cialis (for erectile dysfunction)	Thailand, 2008	Smuggled into Thailand from an unknown source in an unknown country
Xenical (for fighting obesity)	USA, 2007	Contained no active ingredient and sold via internet sites operated outside the USA
Zyprexa (for treating bipolar disorder and schizophrenia)	UK, 2007	Detected in the legal supply chain: lacked sufficient active ingredient
Lipitor (for lowering cholesterol)	UK, 2006	Detected in the legal supply chain: lacked sufficient active ingredient

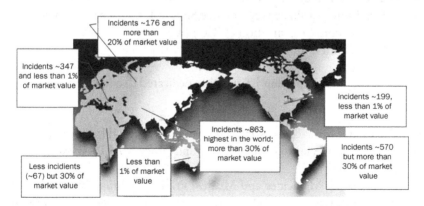

Figure 12.5 Market value of counterfeiting incidents around the world, 2009[5]

Published by Woodhead Publishing Limited

12.2.1 Websites

These are the most important international websites dedicated to counterfeit medicines:

- Australian Therapeutic Goods Administration (TGA) (www.tga.gov.au)
- Business Action to Stop Counterfeiting and Piracy (BASCAP) (www.iccwbo.org/bascap)
- European Alliance for Access to Safe Medicines (EAASM) (www.eaasm.eu)
- German Pharma Health Fund (GPHF) (www.gphf.org)
- Global Congress on Combating Counterfeiting (www.ccapcongress.net)
- International Anti-Counterfeiting Coalition (IACC) (www.iacc.org)
- International Chamber of Commerce (ICC) Commercial Crime Services (www.icc-ccs.org)
- International Chamber of Commerce (ICC) World Business Organization (www.iccwbo.org)
- International Federation of Pharmaceutical Manufacturers (IFPMA) (www.ifpma.org)
- International Pharmaceutical Federation (FIP) (www.fip.org)
- Interpol (www.interpol.int)
- Medicines and Healthcare Products Regulatory Agency (MHRA) (counterfeit@mhra.gsi.gov.uk)
- Organization for Economic Co-operation and Development (OECD) (www.oecd.org)
- Partnership for Safe Medicines (www.safemedicines.org)
- Pharmaceutical Security Institute (PSI) (www.psi-inc.org)
- Verified Internet Pharmacy Practice Sites (VIPPS) (vipps.nabp.net)
- World Custom Organization (WCO) (www.wcoomd.org)
- World Health Organization (WHO) (www.who.int)

These are the most important US websites dedicated to counterfeit medicines:

- BuySafeDrugs.info (www.buysafedrugs.info)
- The Center for Medicines in the Public Interest (CMPI) (www.cmpi.org)
- The Coalition Against Counterfeiting and Piracy (CACP) (www.theglobal ipcenter.com)
- FDA: Buying Medicines and Medical Products Online (http://www.fda .gov/Drugs/ResourcesForYou/Consumers/BuyingUsingMedicineSafely/ BuyingMedicinesOvertheInternet/ucm202675.htm)
- FDA: Center for Biologics Research and Evaluation (CBER) (www.fda .gov/BiologicsBloodVaccines/default.htm)

Published by Woodhead Publishing Limited

- FDA: Center for Drug Evaluation and Research (CDER) (www.fda.gov/Drugs/default.htm)
- FDA: Combating Counterfeit Drugs (www.fda.gov/Drugs/ResourcesForYou/Consumers/BuyingUsingMedicineSafely/CounterfeitMedicine/default.htm)
- FDA: MedWatch (www.fda.gov/Safety/MedWatch/default.htm)
- National Intellectual Property Rights Coordination Center (www.ice.gov/iprcenter)
- Safemedicines.org (www.safemedicines.org)
- StopFakes.gov (www.stopfakes.gov)
- Strategy Targeting Organized Piracy (STOP!) (www.uspto.gov/ip/global/stopfakes.jsp)
- US Chamber Counterfeiting and Piracy Issues Center (www.theglobalipcenter.com)
- US Chamber of Commerce (www.uschamber.com)
- US Customs & Border Protection (CBP) (www.cbp.gov)
- US Department of Commerce (DOC) (www.commerce.gov)
- US Department of Homeland Security (DHS) (www.dhs.gov)
- US Food and Drug Administration (FDA) (www.fda.gov)

12.2.2 Hologram stickers and biotechnological measures

In the past, hologram stickers were an effective way of detecting counterfeit medicines, but because of readily available devices and their low cost, even counterfeiters can use hologram stickers to make products seem legitimate. In future manufacturers will be able to use biotechnological measures to distinguish original medicines from fakes. By this method, the original manufacturer will include some antigens or marker chemicals in the medicine, and supply a testing kit with a specific antibody to detect and confirm authentic products.

12.2.3 Radiofrequency identification

Recent research confirmed that the use of radiofrequency identification (RFID) can track and trace products efficiently for the original manufacturers (Figure 12.6). This wireless device can prevent counterfeiting and diversions of consignment of medicines during transportation. The device includes three important components:

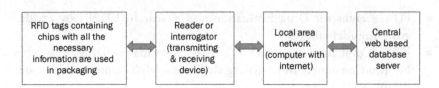

Figure 12.6 RFID network

- *chips* – which contains necessary information, such as the product name, date of manufacturing, place of manufacturing, batch numbers, shipment information
- *a reader* – a device that can transmit as well as receive information from even 20 feet away
- *a database* – a secured server with stored information of the items.

12.2.4 Nuclear quadruple resonance spectroscopy

Research is under way to use nuclear quadruple resonance spectroscopy to detect counterfeit or substandard drugs without removing the product from its packaging. Nuclear quadruple resonance can analyze compounds containing C, Cl, Br, Na, and K atoms, which constitute over 80% of all drugs.

12.3 Risks of internet pharmacies

With the current access provided by the internet and websites, shopping for various items is as easy as clicking a button. Now, e-mails that advertise Lipitor or Viagra tablets at extremely low prices or advertisements on websites that do the same are fairly common. There are two types of internet pharmacies: legitimate and properly licensed pharmacies and unlicensed pharmacies that sell prescription medicines illegally. Most of these websites do not provide a physical address and research suggests that most of them sell counterfeit medicine. People cannot easily assess the quality of medicines from the websites and may ingest them without knowing exactly what they contain. The packaging information and the medicines can be fake. In general, shopping for medicine on the internet poses a serious threat to the health and safety of citizens unless the internet pharmacy is legitimately licensed.

12.4 Drug abuse

Drug abuse is the practice of using drugs in a way that they are not intended for – the drugs are used for a purpose other than the intended therapeutic or medical reasons. Drug abuse sometimes starts with a simple idea: 'Let's see what happens.' Most humans are inquisitive, and if there is a negative warning label on a medicine, especially central nervous system related drugs, young people are sometimes attracted to the drug for recreational purposes.

Alcohol is an example. Doctors never prescribe alcohol for therapeutic purposes, but people do drink alcohol. Some people feel good about drinking or think that drinking makes them sociable or friendly, and relieves anxiety and stress. However, drinking can lead to disorientation and has other side effects that are not pleasant, indeed alcohol consumption can be considered substance abuse. Any drug that affects human feelings in either a depressing or a pleasurable way can be abused. Each drug has a particular dose that achieves the therapeutic response, but the drug is abused when taken in excessive quantities. As a result, side effects become dominant and may lead to dangerous consequences.

Commonly abused drugs are sometimes called club drugs or party drugs, and include psychoactive drugs, which alter moods, thoughts, or perceptions. Psychoactive drugs can be classified into three main categories: stimulants, depressants, and hallucinogens (Figure 12.7).

Commonly abused drugs often have interesting street names, some of which are shown in Table 12.2.

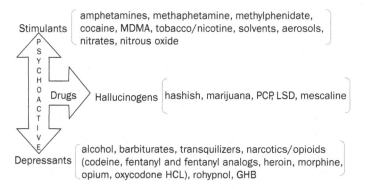

Figure 12.7 The most abused stimulants, hallucinogens, and depressants

Published by Woodhead Publishing Limited

Table 12.2 Some abused drugs and their method of administration and street names

Name of abused drugs	How they are administered	Street names
Methamphetamine	Injected, swallowed, smoked, snorted	Desoxyn, chalk, crank, crystal, fire, glass, go fast, ice, meth, speed
MDMA (methylenedioxy-methamphetamine)	Swallowed	DOB, DOM, MDA; Adam, clarity, ecstasy, Eve, lover's speed, peace, STP, X, XTC
LSD (lysergic acid diethylamide)	Swallowed, absorbed through mouth tissues	Acid, blotter, boomers, cubes, microdot, yellow sunshine
GHB (gamma-hydroxybutyrate)	Swallowed	G, Georgia home boy, grievous bodily harm, liquid ecstasy
Marijuana	Swallowed, smoked	Blunt, dope, ganja, grass, herb, joints, Mary Jane, pot, reefer, sinsemilla, skunk, weed

12.4.1 Stimulants

Stimulants are a class of drugs that increase brain activity. These drugs are thus psychoactive drugs, which are sometimes referred to as 'uppers'. They can temporarily elevate alertness and awareness. Coffee or tea (active ingredient caffeine) and the smoking of tobacco (active ingredient nicotine) are the two most common stimulants; they have been widely accepted in societies throughout the world for centuries. These stimulants have widely known adverse effects.

The two most commonly abused stimulants, amphetamine and cocaine, are not legally accepted in the way coffee or cigarettes are in most societies. Other examples of stimulants include methylphenidate, and 3,4-methylene dioxymethamphetamine (MDMA), better known as 'ecstasy'. Figure 12.8 illustrates the chemical structures of some stimulant drugs.

Amphetamine and amphetamine derivatives, such as dextroamphetamine and methamphetamine, have similar basic structures and thus similar effects. In fact, amphetamine and dextroamphetamine are the same molecule with a stereochemical difference. Amphetamine is a racemic

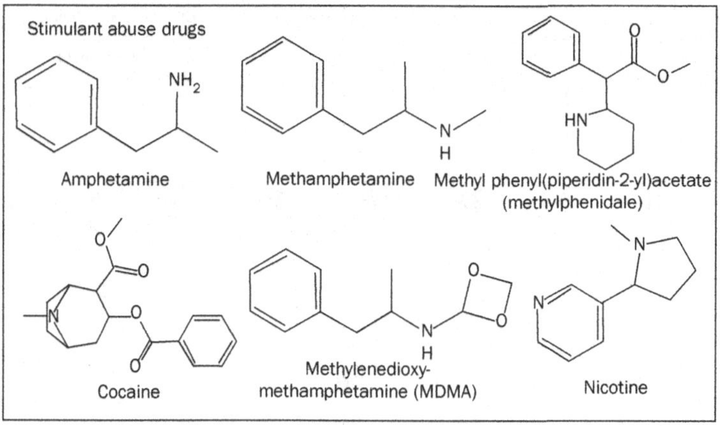

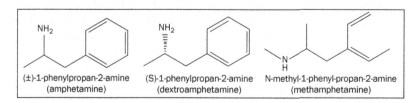

Figure 12.8 The chemical structures of some stimulant drugs

mixture, which means it has both dextro (+) and levo (+) steroisomers. Dextoamphetamine has only the dextro (+) stereoisomer. Methamphetamine is an amphetamine with an extra methyl group attached to an N atom (Figure 12.9).

These amphetamine-type stimulants have been the most commonly abused drugs other than prescription drugs for a long time and are still a growing global problem. A few events in the discovery and uses of amphetamine-type stimulants are shown in Figure 12.10. There is always a potential danger when a medicine is overdosed or abused for a long period of time. In the case of psychoactive medicines, the situation becomes worse. As stimulants, these drugs may produce dose-related symptoms, such as increased alertness, euphoria, hallucinations, heart rate, blood pressure, and violent behavior.

Structurally, methamphetamine is closely related to ephedrine and adrenaline (Figure 12.11). Figure 12.17 illustrates the stereochemical difference between ephedrine and pseudoephedrine.

Figure 12.9 The chemical structure of amphetamine and its derivatives

Published by Woodhead Publishing Limited

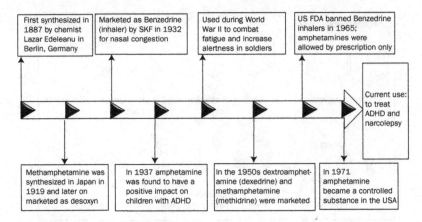

Figure 12.10 The history of the development of amphetamine and its derivatives

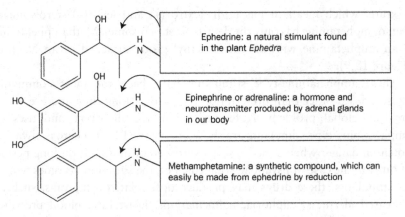

Figure 12.11 The structural relationship between ephedrine, adrenaline, and methamphetamine

12.4.1.1 Synthesis of amphetamine

Amphetamine can be synthesized in one pot reaction, however, isolation and purification of the drug is tedious. A mixture of phenylactone and formamide when heated in the presence of formic acid forms N-formylamphetamine, which in hydrolysis with hydrochloric acid produces amphetamine hydrochloride. After neutralization with a milder base, the oily liquid of amphetamine is produced. The oil of amphetamine is then steam-distilled to get pure amphetamine. The basic amphetamine is then treated with sulfuric acid to get the crystalline salt form of amphetamine (Figure 12.12).

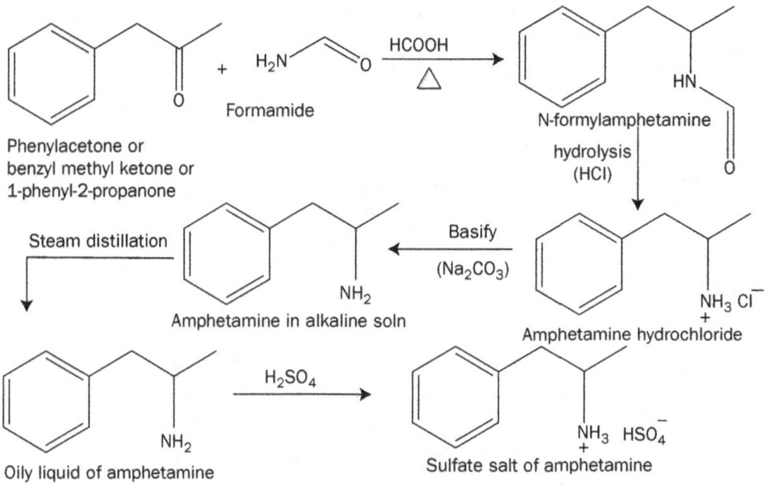

Figure 12.12 Synthesis of amphetamine

Alternatively, amphetamine is synthesized by a reductive amination from phenylacetone. Phenylacetone, when reduced catalytically (Pd/C or Pt_2O) in the presence of ammonia gas, produces amphetamine (Figure 12.13).

12.4.1.2 The synthesis of methamphetamine

Methamphetamine is synthesized starting from either ephedrine or phenylacetone. The reaction sequences are shown in Figure 12.14.

12.4.2 Cocaine

Cocaine is an alkaloid isolated from the coca plant (*Erythroxylon coca*) and a powerful psychostimulant. The effect of cocaine is very quick and

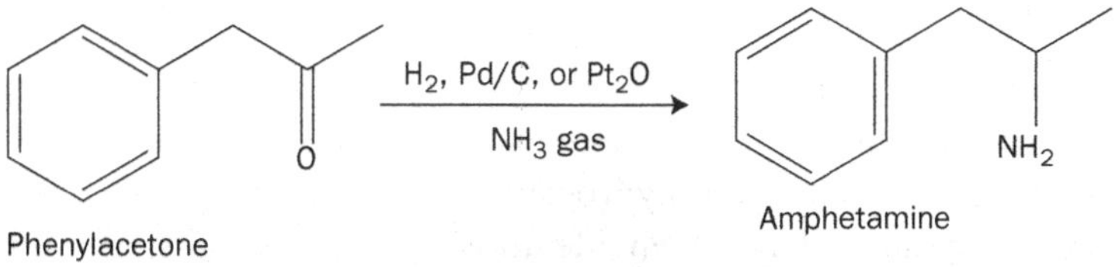

Figure 12.13 Alternative synthesis of amphetamine

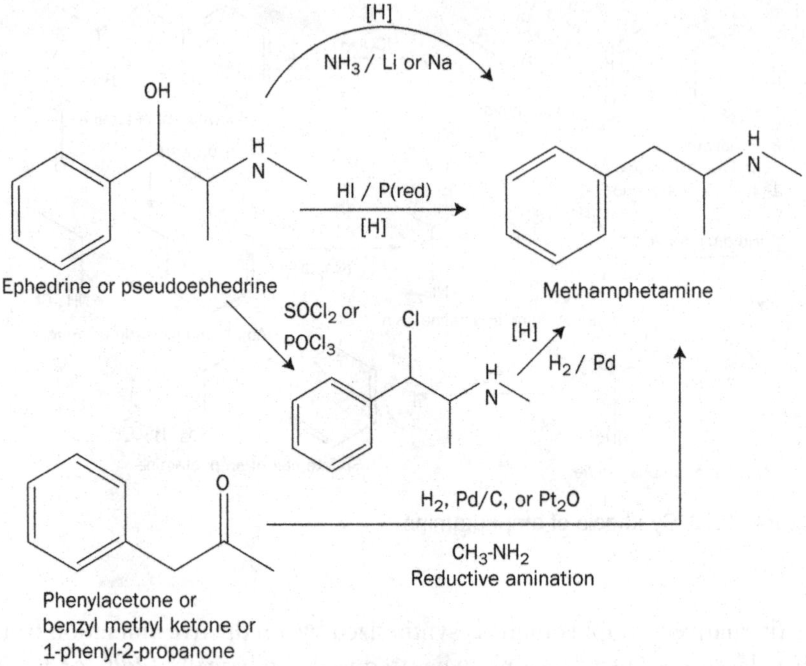

Figure 12.14 Synthesis of methamphetamine

pleasurably euphoric, but ultimately the effects are depressing, and it is one of the most commonly abused drugs. Figure 12.15 shows some important events in the history of cocaine usage.

Chemically, cocaine is isolated as cocaine hydrochloride from which a free base cocaine can be made by neutralizing the hydrochloride salt. The solid form of free base is called 'crack' because it produces a cracking sound when heated and smoked (Figure 12.16).

12.4.3 Hallucinogens

Hashish and marijuana are derived from the cannabis plant (*Cannabis sativa*), which contains variable amounts of tetrahydrocannabinol (THC), more specifically, delta-9-tetrahydrocannabinol ($\triangle$9-THC). More than 60 different compounds have been identified in the extracts of cannabis plant, which as a group are called cannabinoids. The hashish is more

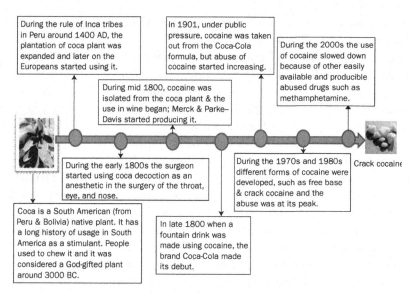

During the rule of Inca tribes in Peru around 1400 AD, the plantation of coca plant was expanded and later on the Europeans started using it.

In 1901, under public pressure, cocaine was taken out from the Coca-Cola formula, but abuse of cocaine started increasing.

During the 2000s the use of cocaine slowed down because of other easily available and producible abused drugs such as methamphetamine.

During mid 1800, cocaine was isolated from the coca plant & the use in wine began; Merck & Parke–Davis started producing it.

During the early 1800s the surgeon started using coca decoction as an anesthetic in the surgery of the throat, eye, and nose.

During the 1970s and 1980s different forms of cocaine were developed, such as free base & crack cocaine and the abuse was at its peak.

Crack cocaine

Coca is a South American (from Peru & Bolivia) native plant. It has a long history of usage in South America as a stimulant. People used to chew it and it was considered a God-gifted plant around 3000 BC.

In late 1800 when a fountain drink was made using cocaine, the brand Coca-Cola made its debut.

Figure 12.15 Important events in the history of cocaine usage

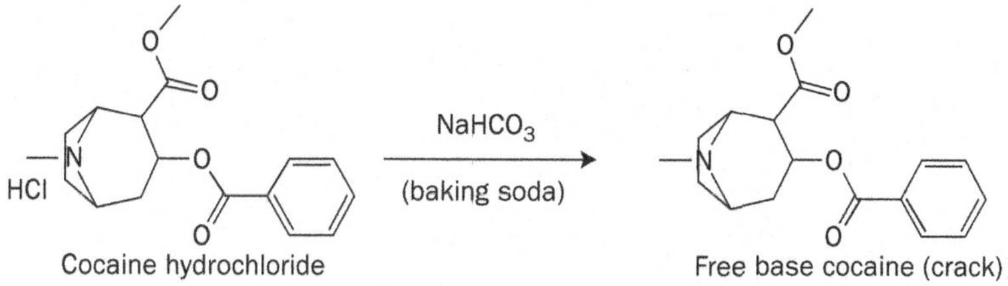

Cocaine hydrochloride

$NaHCO_3$
(baking soda)

Free base cocaine (crack)

Figure 12.16 Free base cocaine (crack) from cocaine hydrochloride

(+) Pseudoephedrine

Ephedrine

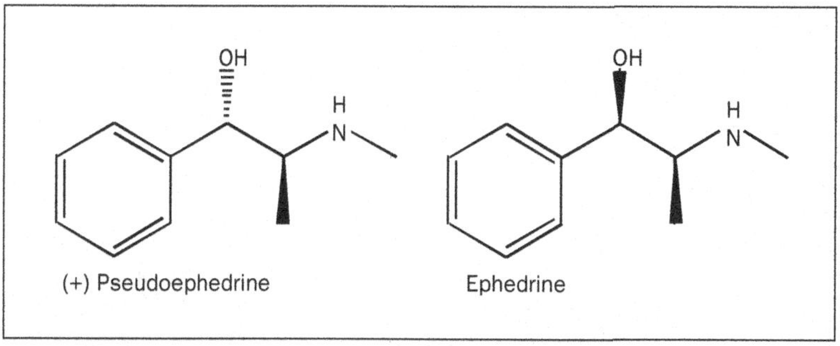

Figure 12.17 The stereochemical difference between ephedrine and pseudoephedrine

potent (containing 40% THC) than marijuana, which contains about 10% THC. Figure 12.18 illustrates the chemical structure of some hallucinogens.

The cannabis plant has been used for thousands of years by almost every culture in the world. Today hashish and marijuana are the most commonly abused drugs in the world aside from alcohol and tobacco because they tend to increase imagination, euphoria, and hallucination, but there are also medical uses for this drug. There is a prescription medication called marinol (generic name, Dronabinol), containing delta 9-tetrahydrocannabinol, which is available for treating nausea and vomiting caused by chemotherapy. This drug is also used to stimulate appetite and prevent weight loss in HIV/AIDS patients. Many states in the USA have legalized medical marijuana for doctors to prescribe in order to reduce pain and suffering in cancer patients.

A common way to consume hashish and marijuana is to smoke it like a cigarette, which results in the peak plasma concentrations taking place within ten minutes, but marinol is available in orally administered tablet form.

One of the most potent hallucinogenic drugs is lysergic acid diethylamide (LSD), which is produced semi-synthetically from ergotamine alkaloids as a water soluble tartrate salt. LSD was first synthesized by Albert Hoffman while working for Sandoz Laboratories in Basel in 1938. One day, Hoffman

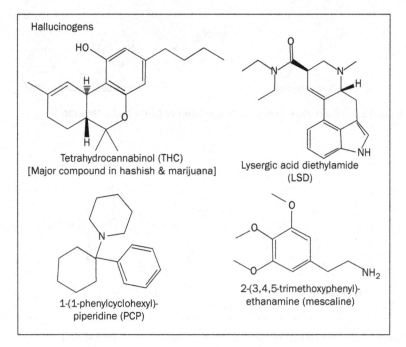

Hallucinogens

Tetrahydrocannabinol (THC)
[Major compound in hashish & marijuana]

Lysergic acid diethylamide
(LSD)

1-(1-phenylcyclohexyl)-
piperidine (PCP)

2-(3,4,5-trimethoxyphenyl)-
ethanamine (mescaline)

Figure 12.18 The chemical structure of some hallucinogens

Published by Woodhead Publishing Limited

accidentally ingested some of LSD, and within 40 minutes he had the first LSD experiences. Hoffman wrote,

> I lay down and sank into a kind of drunkenness which was not unpleasant and which was characterized by extreme activity of imagination. As I lay in a dazed condition with my eyes closed (I experienced daylight as disagreeably bright) there surged upon me an uninterrupted stream of fantastic images of extraordinary plasticity and vividness and accompanied by an intense, kaleidoscope-like play of colors.[6]

Although once marketed under the name Delysid as a psychotherapeutic drug, LSD has no current medical use.

Other hallucinogens have been evaluated. Mescaline, originally isolated from *Peyotl cactus*, was later synthesized. Similarly, in the 1950s Parke Davis developed and marketed phencyclidine (PCP) under the brand name Sernyl as an anesthetic drug, but because it had hallucinogenic effects, it ended up on the street market as a recreationally abused drug.

12.4.4 Depressants

Depressants are medicines that literally depress or slow down the vital physiological activities of the brain. They act as sedatives or in some cases hypnotics on the central nervous system. Alcohol is considered a depressant. The most commonly abused depressant drugs are barbiturates (e.g. Phenobarbital), benzodiazepines (e.g. diazepam, flunitrazepam), and opioids (e.g. codeine, morphine, and heroin). Figure 12.19 shows the chemical structure of some depressant drugs.

Of all these sedatives, hypnotics are the only prescription medicines that are therapeutically useful. Barbiturates are used for seizure disorders; benzodiazepines are useful for anxiety and sleep disorders; opioids are used as pain relievers.

12.4.4.1 *Alcohol – the most abused substance*

Alcohol (ethyl alcohol only, not other alcohols, such as methyl, propyl, or isopropyl alcohol) is a depressant but we should not call it a drug or medicine. Though it does affect our body physiologically, it does not cure or prevent any diseases, so it should not be called a drug or medicine. Alcohol is the most abused drink in most societies of the world.

Published by Woodhead Publishing Limited

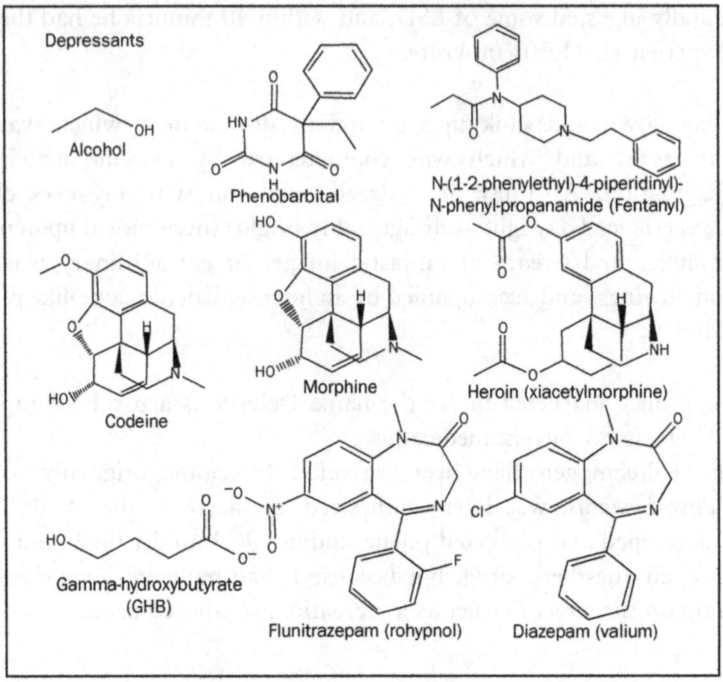

Figure 12.19 The chemical structure of some depressant drugs

The word alcohol has various meanings. Chemically, alcohol is the hydroxyl derivative of alkane, for example, methane to methyl alcohol, and ethane to ethyl alcohol. Whenever we say alcohol, we mean only ethyl alcohol or ethanol. Some alcohols and their names and effects are shown in Table 12.3.

Table 12.3 Some alcohols and their effects

Structure	Name	Effect
CH_3-OH	Methyl alcohol or methanol	Toxic, causes blindness or even death if ingested
CH_3CH_2-OH	Ethyl alcohol or ethanol, commonly known as alcohol	Abused drink, depressant
$CH_3CH_2CH_2$-OH	n-Propyl alcohol or propanol	Harmful if ingested
CH_3-CH(OH)-CH_3	Isopropyl alcohol, isopropanol or rubbing alcohol	Antiseptic, harmful if ingested
$CH_3CH_2CH_2CH_2$-OH	n-Butyl alcohol or butanol	Harmful if ingested

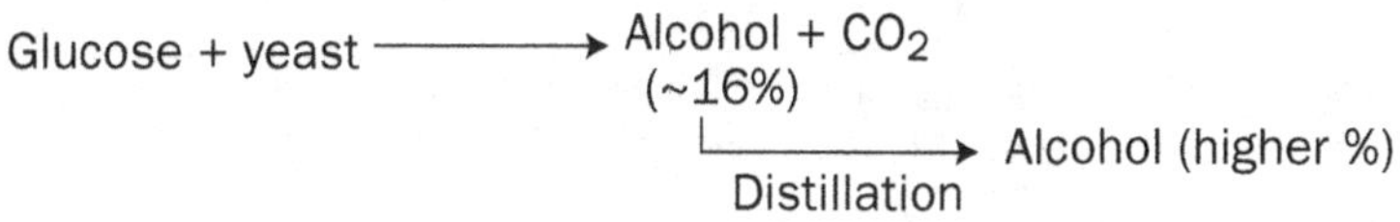

Glucose + yeast $\longrightarrow$ Alcohol + CO_2
(~16%)
$\longrightarrow$ Alcohol (higher %)
Distillation

Figure 12.20 The conversion of glucose and yeast into alcohol

Alcoholic beverages such as beers, wines, and liquors contain varying amounts of alcohol. In general, alcohol is produced by fermentation using glucose or sugar and yeast (Figure 12.20).

12.4.4.2 Non-synthetic narcotic abused drugs

The poppy plant (*Papaver somniferm*) is the source of non-synthetic narcotic drugs, such as morphine, codeine, and papaverine. Narcotics are used therapeutically to treat pain, but they alter mood and behavior significantly, which is why they are sometimes abused. The semisynthetic opioid heroin is made by acetylation of morphine, and is an abused drug. In opium poppy pod extracts, morphine is the main component (4–21%) followed by codeine (0.7–2.5%), but codeine and heroin can be synthesized from morphine (Figure 12.21).

12.4.4.3 Gamma-hydroxybutyric acid or salt

Chemically, γ-hydroxybutyric or gamma-hydroxybutyric acid (GHB) is a very simple molecule. It is a hydroxycarboxylic acid, and used therapeutically to treat depression, insomnia, and narcolepsy. It produces a euphoria in lower doses, and its overdose can lead to death. GHB is known to be a party or club drug and a date-rape drug. It can be synthesized in one step starting with γ-butyrolactone by alkaline hydrolysis (Figure 12.22).

12.4.5 College party drugs

College students often go to parties and usually bring their own alcohol. Whenever alcohol is mixed with drugs there can be very serious health hazards:

> There are more deaths, illnesses, and disabilities from substance abuse than from any other preventable health condition. Today, one in four deaths is attributable to alcohol, tobacco, and illicit drug use.[7]

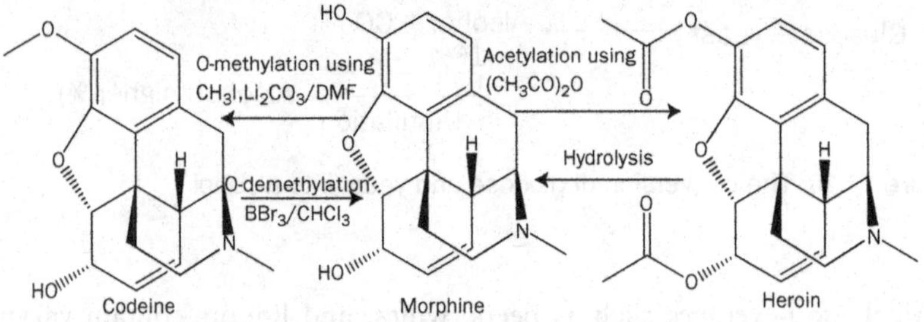

Figure 12.21 Synthetic interconversion of morphine, codeine, and heroin

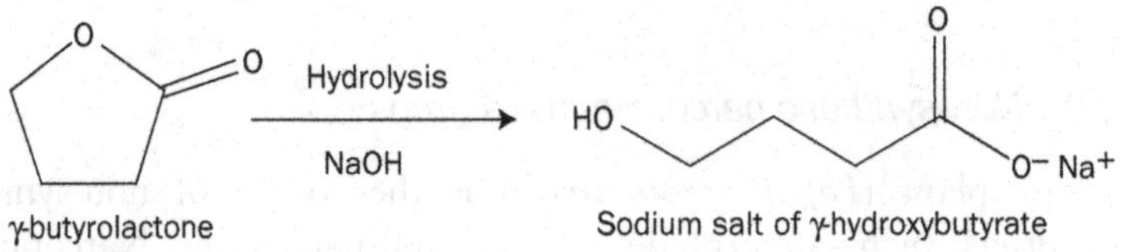

Figure 12.22 Synthesis of GHB

The drugs commonly used in the college parties, also called club drugs, include 3,4-methylenedioxymethamphetamine (MDMA), flunitrazepam, gamma-hydroxybutrate, ketamine hydrochloride, and methamphetamine. The street names or club names of these drugs help explain their effects (Table 12.4).

Table 12.4 Some common party drugs, their street names, and category

Drug	Street names	Therapeutic category
3,4-methylenedioxymethamphetamine	Ecstacy, MDMA, XTC, X, Adam, Clarity	Stimulant
Gamma hydroxybutrate	Liquid X, Georgia Home Boy, Goop, Gamma-oh, Grievous Bodily Harm	Stimulant
Flunitrazepam (Rohypnol)	Roofies, Roach, R-2, 542, Mind Erasers, Roché	Depressant
Ketamine hydrochloride	Special K, Ket, K, Vitamin K, Kit Kat, Keller, Cat Valium, Purple, Super C	Depressant
Methamphetamine	Chalk, Crank, Crystal, Fire, Glass, Go Fast, Ice, Meth, Speed	Stimulant

Practice questions

1. Are there any differences between counterfeit drugs and substandard drugs? Which type is more dangerous? Compare and contrast counterfeit drugs and other consumer goods.
2. Define counterfeit medicine and discuss how it can be identified. How can the production and marketing of counterfeit medicines be stopped?
3. Drug abuse is considered a major social problem. What types of drugs are normally abused? Give a couple of examples from each type.
4. Why is alcohol considered the most abused substance?
5. Most abused drugs are also used therapeutically. Name at least five abused drugs and give their therapeutic uses.
6. Name amphetamines and methamphetamines according to the International Union of Pure and Applied Chemistry (IUPAC) system.
7. Structurally, what is the difference between ephedrine and pseudoephedrine?
8. G-butyrolactone can be hydrolyzed in two ways, through acidic or alkaline hydrolysis. Why is alkaline hydrolysis preferred?
9. GHB and rohypnol (generic-flunitrazepam) are considered to be a date-rape drug. Why?

Answers to some practice questions

6. Amphetamine is 1-methyl-2-phenylethylamine and methampheta mine is N-methyl-N-(1-methyl-2-phenylethyl) amine.
7. The only difference is in the stereochemical configuration (Figure 12.17).
8. Alkaline hydrolysis is irreversible and acidic hydrolysis is reversible.
9. Rohypnol is a very potent tranquilizer, used as sleeping pill. At the same time, it can make the user unconscious and helpless, so the abuser can take the opportunity to rape the user. Similar situations happen to GHB users too.

Notes

1. See S. Kopp, 'WHO survey terminology on "counterfeit" medicines or equivalent', World Health Organization, [2009], www.who.int/medicines/services/counterfeit/Surveyonterminology.pdf (accessed February 16, 2011).
2. Reuters, 'Counterfeit drugs on rise, pose global threat: WHO', May 19, 2010, www.reuters.com/article/2010/05/19/us-drugs-counterfeit-idUSTRE64I6G120100519; '150,000 pounds fake drug stash seized in sting operation, UK', *Medical News Today*, June 10, 2010, www.medicalnewstoday.com/articles/191466.php; 'FDA warns about fraudulent tamiflu', FDA news release, June 17, 2010, www.fda.gov/NewsEvents/Newsroom/PressAnnouncements/ucm216148.htm; 'Fake drugs: a global health threat', PBS Newshour, June 24, 2010, www.pbs.org/newshour/rundown/2010/06/fake-drugs-a-global-health-threat.html; 'Counterfeiting: many risks and many victims', CNBC, July 13, 2010, www.cnbc.com/id/38229835/Counterfeiting_Many_Risks_and_Many_Victims (all accessed September 10, 2010).
3. Pharmaceutical Security Institute, 'Incident trends', 2011, www.psi-inc.org/incidentTrends.cfm (accessed February 16, 2011).
4. International Risk Governance Council, 'Counterfeit prescription drugs', 2010, www.irgc.org/IMG/pdf/Emerging_risks_Counterfeit_drugs.pdf (accessed February 15, 2011).
5. Pharmaceutical Security Institute, 'Geographic distribution', 2011, www.psi-inc.org/geographicDistributions.cfm (accessed February 16, 2011).
6. Albert Hofmann, 'The discovery of LSD and subsequent investigations on naturally occurring hallucinogens' in Frank J. Ayd, Jr. and Barry Blackwell (eds), *Discoveries in Biological Psychiatry*, Philadelphia: J.B. Lippincott Company, 1970, www.psychedelic-library.org/hofmann.htm (accessed February 16, 2011).
7. National Institute on Drug Abuse, 'Mortality', www.nida.nih.gov/consequences/mortality/ (accessed February 23, 2011).

13

New pharmaceutical technology and pharmaceuticals

Learning objective

This chapter will briefly introduce some new and evolving pharmaceutical technologies and pharmaceuticals. There is a discussion of the current situation of established and prospective technologies.

Published by Woodhead Publishing Limited

Key concept terms

API: active pharmaceutical ingredient

Biologic: a therapeutic, prophylactic and *in-vivo* diagnostic substance made from a living system; biologics include vaccines, blood products, recombinant therapeutic proteins, gene therapy, and biotechnology products

Biopharmaceutical: biologic or biotechnology product

Biotechnology: the technology that produces biologics, e.g. fermentation

Nanomedicine: the medical application of nanotechnology

Nanotechnology: the study of manipulating matter on an atomic and molecular scale; nano means extremely small in size – one-billionth $(1/10^9)$; APIs are made to nanometer size ($< 1,000$ nm); nanotechnology is used to produce nanomedicines

rDNA: recombinant DNA technology; the desired DNA is inserted into plasmid and transferred to a host cell to make clones

Regenerative medicine: the ultimate dream medicine that will repair, replace, restore, or regenerate the cellular, tissue, or organ systems in the human body

Transdermal patch: a medicated patch that can deliver drugs through skin portals directly to the bloodstream at a predetermined rate

13.1 Biologics

The vaccines that saved and are still saving many lives around the world are biologics. Vaccines are prophylactic biologics, and there are also *in-vivo* diagnostic biologics and therapeutic biologics.

Biologic technology has been in practice for thousands of years, and products such as beer, wine, cheese, and bread are biotechnological or fermentation products. Biological research started in the nineteenth century during the time of Robert Koch in Germany and Louis Pasteur in France. Over the years, the technology has made great advancements. Pharmaceutical biologics include vaccines, blood and blood components, allergenics, somatic cells, gene therapy, tissues, and recombinant therapeutic proteins.

The US Food and Drug Administration (FDA) created its Center for Biologics Research and Evaluation (CBER) in 1988. The first three successful biologics were insulin, growth hormones, and erythropoietin. The purposes of pharmaceutical drugs and biologics are the same (to cure diseases) but their nature and products are completely different. Table 13.1 lists the characteristics of drugs and biologics and Figure 13.1 shows an example of each.

There are currently more than a 100 biologics on the market and more than 500 in the pipeline, from which more biologics are being researched

Table 13.1 Characteristics of pharmaceutical drugs and biologics

Characteristics	Drugs (pharmaceuticals)	Biologics (biopharmaceuticals)
Basic nature	Simple	Complex
Size	Small (low molecular weight)	Thousand times larger (very high molecular weight)
Example	Aspirin	Insulin
Production process	Developed by chemical synthesis	Developed by biological process (fermentation)
Route of administration	Oral	Injection (or shot)
Stability	Stable in stomach acid	Unstable in stomach acid
Batch to batch products	Homogenous	Heterogenous
Off-patented name	Generic drug	Biosimilar or follow-on biologics

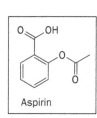

Aspirin

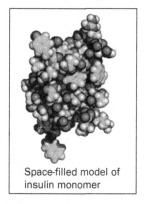

Space-filled model of insulin monomer

Figure 13.1 An example of a pharmaceutical (aspirin) and a biopharmaceutical (insulin)

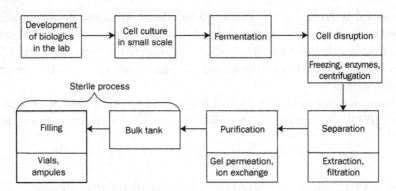

Figure 13.2 Production schematics of biopharmaceuticals

as cures for cancer and infectious diseases. Figure 13.2 illustrates the production of biopharmaceuticals.

In the field of biotechnology (the technology that produces biologics), recombinant DNA (rDNA) is now an established technique of producing biologics since the process was successfully developed and used by Boyer and Cohen in 1973 to produce insulin. The technique of rDNA is illustrated in Figure 13.3.

13.2　Nanomedicines by nanotechnology

The word 'nano' means extremely small in size – one-billionth of the whole. For example, 1 nanometer is one-billionth ($1/10^9$) of a meter. More simply, 1 nanometer is about 1/80,000 the width of the diameter of a human hair.

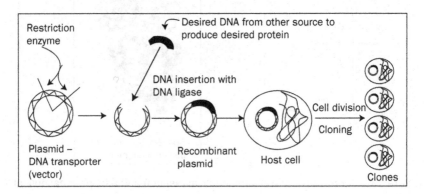

Figure 13.3 Recombinant DNA technology to produce biologics

Published by Woodhead Publishing Limited

The technology that works with this level of sizes is known as nanotechnology.

In nanomedicines, the active pharmaceutical ingredient (API) is used at a nanosize level (< 1,000 nm), which is equivalent to colloids. Smoke is an example of a colloid where nano-solid particles are dispersed in air. In pharmaceuticals, nanosized drugs are carried by nano vehicles inside the body to a specific target. The interaction between drug and cells happens on the molecular level. The nanosize is important to pharmaceuticals because researchers expect a better therapeutic benefit out of nanomedicines. Conventional and nano-treatment approaches are shown in Figure 13.4.

Nanotransporters are needed to carry nano-drugs to the target, and there are numerous nanotransporters in development (Figure 13.5).

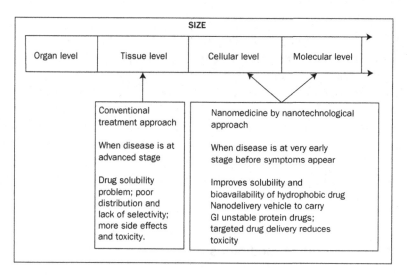

Figure 13.4 Conventional and nano-treatment approaches

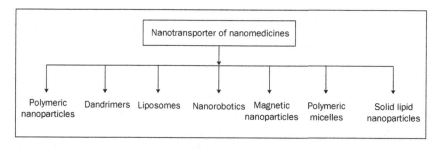

Figure 13.5 Examples of nanotransporters

Published by Woodhead Publishing Limited

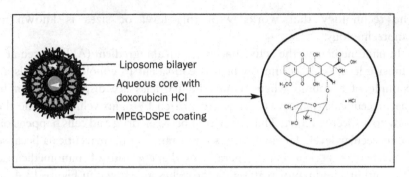

Figure 13.6 Representation of doxorubicin liposome

Source: Doxil website[1]

There are some nanotechnologies available on the market, such as doxorubicin (Doxil) liposome injection and the polymer-drug conjugate Oncaspar. There are many more being developed.

The drug doxorubicin is used to treat ovarian cancer, AIDS-related Kaposi's sarcoma, and multiple myeloma. The API of doxorubicin, doxorubicin HCl, is encapsulated in long circulating 'STEALTH' liposomes, which are formulated with a surface bound carrier composed of N-(carbonyl-methoxypolyethylene glycol 2000)-1,2-distearoyl-sn-glycero3-phosphoethanolamine sodium salt (MPEG-DSPE) (Figure 13.6). Researchers believe that because of its nanosize, the drug can easily penetrate the tumor.

13.3   Regenerative medicines

The function of regenerative medicines is to enhance the body's own regeneration of tissues and organs. Dr Steven Bauer of CBER and the US FDA described regenerative medicines as medicines that repair, replace, restore, or regenerate the cellular, tissue, or organ systems in the human body.[2] It would be the ultimate medicine if it could carry out all of these four functions. Medicines can stimulate the tissue at a cell, molecular, or even DNA level to repair it. At the extreme level, a laboratory-made substitute could replace tissues or organs, and regenerative medicines could restore youthful organs or regenerate a particular organ, such as a heart, after infarctions. This would be very exciting.

Tissue engineering research is continuing to build products in different categories:

- biological parts such as cells that can be genetically modified to carry out particular functions
- chemical products that can signal the tissue to regenerate
- polymeric materials such as fibers and plastics for replacement.

The world's first clinical trial of a human embryonic stem cell in patients with acute spinal cord injury began in 2010.

13.4 Transdermal patch technology

The transdermal patch or transdermal drug delivery system is a medicated patch that can deliver drugs through skin portals directly to the bloodstream at a predetermined rate. This is the most comfortable dosage form – it is non-invasive, avoids the gastrointestinal tract and bypasses first-pass metabolism, can have multiday therapy, and can be terminated at any time. The site of application should be clean, not oily, and hairless, and the location may vary with the therapeutic category of drug, such as nitroglycerin around the chest, estradiol around the buttocks or abdomen, and nicotine around the upper torso or upper outer arm.

The system consists of several layers:

- a backing layer to protect from the outside environment and water
- a drug reservoir on a semipermeable membrane to control the release of the drug
- an adhesive to glue onto skin
- a liner to protect the patch and adhesive.

The liner has to be taken out before putting the patch on the skin surface. Figure 13.7 illustrates the makeup of a medicated patch.

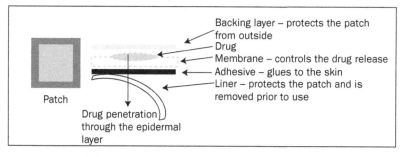

Figure 13.7 The makeup of a medicated patch

Practice questions

1. What are the differences between pharmaceuticals and biopharmaceuticals?
2. What does 'biologics' mean? Are there any biologics on the market?
3. Briefly discuss regenerative medicines. Are you optimistic that one day we will be able to see regenerative medicines on the market?
4. Biologics are essentially very large size molecules. Nanotechnology deals with nanosizes. Is this a physical size? Describe one nanomedicine available on the market.

Notes

1. Redrawn from www.doxil.com (accessed December 22, 2010).
2. Steven R. Bauer, 'Potential use of tissue gene, and cell therapy products: repair, replace, restore, regenerate', 2002, www.bcg-usa.com/regulatory/docs/2003/WSP20031023I.pdf (accessed December 10, 2010).

14

Future prospects for the pharmaceutical industry

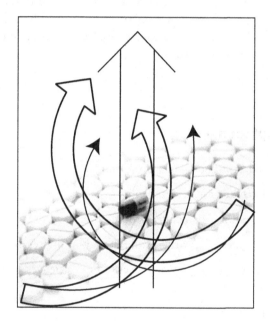

Learning objective

This chapter discusses the future prospects of the pharmaceutical industry, especially in the way it affects:

- the chemistry of carbon and silicon
- the impact of pharmaceuticals on longevity

Published by Woodhead Publishing Limited

- employment opportunities and world market analysis
- drug discovery and drug delivery systems
- personalized medicine
- drug development, especially for an ageing population around the world
- the emerging drug market in the world
- how advanced technology is helping to shape the twenty-first-century pharmaceutical industry.

As discussed in the first chapter, the pharmaceutical industry is highly research based, and there is little to inhibit research. This chapter looks at how future pharmaceutical research will move in different directions, including looking for new molecular entities in pharmaceuticals or biopharmaceuticals, regenerative medicines, personalized medicines, and newer and better drug deliveries.

Key concept terms

AIDS: Acquired Immune Deficiency Syndrome

API: active pharmaceutical ingredient

AZT: azidothymidine, also called zidovudine; drug to treat AIDS

Bioavailability: amount of drug available in blood after administration

Bioinformatics: use of statistics and computer sciences to understand molecular biological processes

Biologic: biotechnology-based drug

Biomarker: indicator of biological state; biochemical characteristics used to measure disease or treatment stage

Biopharmaceutical: drug produced using biotechnological processes

Biosimilar: generic version of a biotechnology drug

Biotechnology: use of living organisms or their products for therapeutic purposes

Brand name: trade name of a drug given by the originator

Carbon and silicon: elements in the periodic table (C and Si)

Controlled release drug: drug that releases over time

DNA: Deoxyribonucleic acid

Enzyme: biocatalyst made of proteins

Excipient: inactive or inert material other than API in medicine

Follow-on biologic: generic version of a biotechnology drug; biosimilar

Gene: functional unit of our heredity (genetic materials)

Gene technology: technology for manipulating genetic material or DNA

Generic name: international nonproprietary name for a drug

Genome: the entirety of an organism's hereditary information

Genomics: study of genes and their functions

HIV: Human Immunodeficiency Virus

Lipophilic drug: a lipid soluble drug

Mab: monoclonal antibody

Metabolomics: study of metabolites of cellular processes in a biological cell, tissue, or organ

Monoclonal antibody: protein produced from a single clone of B cells

Off-patented: after the expiration of patent

Pharmacogenomics: pharmacology of drugs based on genetic variation

Proteomics: study of proteins expressed by gene, cell, tissue, or organism

RNAi: ribonucleic acid interference

Stem cells: our body's master cells, which have the ability to grow into more than 200 cell types

Therapeutic: related to treatment of diseases

Vaccine: biological preparation that improves the body's immunity to fight a particular disease

Published by Woodhead Publishing Limited

14.1   Introduction

As long as we are alive, we will be susceptible to diseases. We may eliminate some diseases, but newer ones will come up. Diseases are a part of life, so we will always search for new medicines to treat or prevent new diseases. We need medicines to save injured people because of accidents or natural disasters, and to treat older people whose bodies become more susceptible to illness and injury. The pharmaceutical industry is thus an integral part of our lives (Figure 14.1).

14.2   Carbon and silicon

Carbon (chemical symbol C) and silicon (chemical symbol Si) belong to the same family in the chemistry periodic table. Humans are carbon based and the pharmaceutical industry keeps this carbon factory alive and active.

The chemistry of carbon and silicon are similar but somewhat different (Figure 14.2). Both are in the same group IV of p-block in the periodic table but the property of carbon is more diversified than that of silicon. Carbon is nonmetal and silicon is metalloid. The silicon in computers can contain some manmade viruses, but carbon in humans has natural viruses. It is possible to prevent or protect carbon-based humans from these natural bacteria or viruses, which are also carbon based and often pathogenic and life threatening.

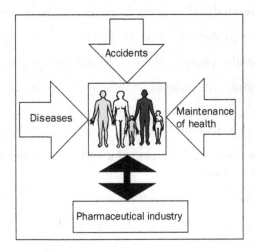

Figure 14.1 The relationship between pharmaceutical industry and human needs

Published by Woodhead Publishing Limited

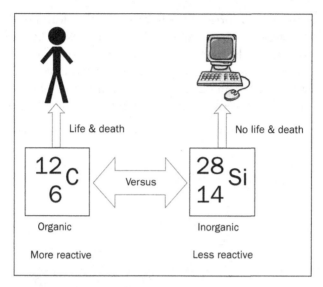

Figure 14.2 The distinction between carbon and silicon

Carbon-based microorganisms and/or their products are the most deadly threat to the healthy living of larger animals including humans. Carbon is the building element of all life forms on this planet and can build biomolecules, such as carbohydrates, proteins, fats, and nucleic acid, but at the end of life these biomolecules degenerate and convert to non-living molecules. As long as we live, we have to fight against diseases using medicines that the pharmaceutical industries discover, develop, produce, and deliver to consumers.

14.3 The role of the pharmaceutical industry in increasing longevity

The average life expectancy around the world is now twice what it was 200 years ago.[1] The world became a healthier place because of improvements in public health because of sanitation and clean drinking water, and the number of vaccines, antibiotics, and other medications produced on a mass scale and distributed to a growing market. The pharmaceutical industry is responsible for these medications. Although many medicines and cures exist in nature and will continue to be discovered, they can only be harnessed to their full potential with the innovation and technology of industry.

Published by Woodhead Publishing Limited

The geneticist Chris Morris of the Institute for the Health of the Elderly in Newcastle, England, estimates there will be an increase in life expectancies of five to ten years in the next 30 years, as a result of improved diet and medication.[2] Life expectancies in developed and developing regions around the world between 1950 and 2000 are shown in Figure 14.3, and the life expectancy in the USA between 1950 and 2007 is shown in Figure 14.4.

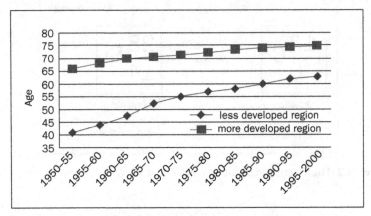

Figure 14.3 Life expectancy by birth 1950–2000 around the world by more developed versus less developed region

Source: US Department of Health and Human Services, Centers for Disease Control and Prevention, National Center for Health

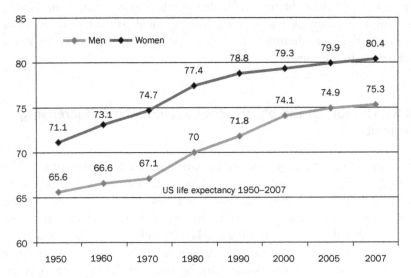

Figure 14.4 US life expectancy 1950–2007

Sources: Department of Health and Human Services, CDC, US, and Innovation.org

Commenting on increased longevity, the former commissioner of the US Food and Drug Administration (FDA), Mark McClellan, said, 'New drugs are no small part of this medical miracle.'[3]

14.4 Aspirin to Avastin

The pharmaceutical industry is developing to meet the need for new medicines to treat more complicated diseases and newer forms of diseases. The synthetic drugs developed in the early twentieth century (e.g. acetylsalicylic acid or aspirin) were simple in structure, but nowadays drugs are more complex (e.g. atorvastatin or Lipitor) and recently even more complex synthetic biologics (e.g. bevacizumab or Avastin) have been introduced to the market (Figure 14.5).

Aspirin has been in use for years as a traditional non-steroidal, anti-inflammatory agent and more recently in low doses as a blood thinner. Aspirin helps maintain blood flow by reducing platelet aggregation or coagulation, which in turn helps prevent heart attacks. Recently developed atorvastatin helps patients with heart diseases by reducing their cholesterol level, thus targeting the root cause of the disease.

The introduction of biopharmaceuticals such as Avastin is a breakthrough development in treatment. Avastin is a monoclonal antibody so can

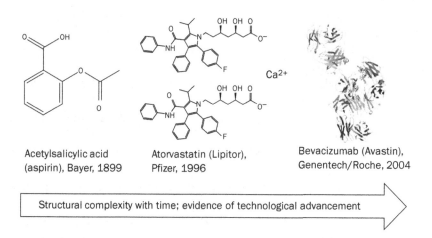

Acetylsalicylic acid (aspirin), Bayer, 1899

Atorvastatin (Lipitor), Pfizer, 1996

Bevacizumab (Avastin), Genentech/Roche, 2004

Structural complexity with time; evidence of technological advancement

Figure 14.5 The structure of acetylsalicylic acid (aspirin), atorvastatin (Lipitor), and bevacizumab (Avastin)

specifically bind with its targeted protein, in this case vascular endothelial growth factor-A (VEGF-A), and inhibits its activity. VEGF-A is a necessary factor for the growth of blood vessel (angiogenesis). Cancerous tissues need and develop more blood vessels to survive and grow, and Avastin inhibits angiogenesis by selective blocking of VEGF-A, thereby helps controlling cancer. The journey from aspirin to Avastin shows the significant advancement of science and technology in the pharmaceutical industry.

As newer diseases or old diseases in newer forms emerge periodically, such as severe acute respiratory syndrome (SARS), multi-drug resistant tuberculosis, Ebola fever, and hepatitis C, pharmaceutical research is directed to develop newer and better drugs to fight them. However, no anticancer drug yet exists that acts as a magic bullet – as is the case with penicillin and infectious diseases – although drugs are used to treat cancer patients, and in some cases lives have been extended through their use. Nonetheless, the future for developing anticancer drugs looks very bright; one of these is the monoclonal antibody Avastin.

14.5 Monoclonal antibody drugs

An antibody is an immunoglobulin, an immune protein produced when an antigen is introduced into the body; monoclonal means produced from a single clone.

Our white blood cells, called B-cells, produce antibodies whenever there are foreign organisms in our bodies, which is how our bodies' immune systems work. A monoclonal antibody can be made in the laboratory with a specific protein, which can also be used alone or to carry certain drugs or radioactive particles to kill cancer cells. The production of a monoclonal antibody is shown in Figure 14.6.

Monoclonal antibody (mab) drugs are anticancer drugs developed and marketed by biotechnology companies. One innovative idea is to use them to make cancer cells more recognizable as foreign by our bodies' immune systems, so they can fight against the cancer cells. Rituximab (brand name Rituxan) is a specific monoclonal antibody drug that attaches to a protein CD20 receptor found on B-cells and causes the tumor cells to disintegrate. Certain mab drugs can block the growth signal to cancer cells. Cetuximab (brand name Erbitux) attaches to the receptor of cancer cells, so they do not get the growth signal to multiply. Another mab drug, ibritumomab (brand

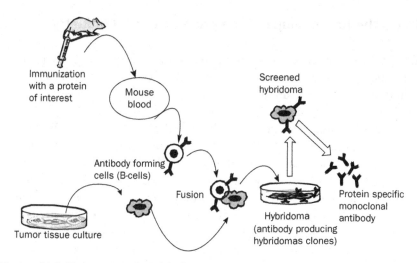

Figure 14.6 How a monoclonal antibody is produced

name Zevalin), is tagged with a radioactive particle so it can give radiation to the cancerous cells without affecting the normal cells.

These ideas all uniquely reach only the target cancer cells, so are commonly known as targeted therapies. The US FDA has approved a number of monoclonal antibody drugs (Table 14.1) and hundreds more are in clinical trials.

Table 14.1 US FDA approved monoclonal antibody drugs and their uses

Drug (generic)	Company	Uses
Alemtuzumab (Campath)	Genzyme	Chronic lymphocytic leukemia
Bevacizumab (Avastin)	Genentech and Roche	Breast cancer, colon cancer, lung cancer
Ibritumomab (Zevalin)	Spectrum Pharmaceuticals	Non-Hodgkin's lymphoma
Panitumumab (Vectibix)	Amgen	Colon cancer
Rituximab (Rituxan)	Genentech and Biogen Ideac	Non-Hodgkin's lymphoma
Cetuximab (Erbitux)	ImClone Systems	Colon cancer, head cancer, and neck cancer
Trastuzumab (Herceptin)	Genentech and Roche	Breast cancer

Published by Woodhead Publishing Limited

14.6   The future shape of the pharmaceutical industry

When there is a pandemic, or when apparently incurable diseases affect a human population, the pharmaceutical industry has the ability to develop medicines to fight these diseases. It takes time, but ultimately companies are able to develop medicines that can extend longevity if not cure the disease completely.

Acquired Immune Deficiency Syndrome (AIDS) is an example. When this disease began causing health problems and deaths, people were scared, and some thought the world was ending. But the pharmaceutical industry developed a number of medicines and antiretroviral drugs, such as emtricitabine, tenofovir, ritonavir, atazanavir, efavirenz, and AZT, which can prolong lives of AIDS patients when are taken in combination; this strategy is recognized as a highly active antiretroviral therapy (HAART) (Figure 14.7). It is expected that there will be an AIDS vaccine on the market within the next few years.

It takes a long time, considerable staff resources, and therefore huge money to develop a drug. According to Roche, drug research and development resembles a big number game (Figure 14.8).

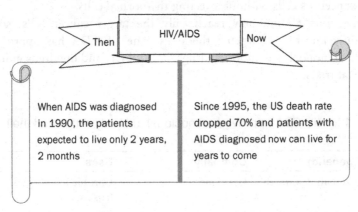

Figure 14.7 Longevity of people with HIV/AIDS, 1990s and 2000s

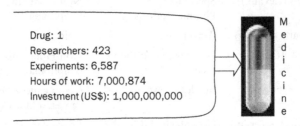

Figure 14.8 Statistics of the cost of developing a new drug[4]

Published by Woodhead Publishing Limited

Because of the long time (10–15 years on average) it takes to develop a new medicine to treat a particular disease, millions of people can die before treatment is available. This is what happened to people with HIV/AIDS before AIDS drugs began to be marketed in 1996: about 25 million people died around the world.

14.7 Personalized medicine

People don't always respond to drugs in the same way. One drug does not fit everyone. Recently the US FDA announced a new boxed warning on the anticlotting drug clopidogrel (Plavix), explaining that it can be less effective in people who cannot metabolize the drug to convert it to its active form. So this drug is less effective for people with a variant gene for a liver enzyme, which catalyzes clopidogrel to its active form.

The situation is similar to people who are lactose intolerant. Those who have lactase enzyme deficiency cannot digest cow's milk. The genes control so many things in our bodies' functions. An analysis of an individual's genomic data can show possible responses to a particular drug. The future of the pharmaceutical industry depends on who can provide personalized medicine.

Personalized medicine is custom or tailor-made medicine. Treatment or appropriate medicine can be selected to provide the optimum therapeutic value for an individual patient according to their genomic makeup (Figure 14.9).

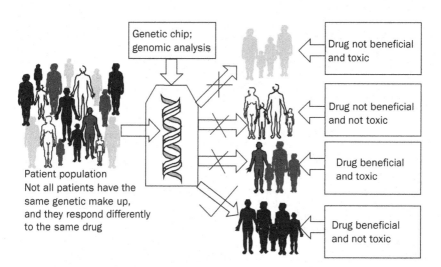

Figure 14.9 How a personalized medicine benefits some patients but not others

Published by Woodhead Publishing Limited

Personalized medicines can ensure personal wellness. Pharmacogenomic analysis can predict health risks for every individual, and manage life styles through:

- early diagnosis of certain chronic diseases
- better diagnosis and choosing the best course of treatment.

It might be possible to provide the right treatment for the right person at the right time in the near future. Before giving a prescription, physicians need to determine a patient's single nucleotide polymorphism (SNP) profile, compare it with the data bank, and figure out the drug that will work best for the patient. For example, for cancer patients the physician can determine the right dosage of a specific chemotherapeutic drug without using trial and error methods (Figure 14.10). Trastuzumab (Herceptin) is a kind of personalized medicine as the treatment works for a breast cancer patient who has too much HER2 protein in the tumors.

The genetic variant of the enzyme, which is responsible for deactivating the cancer drug, can determine the level of that enzyme. To do this, a DNA sample of the patient has to be analyzed based on SNP profiling. Similarly, cytochrome P450 enzymes are responsible for metabolizing many drugs, such as antidepressants, anticoagulants, and proton pump inhibitors. Some people can metabolize these drugs very quickly; others metabolize them more slowly. The CYP450 test identifies people with genetic

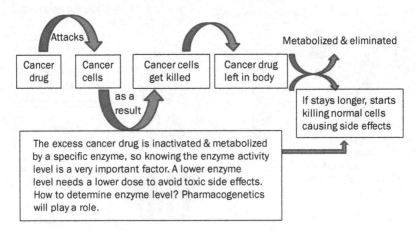

Figure 14.10 The role of genomics in avoiding side effects of cancer drugs

variations and physicians can make the correct decision in prescribing drugs and doses.

For tailored treatment or medicine, diagnostic advancement and affordability are very important before personalized medicines are used. Future generations of pharmaceutical and medical students need to understand genome sequencing data. Dr Jeremy Berg, director of the US National Institute of General Medical Sciences, describes this as, 'when combined with other sources, [having] the power to predict the diseases a person is most likely to develop and how he or she might respond to certain medicines'.[5]

14.8   Treatment of the increasing ageing population

As the population's longevity increases, so does the healthcare burden, but some older people are more of a burden than others, depending on how active they are. When they are less active it is usually because they have an age-related chronic illness, such as Alzheimer's disease, Parkinson's disease, dementia, arthritis, cancer, a destructive eye disease, or type II diabetes (Figure 14.11). There is no doubt that the demand for better drugs in those areas will continue to be a priority.

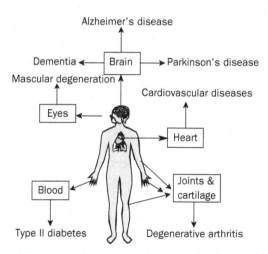

Figure 14.11 Diseases commonly found in elderly people

Published by Woodhead Publishing Limited

The objective of advancing drug delivery technology is to improve patient compliance and produce better clinical outcomes. An example of this is the needleless injection – many people are afraid of needles so prefer needleless injections, which are now a reality. Another example is the sustained release tablet. At one time, only simple tablets were available, but now there are sustained release tablets, half of which are released immediately on consumption and the other half released over a longer period. In the near future there will be advancements in nanotechnology-controlled release drugs, especially for orally administered lipophilic drugs. In general these are not very water-soluble, so bioavailability of the drugs is limited.

One of the major possible advancements in drug development and delivery in future relates to gene silencing pathways or ribonucleic acid interference (RNAi) technology. It is known that our messenger RNA (mRNA) carries instructions from the DNA of the cell's nucleus to build proteins, and all the diseases are linked with either mutated or abnormally regulated gene products.

In 1998 Andrew Fire and Craig Mello discovered a novel phenomenon: short double-stranded RNA can fool the cell to destroy the relevant mRNA before translating its protein. This discovery opened up a new dimension in health science where scientists can selectively eliminate a mutated or unwanted protein that is the root cause of a disease. This discovery won Fire and Mello the Nobel Prize in Physiology and Medicine in 2006. The pharmaceutical industry immediately considered the RNAi as a superior therapeutic modality over the small molecule-based conventional drug discovery protocol because many of the gene targets are not selectively controllable by conventional small molecule drugs, whereas RNAi can selectively remove the disease-causing gene from the system.

RNAi activity is mainly achieved through two pathways: short interfering RNA (siRNA) and miRNA. siRNA are double stranded, and can selectively shut down a gene by cleaving the relevant mRNA. miRNA are single stranded, and cannot eliminate a specific mRNA but can inhibit translation of several mRNAs. Many RNAi products are in clinical trial stages and will be on the market in the near future. Figure 14.12 illustrates RNA interference in the body.

Recently Mayo researchers have used RNAi methods in mice models to demonstrate that it is possible to silence the gene that produces alpha-synuclein, which is believed to be the primary cause of Parkinson's disease.

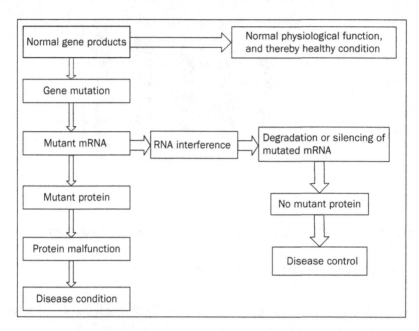

Figure 14.12 RNA interference and our body's natural defense mechanism[6]

14.9   Controlled-release drugs using a magnetic field switch

Boston Children's Hospital has developed a completely new approach to drug delivery systems. Researchers used a tiny, subcutaneous implantable device containing a membrane-based nanogel embedded with magnetite nanoparticles, which releases the drug by turning a magnetic field on or off. In an article in *Nano Letter*, the researchers showed that the drug dose delivered was directly proportional to the duration of the 'on' pulse.[7] The main objective of drug delivery systems is to deliver the intact medication to specifically targeted parts while causing little toxicity. The pharmaceutical researchers are now trying to use nanotechnology to target specific drug delivery using different vehicles, such as biodegradable polymers, dendrimers, electroactive polymers, and modified C-60 fullerenes.

14.10   The world pharmaceutical market and employment

The pharmaceutical market is growing every year (Figure 14.13). According to the forecasts of the Intercontinental Marketing Services (IMS), the world

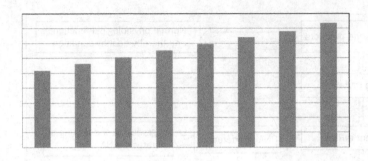

Figure 14.13 Yearly growth of global pharmaceutical market, 2002–2009 (US$ billion)

Source: IMS Health Market Prognosis, March 2010

pharmaceutical market will grow 5–8% annually through 2014 and sales will reach US$1.1 trillion in 2014 from US$808 billion in 2009.

As the market is steadily growing, we should be able to expect more employment opportunities in this industry, but the world economic crisis may lead to job cuts. Figure 14.14 shows the number of people employed

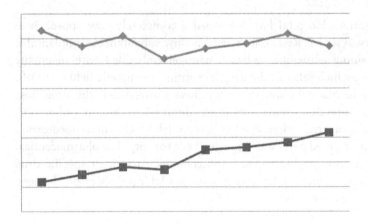

Figure 14.14 Number employed in the UK pharmaceutical industry, 1980–2007

Source: The Association of British Pharmaceutical industry

Published by Woodhead Publishing Limited

in the UK pharmaceutical industry from 1980 until 2007. Though there is a steady increase in R&D employment, the numbers employed in the industry overall changed little.

The US Bureau of Labor Statistics reported that there were 289,800 pharmaceutical employees in the USA in 2008, and this number is expected to increase by 6% between 2008 and 2018.[8] As a result of the economic crisis that started in early 2008, several industries have down-sized; the pharmaceutical sector has not down-sized but there have been job cuts in the sector.

14.11 Stronger generics markets in future

Saving costs on healthcare is an important concern in developing countries and developed countries. Though the cost of medicines is not a major part of the overall healthcare cost in developed countries, it is significant, especially for those who are chronically dependent on them.

Generic drugs are exact copies of the original brand name drugs in their active ingredient(s), strength, dosage form, purity, quality, stability, safety, and efficacy, but excipients such as colors, flavors, and fillers may be different. IMS Health figures show there has been a steady growth of generic markets from 2004 to 2009 (Figure 14.15).

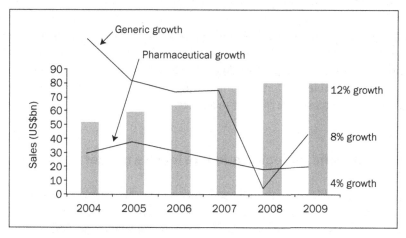

Figure 14.15 Global generic market sales (US$ billion) and generic and pharmaceutical growth, 2004–2009

Source: Redrawn with permission from IMS Health[9]

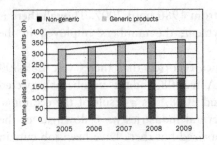
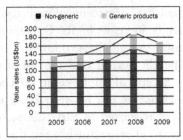

Figure 14.16 Market for generic drugs in Europe by volume sales and value sales

Source: Redrawn with permission from IMS Health[10]

As a result of the economic crisis in early 2008, the growth of generic markets dropped significantly, but generic markets will be stronger in future because some of the blockbuster drugs will soon be off-patented. Once the patent is off, generic companies launch generic equivalents. In Europe, a generic market is growing, and generics make up almost 50% of volume sales with a fraction of the dollar value of non-generic drugs (Figure 14.16).

The British Generic Manufacturers Association estimates that the price of the generic version of a drug often undergoes a reduction of 90% of the original cost of the brand name drug within a few weeks.[11] Two factors gain generic drugs immediate access to the market: reduced cost for consumers, and guarantee by a drug control authority of their safety, quality, and efficacy. For example, the US FDA and the Medicines and Healthcare Products Regulatory Agency (MHRA) in the UK are government bodies responsible for approving generic versions of medicines after carrying out extensive reviewing processes.

14.12   Generic biologics and biosimilars market potential

Biologics are biotechnology-based drugs or the generic versions of biotechnology-based drugs, known as biosimilars or follow-on biologics. Most biologics are very large and complex molecules or a mixture of molecules. There are debates about whether it would be difficult to make the equivalent generic versions of biologics because, unlike small molecule drugs, they are usually protein, and even a minor variation in the production and processing procedure affects the final 3D conformation and thereby their functionality. This also affects the efficacy and safety of the relevant biosimilar.

More than 150 biopharmaceutical products, including cytokines, hormones, clotting factors, vaccines, and antibodies, have been marketed around the world, but patents on some of the biologics have already expired or will expire in 2011, and the introduction of generic versions to the market is fast approaching. Currently, biotechnology-based drugs, especially large molecules such as monoclonal antibodies, are very expensive and not affordable for many patients. Prices can be reduced if the regular approval process is carried out for biosimilar products after their patents expire.

The patent of Amgen's blockbuster biologic epoetin alfa (brand name Epogen, known as EPO) expired in the European market in 2004, and the company's US patent will expire in 2013. Generic versions of EPO are available in China, India, Peru, and Brazil, and Amgen itself is selling generic EPO in China and South America. Biosimilars are also available for GSK's Engirix B, a hepatitis B vaccine, and Eli Lilly's Humulin, a human insulin. Developing countries will be a big market for future biosimilar products because of the low cost of the biologics. Figure 14.17 shows some blockbuster biopharmaceuticals with high market potential as biosimilar products. Table 14.2 lists the differences between pharmaceuticals and biopharmaceuticals.

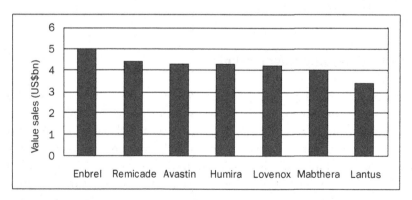

Figure 14.17 Blockbuster biopharmaceuticals with high biosimilar market potential

Table 14.2 Differences between pharmaceuticals and biopharmaceuticals

Characteristic	Pharmaceuticals	Biopharmaceuticals
Active ingredient	Simple molecule, any chemical compound	Large and complex molecule, protein
Sources	Chemicals	Living organism, plants, animals
Structure and characterization	Well defined chemical structure and finished products can be analyzed	Not well defined structure and very difficult to characterize
Compound's integrity	Chemically synthesized, always the same compound, and can be identified analytically	Activity affected by the production cell system, fermentation media, and operating conditions
Impurity	Predictable impurity	Unpredictable and difficult to identify
Production process	Simple, well defined synthetic routes; can be produced in large quantities	Complex production routes; produced in small quantities
Dosage forms	Variable	Usually injectable
Variations among manufacturers	No variation among different manufacturers	Manufacturer to manufacturer variation is possible
Bioequivalence	Criteria defined	Unknown, hard to define

14.13 Emerging new markets

For many years, the USA, European countries such as Germany, UK, France, Italy, and Spain, and Japan were the leading global pharmaceutical markets, but more recently countries from Asia and Latin America have emerged with remarkable market growths. IMS figures show that China, Brazil, Russia, and India in particular have emerging new markets.[12] In 2009, the pharmaceutical markets of Asia, Africa, and Australia grew by nearly 16% whereas those in North America and Europe grew by only about 5% (Figure 14.18).

China and India both have populations of more than one billion people, and as the countries develop economically the 'pharmerging'

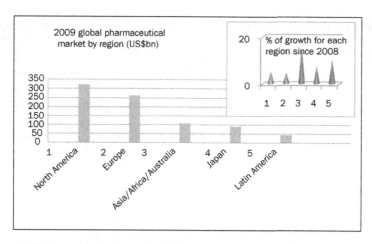

Figure 14.18 The global pharmaceutical market by region (US$bn) and percentage of growth in 2009

Source: IMS Health Market Prognosis[13]

(pharma-emerging) markets are poised for significant growth. According to a report by PricewaterhouseCoopers, India will join the top ten countries by 2020 with a market value of US$50 billion.[14]

14.14 Biotechnology – a way forward

Modern biotechnology has widespread applications in the production of biopharmaceuticals, vaccines, and diagnostics. In the field of biopharmaceuticals, biotechnology applications include drug development, genetic testing, gene therapy, and pharmacogenomics. Human insulin was the first biotechnologically produced medicine, developed and produced by Genentech and marketed by Eli Lilly. The first modern biotechnology company, Genentech (acquired by Roche in 1999), had great success in producing a number of biopharmaceutical products (Table 14.3).

According to a report by the Pharmaceutical Research and Manufacturers of America (PhRMA), in 2008 there were 633 new biotechnology medicines under development. These included 254 medicines for cancer, 162 for infectious diseases, 59 for autoimmune diseases, 34 for HIV/AIDS and related conditions, 25 for cardiovascular disease, and 19 for diabetes and related conditions. Most were waiting for the US FDA's approval.[15]

Published by Woodhead Publishing Limited

Table 14.3 Biopharmaceuticals developed by Genentech and/or Roche

Generic (brand name)	Year introduced	Uses
Human insulin	1982	To treat diabetes
Somatrem (Protropin)	1985	Growth hormone for children
Interferon alfa-2a, recombinant (Roferon-A)	1986	To treat life-threatening neuropsychiatric, autoimmune, ischemic, and infectious disorders
Alteplase (Activase)	1987	To treat dissolving blood clots in myocardial infarction
Interferon gamma-1b (Actimmune)	1990	To treat chronic immunodeficiency
Dornase alfa (Pulmozyme)	1992	To treat asthma; cooperative project with Roche
Somatropin (Nutropin)	1993	A growth hormone
Rituximab (Rituxan)	1997	To treat non-Hodgkin's lymphoma; cooperative project with Idec
Trastuzumab (Herceptin)	1998	To treat particular type of breast cancer
Bevacizumab (Avastin)	2003–2004	To treat cancer
Omalizumab (Xolair)		To treat asthma
Efalizumab (Raptiva)		To treat psoriasis

14.15   Stem cell therapy – hope for the future

Every cell in the body originates or stems from stem cells. After receiving instructions from the body, stem cells start to divide to make certain genes or new proteins. This process is how different types of cells, such as nerve, blood, muscle, bone, and skin cells, are produced during early life and growth (Figure 14.19). A cell's gene controls the internal signals and external signals come from chemicals, such as hormones secreted by other cells.

There are two types of natural stem cells: embryonic and adult stem cells. Embryonic stem cells are extracted from the embryo right after fertilization and are pluripotent, which means they can produce any types of fetal or adult cell of the animal under investigation. In contrast, adult stem cells are isolated from mature tissues and are multipotent, which means they can produce limited types of cells. The first human clinical trial using stem cells began in October 2010. The US FDA has approved a study by the biotech

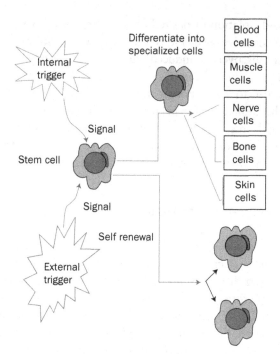

Figure 14.19 How stem cells are differentiated

company Gernon to investigate the injection of embryonic stem cells into patients with spinal injuries to restore their motor functions.

Medical and pharmaceutical researchers believe that stem cell therapy has the potential to cure chronic diseases. Current stem cell therapies include bone marrow transplants to treat leukemia and other cancers. Leukemia is a cancer of white blood cells, leukocytes, made up of bone marrow; these cancerous leukocytes grow abnormally and cannot fight against infections. The treatment includes chemotherapy and/or bone marrow transplant, where healthy bone marrow from donors is given to the patient.

In future researchers expect to use this technology to treat different cancers, Parkinson's disease, spinal cord injuries, Alzheimer's disease, multiple sclerosis and muscle damage, diabetes, burns, osteoarthritis, rheumatoid arthritis, and heart diseases. Current stem cell transplant methods have one major drawback, however: the patient's body can reject donor stem cells, even though they are screened for matching.

Scientists are conducting research to regenerate new tissues in the laboratory after collecting healthy adult stem cells from the patient and then transplanting the cells back into the same patient. As the regenerated tissue is genetically identical to the recipient's cells, graft rejection will not occur.

The availability and isolation of desired adult stem cells are very restricted, so this kind of regenerative medicine is practically very restrictive for many diseases. The recent discovery of induced pluripotent stem cell has shown the light to overcome this limitation. In this process, any cell, such as a fibroblast, can be reprogrammed to a pluripotent stem cell, which then can be used to differentiate to the desired cell type for the treatment of a patient. The technology is not risk free, however. The cells may divide in an uncontrolled manner and generate tumors. Scientists are working to fine tune the process of this type of treatment so this technology can be used clinically.

14.16 Technology and automation

In 2010 television news programs showed how robots were used at a depth of 5,000 ft below the surface of the ocean to stop the gushing oil spill in the Gulf of Mexico. Drug discovery processes in the pharmaceutical industry have also greatly benefitted because of the introduction of automation and robotics with the ability to identify new drug candidates out of millions of compounds. In addition, the use of advanced bioinformatics helps scientists create computer-aided design of new drugs, and understand the molecular pathways of diseases and the three-dimensional structure of proteins.

General practitioners are pleased whenever they find a broad spectrum drug (one that has wide coverage) because they can prescribe it based on symptoms without any clinical diagnosis. Patients can save money and time in such a situation. However, if a patient's treatment using broad spectrum drugs is to be effective and free from side effects it is essential that the disease is detected at its earliest stages, before symptoms appear, with an extremely accurate diagnosis.

Biomarkers are biochemical characteristics used to a measure disease or treatment stage. They are powerful tools, which could be used in future to diagnose, treat, monitor, and prevent diseases. Diagnostic tests currently used to identify a disease need to offer a more precise assessment for specific personalized treatments. The early detection of diseases and an understanding of their causes may help physicians start a new form of treatment. Once biomarkers for chronic diseases, such as cancer, HIV, cardiovascular diseases, Alzheimer's and Parkinson's, are developed and validated, drugs can be developed more specifically and effectively for a particular genetic trait.

The science of nanotechnology, using microscopic devices at the atomic and molecular levels, is soon going to revolutionize the diagnosis and treatment of diseases. Gene chip technology, which is already in use, can examine and analyze genetic sequences very quickly, and identify active genes in diseased tissue.

Published by Woodhead Publishing Limited

14.17   The future pharmaceutical R&D work force

R&D has always been a primary sector in the development of the pharmaceutical industry and will remain so. Medical treatments will gradually shift from the traditional towards personalized treatments. Pharmacogenetics will replace the conventional path of diagnosing diseases, and there will be an evolution of newer drug development strategies and screening methods towards making the right kind of biopharmaceuticals. The future pharmaceutical R&D work force will remain multidisciplinary but more inclined towards areas related to molecular genetics (Figure 14.20).

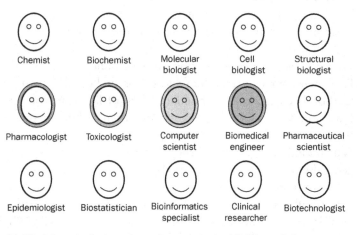

Figure 14.20 A twenty-first-century pharmaceutical R&D work force

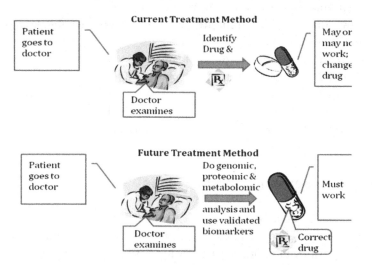

Figure 14.21 Current and future treatment methods in medicine

Published by Woodhead Publishing Limited

Practice questions

1. Is DNA a monomer or polymer? If a polymer, what is its monomer, or vice versa?
2. What are the nucleotides in DNA and RNA? Mention the base pairs for both.
3. Which of the following are biotechnology products?
   (a) bread (b) beer (c) yogurt (d) wine?
4. Can fermentation be considered the same as biotechnology?
5. What was the first successful biotechnology medicine?
6. Name a few biotech companies.
7. How many electrons, protons, and neutrons are there in carbon and silicon?
8. Write the electron configuration of carbon and silicon.
9. How many bonds can carbon and silicon make? Give examples.
10. Carbon is considered the building block of life. Can you name a few biomolecules? What elements other than carbon are present in those biomolecues?
11. Which kind of molecules, carbonaceous or non-carbonaceous, can generally be disease-causing? Explain with examples.
12. Why are there two molecules in the structure of atorvastatin?
13. Structurally, what kind of molecule is bevacizumab (Avastin)? The generic name of this kind of drug always ends with mab. Why?
14. What is the basic difference between an aspirin and Avastin molecule?
15. What kind of side effects can Avastin produce?
16. How do you differentiate between pharmaceuticals and biopharmaceuticals?
17. Are there any biosimilar products on the market?
18. Were there any blockbuster biologics in 2009?
19. Why are generic biologics called biosimilars and not biogenerics?
20. Explain your ideas about courses you should take to prepare yourself for a potential pharmaceutical career.

Answers to some practice questions

2. For DNA, adenine, thymine, guanine, and cytosine are the nucleotides. The base pairs are adenine and thymine, and guanine and cytosine. Find out the answer for RNA.

Published by Woodhead Publishing Limited

3. They are all biotechnological products.
5. Human insulin is the first biotechnologically manufactured medicine developed by Genentech in bacterial cells.
6. Amgen, Biogen Idec, Cephalon, Chiron, Eli Lilly, Genentech, Genzyme, Invitrogen, J & J (USA); Seron and Roche Group (Switzerland); GSK (UK); Novo Nordisk (Denmark); Boehringer Mannheim (Germany); Chugai (Japan).
7. Look at Figure 14.2. Carbon has atomic number 6 and atomic mass 12. Therefore, carbon has 6 protons, 6 electrons, and 6 neutrons. Now figure out those numbers for silicon.
8. Electron configuration of Si is 14 = $1s^22s^22p^63s^23p^2$. Find out electron configuration for carbon.
9. Both are tetravalent. Find out examples.
10. Carbohydrates, proteins, fats, and nucleic acids; figure out their composition.
12. Atorvastatin is produced as calcium salt and calcium is +2 positively charged.
13. Protein molecules are drawn this way. 'Mab' is abbreviated from monoclonal antibody.
14. Aspirin is a pharmaceutical and synthetic drug but Avastin is a biopharmaceutical and biologic.
15. It can inhibit normal blood vessel growth.
16. The answer is given in tabular form in Table 14.2.
17. Recombinant human insulin is on the market.
18. Find out from Chapter 1.
19. Biologics are produced from biological sources or using recombinant DNA engineering. They are complex protein molecules and very difficult to duplicate exactly. It could be similar and not an exact duplication of the originator.
20. Traditionally chemists, biochemists, biologists, and microbiologists with some pharmaceutical background used to have easy access to the pharmaceutical industry and its marketing and sales jobs. To make a career in twenty-first-century pharmaceutical jobs, students need to equip themselves with further knowledge of emerging sciences, especially 'omics' such as genomics, proteomics, and metabolomics, because treatment methods will change (Figure 14.21).

Notes

1. Central Intelligence Agency, *The World Factbook*, 2008, https://www.cia.gov/library/publications/the-world-factbook/geos/xx.html (accessed December 20, 2010); Oded Galor and Omer Moav, 'Natural selection and the evolution of life expectancy', http://sticerd.lse.ac.uk/seminarpapers/dg09102006.pdf (accessed December 20, 2010).

2. BBC News, 'Children could "live to 100"', December 26, 1999, http://news.bbc.co.uk/2/hi/health/578701.stm (accessed November 25, 2010).

3. Quoted on PhRMA, 'New medicines transforming patient care', 2003, www.phrma.org/new-medicines-transforming-patient-care (accessed October 10, 2010).

4. Roche, *Life Writes the Questions, We Pursue the Answers*, 2008, www.roche.com/corporate_brochure.pdf (accessed December 15, 2010).

5. Krista Conger, 'Study first to analyze individual's genome for risk of dozens of diseases, potential responses to treatment', Stanford School of Medicine, April 29, 2010, http://med.stanford.edu/ism/2010/april/genome.html (accessed October 15, 2010).

6. I appreciate the help given to me by Kakon Nag in creating this figure.

7. Todd Hoare et al., 'A magnetically triggered composite membrane for on-demand drug delivery', *Nano Letters*, Vol. 9, Issue 10, October 14, 2009, pp. 3651–57.

8. See US Bureau of Labor Statistics website, www.bls.gov/oco/cg/cgs009.htm (accessed October 10, 2010).

9. IMS Health, Midas, 'Market segmentation', September 2009, prescription-only medicines.

10. Ibid.

11. British Generic Manufacturers Association, 'Generic medicines and the market', 2010, www.britishgenerics.co.uk/about-generics/generic-medicines (accessed November 11, 2010).

12. Strategies for Emerging Markets, *The Business Magazine of Phama*, Vol. 30, No. 8, August 2010.

13. IMS Health, 'Total unaudited and audited global pharmaceutical market by region', March 2010, www.imshealth.com/deployedfiles/imshealth/Global/Content/StaticFile/Top_Line_Data/Global%20Pharmaceutical%20Market%20By%20Region_April_2009.pdf (accessed November 15, 2010).

14. PWC, 'Global pharmaceutical companies need to take an even closer look at India', PricewaterhouseCoopers, 2010, www.pwc.com/gx/en/press-room/2010/global-pharma-cos-need-to-take-closer-look-at-India.jhtml (accessed October 10, 2010).

15. America's Pharmaceutical Research Companies, *Medicines in Development: Biotechnology*, 2008, www.phrma.org/sites/default/files/422/biotech2008.pdf (accessed April 19, 2011).

Published by Woodhead Publishing Limited

15

Pharmaceutical case studies

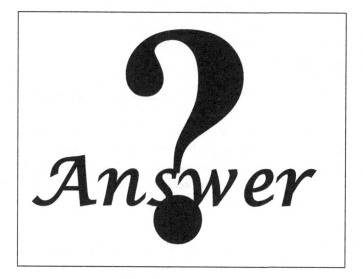

Learning objective

This chapter presents some case studies, which serve to answer some
frequently asked questions about medicine. You will find out what, why,
and how the medicines are used from the discussion of three important
questions on pre- and post-operative medicines, drug–food interaction, and
effervescent tablets.

Published by Woodhead Publishing Limited

15.1 Medicines given to an 11-year-old girl following adenoidectomy and tonsillectomy

An 11-year-old girl had an adenoidectomy and tonsillectomy in November 2010. Figure 15.1 illustrates the pre- and post-operative medicines she received and Figure 15.2 lists the questions that had to be asked before these drugs were administered. The rationalization for using these medicines is described below.

Saline solution is a large volume parenteral product given intravenously. It is a sterile, non-pyrogenic isotonic solution of 0.9% w/v of sodium chloride (NaCl). The practice of using pre- and post-operative saline infusions has been well established over a long period. A paper published in 1937 in the *British Medical Journal* on continuous intravenous saline infusion listed the following benefits of using these infusions:

- for fluid and electrolyte replenishment
- to prevent post-operative shock
- useful when treating thyrotoxicosis
- a convenient means of inducing medication, such as anesthesia.[1]

The patient was given midazolam, which is a short-acting benzodiazepine class drug for inducing sedation before medical procedures.

Propofol is a simple phenolic compound (2,6-diisopropylphenol) used as a short-acting, intraenously administered general anesthesia – the surgery was completed in approximately 30 minutes.

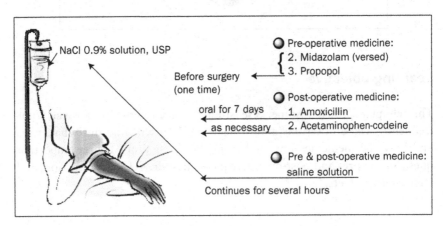

Figure 15.1 Pre- and post-operative medicines given to an 11-year-old girl following adenoidectomy and tonsillectomy

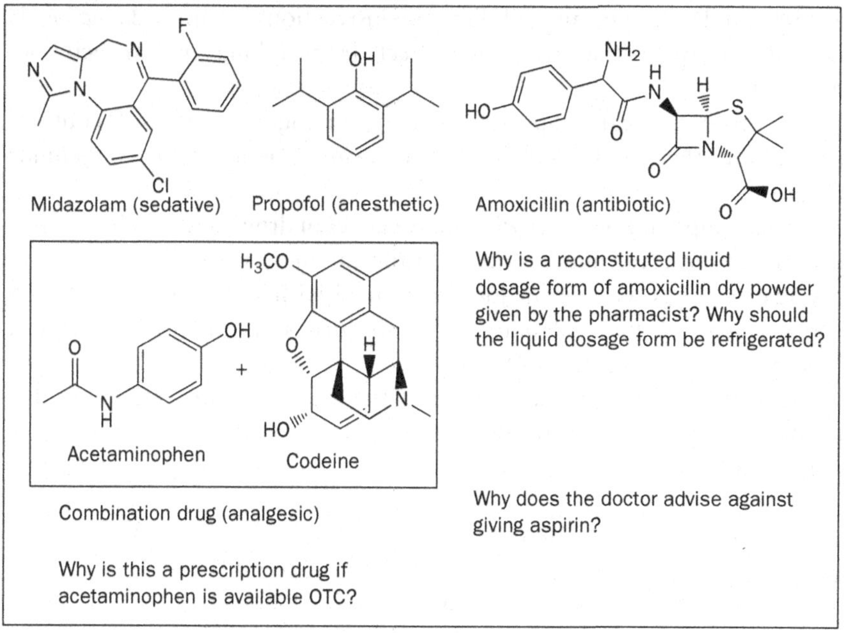

Figure 15.2 Medicines used during pre- and post-operative surgery and questions to be asked

The antibiotic amoxicillin is given to prevent any infection at the operation site. Amoxicillin in aqueous solution degrades quickly at high temperatures, and there is less hydrolysis at refrigeration temperatures.

Finally, a combination drug of acetaminophen (non-narcotic analgesic) and codeine (narcotic analgesic) is given to suppress pain. As codeine is a drug in the narcotics category with a history of being abused, this combination is a prescription-only medicine. Aspirin also works as a pain reliever, but aspirin is also a blood thinner, so if taken there is a high probability that bleeding may continue at the operation site.

15.2   Drug–food interactions

Certain drugs, such as non-steroidal anti-inflammatory drugs (NSAIDs; for example ibuprofen, aspirin, and naproxen), should be taken on a full stomach. These drugs may upset the stomach, and food can help by acting as a buffer. In contrast, certain drugs such as acetaminophen and Claritin are taken on an empty stomach because food can delay and decrease absorption. It is important to follow the instructions on all medicine labels in order to gain the maximum effect from taking the medicine in question.

Grapefruit juice can enhance the effect of taking many drugs. It contains naringenin (flavonoid) and furanocoumarins among other compounds (Figure 15.3).

These compounds interact with many classes of drugs, such as cholesterol-lowering drugs, calcium blockers, antihistamines, benzodiazepines, and psychiatric drugs. Grapefruit juice combined with statin drugs creates an enhancement of bioavailability of statin drugs in the body, called a synergistic effect (Figure 15.4).

These are the experimental results of the increase of bioavailability due to the synergistic effect of the compounds (especially bergamottin) in grapefruit juice:

- *lovastatin* – increase of 1,400%
- *atorvastatin* – increase of 200%
- *simvastatin* – increase of 1,500%.

This enhancement of bioavailability takes place in the following way. Drugs undergo absorption, distribution, metabolism, and elimination in the body, and in most cases, the drug starts to be eliminated from the body immediately after metabolism. If metabolism can be delayed, the drug will stay in the blood stream longer, which is what happens when statin drugs are combined with grapefruit juice.

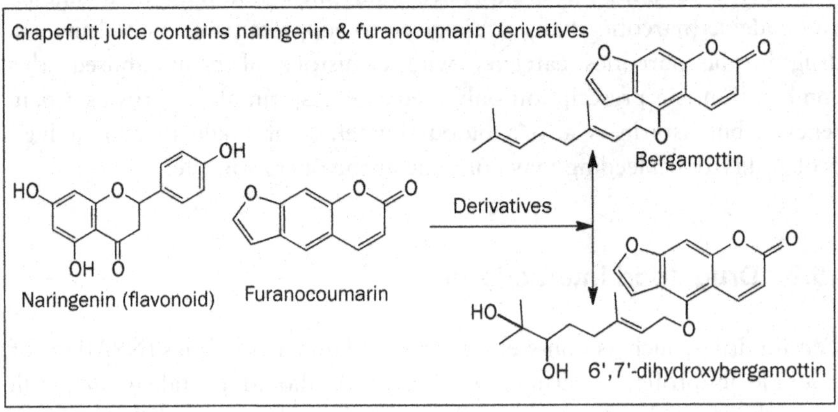

Grapefruit juice contains naringenin & furancoumarin derivatives

Naringenin (flavonoid) Furanocoumarin

Derivatives

Bergamottin

6',7'-dihydroxybergamottin

Figure 15.3 Compounds in grapefruit juice responsible for drug interactions

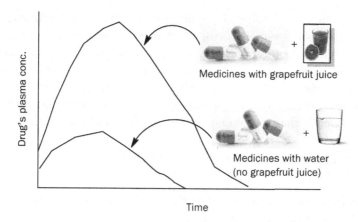

Figure 15.4 Enhancement of bioavailability of statin drugs due to grapefruit juice

More specifically, statin drugs lower the production of cholesterol by inhibiting HMG CoA reductase, which is the key enzyme for cholesterol production. However, statin drugs are metabolized by a specific cytochrome P450 called CYP3A4. The compounds in grapefruit juice, especially bergamottin, deactivate or decrease the activities of the enzyme CYP3A4. As a result, the statin is not metabolized and will accumulate in high amounts in the blood stream, and there will be greater inhibition of HMG CoA. Excessive inhibition is undesirable and can cause many side effects and complications.

15.3 Effervescent tablets

The Zantac website provides the following information about effervescent tablets:

Each individual tablet contains 28 mg of ranitidine HCl equivalent to 25 mg of ranitidine and the following inactive ingredients: aspartame, monosodium citrate anhydrous, povidone, and sodium bicarbonate. Each tablet also contains sodium benzoate. The total sodium content of each tablet is 30.52 mg (1.33 mEq) per 25 mg of ranitidine.[2]

Published by Woodhead Publishing Limited

How is 28 mg of ranitidine HCl equivalent to 25 mg of ranitidine, and which excipients are responsible for the effervescent (bubbling) action? The actual active ingredient is ranitidine, but the compound is used as ranitidine hydrochloride because it provides many pharmaceutical advantages. To get 25 mg of ranitidine (not ranitidine HCl), more than 25 mg of ranitidine hydrochloride is required because ranitidine hydrochloride has a greater molecular weight than a ranitidine molecule. This is the calculation:

Molecular formula of ranitidine = $C_{13}H_{22}N_4O_3S$ = Molecular weight = 314.4 g/mol

Molecular formula of ranitidine hydrochloride = $C_{13}H_{22}N_4O_3S \bullet HCl$ Molecular weight = 350.87 g/mol

Therefore for 25 mg of ranitidine = 350.87 X 25/314.4 = 28 mg

The effervescent action comes from an acid-base reaction of excipients used in the formulation. As soon as the effervescent tablet is put in water, the monosodium citrate anhydrous reacts with sodium bicarbonate, producing carbon dioxide gas and other products, which causes the fizzing (Figure 15.5).

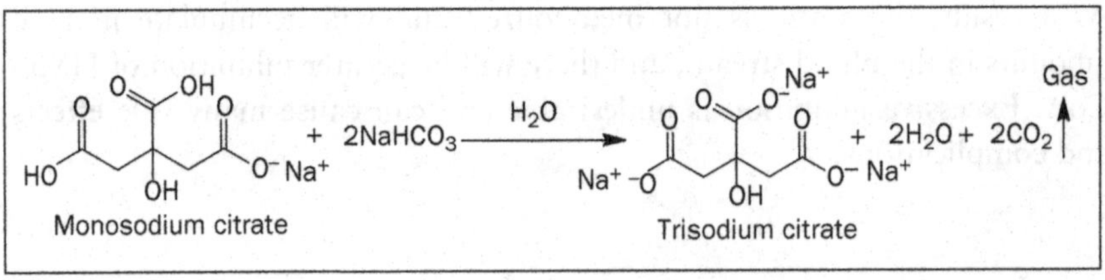

Figure 15.5 Reaction that produces CO_2 gas for effervescent action

Notes

1. Hamilton Bailey, Wilfred I. B. Stringer, and Kenneth D. Keele, 'Continuous intravenous saline infusion', *British Medical Journal*, Vol. 1, No. 3975, March 13, 1937, pp. 552–54.
2. See GlaxoSmithKline, 'Prescribing information: Zantac', 2011, http://us.gsk .com/products/assets/us_zantac.pdf (accessed February 23, 2011).

Index

Published by Woodhead Publishing Limited

Published by Woodhead Publishing Limited

sildenafil citrate. *See* Viagra
silicon, 360–1
simvastatin, 89, 309, 316, 388
solid dosage forms, 47, 56–8, 114–15,
   117, 124–5, 139, 157
   excipients, 117–19
   see also excipients
solvents, 119, 134
staccato system, 150
statin drugs, 308–18
   atorvastatin, 308–17
   see also atorvastatin
   bioavailability, 388–9
   development, 309, 315
   fluvastatin, 309, 316
   see also fluvastatin
   lovastatin, 309–10, 315–16
   see also lovastatin
   metabolism, 389
   mevastatin, 309, 315–16
   see also mevastatin
   pravastatin, 316
   see also pravastatin
   simvastatin, 309, 316
   see also simvastatin
stem cell therapy, 378–80
   future, 379–80
   leukemia, 379
stereochemistry
   definition, 82, 313
   dextro-rotatory (+), 313
   drug interaction, 313
   levo-rotatory (–), 313
stereoisomerism
   nitrogen atoms, 84
   sulfur atoms, 84
sterile production, 191–6
   solution, 193
sterilization methods, 193–5
stimulants, 336–40
   amphetamine, 336–9
   see also amphetamine
   chemical structure, 337
   cocaine, 336, 339–41

dextroamphetamine, 336–7
   see also dextroamphetamine
   methamphetamine, 336–40
sugar coating, 118
suspension agent, 120
sweetening agent, 116–17, 120 , 135
syrup
   production process, 137
systemic circulation, 208, 213–14, 222
systemic effects, 219

tablets, 20–1, 70
   chewable, 139
   control checks, 129–33
   disintegration, 216
   excipients, 117–21
   see also excipients
   formulation, 126
   in-process controls, 129–30
   machinery, 126
   manufacturing, 126–33
   manufacturing problems, 128–9
   manufacturing process, 127
   materials, 126
tadalafil, 298–9
taxol, 17
terminal sterilization, 184, 192–5
tetracycline
   dehydration, 160–1
   epimerization, 160–1
tetrahydrocannabinol, 18
thalidomide
   side effects, 87
   stereoisomer, 86
   tragedy, 184, 188
therapeutic window, 227
therapeutical stability, 162–3
thromboxanes, 320
tonsillectomy
   case study, 386
toxicological stability, 163
transdermal patch technology, 355
trastuzumab, 365, 368, 378
Tylenol. *See* paracetamol